Interpersonal Psychoanalytic Theory for the 21st Century

Evolving Self

Sue Harris, Janet R. Mayes,
Marilyn Miller, and David Singer

LEXINGTON BOOKS
Lanham • Boulder • New York • London

Published by Lexington Books
An imprint of The Rowman & Littlefield Publishing Group, Inc.
4501 Forbes Boulevard, Suite 200, Lanham, Maryland 20706
www.rowman.com

86-90 Paul Street, London EC2A 4NE

British Library Cataloguing in Publication Information Available

Library of Congress Cataloging-in-Publication Data

Names: Harris, Sue Ellen, 1939- author. | Mayes, Janet R., author. | Miller, Marilyn, author. | Singer, David, author.
Title: Interpersonal psychoanalytic theory for the 21st century : evolving self / Sue Harris, Janet R. Mayes, Marilyn Miller and David Singer.
Description: Lanham : Lexington Books, [2023] | Includes bibliographical references and index. | Summary: "This book examines relevant social/political issues while analyzing how repetitive patterns of interactions with significant people and the wider world develop one's expanding personality and how some repetitive patterns create 'problems in living.' The authors argue that people evolve by comprehending and challenging those patterns"– Provided by publisher.
Identifiers: LCCN 2022054395 (print) | LCCN 2022054396 (ebook) | ISBN 9781666927504 (cloth ; alk. paper) | ISBN 9781666927511 (ebook)
Subjects: LCSH: Psychoanalysis. | Interpersonal relations. | Self. | Personality.
Classification: LCC RC506 .H2825 2023 (print) | LCC RC506 (ebook) | DDC 616.89/17--dc23/eng/20221117
LC record available at https://lccn.loc.gov/2022054395
LC ebook record available at https://lccn.loc.gov/2022054396

To our cherished validators: Joan Harvey, Ralph Klein, and Jane Pearce

Contents

Preface

Evolving Self is a reintroduction, exposition and elaboration of interpersonal psychoanalytic theory, developed by Harry Stack Sullivan in the early 20th century. It focuses on and modernizes his original theoretical constructs as interpreted and enhanced at The Sullivan Institute for Research in Psychoanalysis in the mid-20th century. Jane Pearce, a founder of the institute, was a student of Sullivan as well as interpersonal theorists Frieda Fromm-Reichmann and Clara Thompson. In the spirit of Sullivan and the institute, our book reinterprets the theory, rendering it applicable to the 21st century.

We humbly assert that the theory espoused in *Evolving Self* stands on their shoulders. They stand on the shoulders of and depart from the original teachings of Sigmund Freud. We make use of neurological and observational research on infancy and empathy over the past 40 years to bring the theory up to date. Our volume represents another chapter in the evolution of psychoanalytic theories.

Interpersonal psychoanalytic theory assumes that people can achieve insight into how, within their interactions with people, they become who they are, and how they can change patterns of living that impede need fulfillment. People are born with a blueprint for growth and development that includes self-respect, self-fulfillment, expansion of experiences, and ever widening and deepening human interactions. It is similar to a seedling, which possesses the potential for growing into a flourishing tree.

Our book is timely and urgent. We were driven to write it because of the pressing need for interpersonal theories to be restated and reinforced in the context of current socio-economic conditions. With some exceptions, the mental health profession in the United States tends to be dictated by insurance and pharmaceutical companies, focusing primarily on symptom reduction and social conformity. These goals are inadequate. The goal of interpersonal therapy, as elucidated in this volume, is maximizing one's human potential.

This mental health crisis makes it even more imperative that we present a strong case for a theory that employs long-term interpersonal psychotherapy. Short-term interventions, even those utilizing some aspect of the concept of "interpersonal," do not accomplish an incisive, comprehensive, and enduring reorganization of people's orientation to themselves and their interpersonal milieu. Additionally, short-term interventions do not comprehensively aid people in understanding how past interpersonal experiences, primarily those early in life, can impact their current struggles in daily life. We live in a complicated and troubled world. We must continue to grow despite unforeseen obstacles. Our primary aim is to encourage readers to embrace this expansive and hopeful view of human potential.

Evolving Self is written for practitioners in all areas of mental health and pedagogy, whether or not they can explore a person's deep interpersonal history or engage in comprehensive interpersonal interventions within the constraints of their work. We hope that our book not only supports and enhances the resurrection of interpersonal perspectives but also opens new research topics within scientific/academic communities. Although not intended as a self-help book, we honed our prose so laypeople could make use of it. It is for people interested in understanding themselves and other people. Finally, this volume also addresses some pressing issues relevant to interpersonal theory and practice in the 21st-century social/economic/political milieu.

It has been a long, arduous, and rewarding learning experience over the last decade as we hashed out our diverse conceptualizations of theory and practice.

Acknowledgments

We are deeply grateful to the faculty of The Sullivan Institute for Research in Psychoanalysis, particularly the late Ralph Klein for his witty, insightful critiques of our work, and the late Joan Harvey for her unwavering encouragement and invaluable contribution to the chapter on dreams. We are humbly appreciative to Colwyn Trevarthen, professor emeritus of child psychology and psychobiology at the University of Edinburgh, for his warm support and for critiquing the chapter "Early Infancy: The Development of Initial Blueprints for Later Experience"; to Namratha Boda, MD, attending psychiatrist, Maimonides Medical Center; Brooklyn, New York, for her close review of our book and insightful comments; to LeiLani Dowell for her meticulous copyediting and critiquing of the manuscript; to Sara Flounders, co-director of the International Action Center, for critiquing the chapter "A Comparison of Revolutionary and Interpersonal Theories"; to Ben Caroll for designing and developing our website; and to photographer Rain Bengis for "evolving" the photo on the site's homepage. Because we have been living and breathing our work for over 50 years, terminology and concepts that felt obvious were not always obvious to laypeople. We rewrote based on the tender, critical suggestions of the late Susan E. Davis, the late Josephine Diamond, Loretta Goldberg, Jeri Hilderley, and Caroline Thomas. We are so appreciative to our agent, Nancy Rosenfeld, AAA Books Unlimited, who meticulously, patiently, and enthusiastically ushered us every step of the way toward publication. We extend our deepest appreciation to Jasper Mislak, associate acquisitions editor for Slavic studies and psychology, Rowman & Littlefield, for his enthusiastic dedication to guiding our project to completion. We also thank our readers in advance and look forward to their comments and critiques; please find us at interpersonaltheory.com. Finally, we are grateful to those in our practices, whose responses to our therapeutic and supervisory efforts always challenge and make us grow personally and professionally.

Introduction

A person's first intimate connection is with those responsible for their very survival. They are completely dependent on their interpersonal environment. As children develop, to the extent their primary parenting one(s) can validate experiences with people and phenomena outside their immediate orbit, they are also influenced by the wider world. This confluence defines our humanness and unique personalities, which, in their complexities navigate with varying degrees of success a satisfying or not-so-satisfying life.

Evolving Self examines how repetitive patterns of interactions with significant people and the wider world, particularly but not exclusively in the formative years,[1] are primarily responsible for one's ever-expanding personality, and how some repetitive patterns can also create debilitating "problems in living."[2]

The book is rooted in interpersonal[3] theory, developed by Harry Stack Sullivan (1953), Frieda Fromm-Reichmann (1960), and their colleagues and students, and further interpreted and enhanced by The Sullivan Institute for Research in Psychoanalysis.[4] It is also grounded in more than 50 years of clinical experience in the practice of interpersonal psychotherapy by each of the authors.

The dominant orientation of psychiatry and most related mental health professions is that, with some exceptions, most problems in living (depression, psychoses, attention deficits, etc.) are based in aberrations which can be addressed with medication[5] and/or short-term psychotherapy.[6] That orientation is closely tied to the *Diagnostic and Statistical Manual of Mental Disorders (DSM)* (American Psychiatric Association, 2013), which classifies mental disorders via a listing of symptomatology. Unless diagnoses can be presented within *DSM* criteria, issues such as an unhappy marriage, an unsatisfying career, or despair about one's capacity for intimacy are often not covered by insurance.[7]

Fusing his theory of human development with the socio-economic climate of his time, Sullivan wrote about race, war, and poverty in 20th-century terms. The fusion is even more urgent now, as the world faces ever-increasing oppression and devastating international conflict. Paralleling these developments, the mental health field focuses less on human need and more on solutions based on corporate profit and behavioral conformity.

Evolving Self was written against the current backdrop of psychiatric perspectives devoted to "curing." These include short-term quick fixes designed to be consistent with "evidence-based" criteria. Focusing on narrow measurable indices, such as number of positive or negative interactions, the approach usually omits the broader context of a person's life. For changes to be long-lasting, people must understand symptoms in the context of their historical interpersonal development and incorporate strategies to mitigate them.

The American Psychological Association's (2002) standard of successful treatment is to bring a person back to "functioning within normal limits," which is considered the "actual clinical benefit."[8] Besides obvious difficulties of researching outcomes and defining "normal" (American Psychological Association, 2002), the orientation is superficial, constrained by an arbitrary definition of "mental health" plaguing psychology and other social sciences. Rather than return to "normal" functioning, "mental health" is an open-ended process of continual personality growth.

The mainstream mental health community still promotes "talk therapy," not only for people seeking help with their problems in living, but often as an ancillary to medical management and/or post-psychiatric hospitalization. Among the most popular is "Interpersonal Psychotherapy" (IPT). Although "interpersonal," the short-term treatment is different from the longer-term interpersonal psychoanalytic treatment delineated in this volume. IPT is defined as

> a time-limited psychotherapy that focuses on interpersonal issues, which are understood to be a factor in the genesis and maintenance of psychological distress. The targets of IPT are symptom resolution, improved interpersonal functioning, and increased social support. Typical courses of IPT range from 6–20 sessions with provision for maintenance treatment as necessary. (Interpersonal Psychotherapy Institute, 2016)

Its popularity, however, makes it obvious that talk therapy is recognized as part of a treatment plan. More traditional talk therapy modalities are indeed back on the table, and, in many instances, have never really left the table.

However, in today's mental health environment, crucial clinical decisions are often made based on short-term symptom reduction and diagnostic categories. Because of pressure from insurance companies, including ones provided by the government, many psychiatric hospitalizations consist of rapid diagnosis formulation, regulating people via medications to stabilize and discharge them in the shortest time possible, without ample opportunity to work through very strenuous issues in a protected, closed environment.[9] They are often discharged to outpatient clinics where psychotropic treatment (medication maintenance) is usually continued. Perhaps people receive "long-term" talk therapy, perhaps six months to a year, which may or may not provoke insight into the developmental history of life-restricting patterns of living and may or may not validate attempts to change those patterns. In addition, many therapists and the people they work with assume that mental health problems constitute symptoms of "chronic diseases" that must be regulated, not unlike diabetes or a thyroid condition.

Some schools of thought consistent with the perspective in this volume are gaining recognition. Developed over the past 50 years, some are contemporaneous with, but not related to, the rise of the marriage between pharmaceutical and insurance companies. These include psychobiologists, who study human nervous system development from one-celled organisms.[10] Through videotaped mother-infant interactions in the first hours of birth and beyond,[11] researchers also demonstrate the importance of early relationships in developing human personality, including the infant's persistent drive to relate. Based on these studies, some have coined the term "intersubjective" (Trevarthen, 1980) to describe a theory about the development of human personality and the treatment of problems in living. Many other developments in psychiatric research and theory that focus on interpersonal interactions are compiled in the *Handbook of Interpersonal Psychoanalysis* (Lionells et al., 2015).

The time is ripe for *Evolving Self* because it belongs among resources available to practitioners who grope for treatment modalities satisfying insurance requirements while retaining a larger human perspective. In cogent, easy-to-read detail, the approach in *Evolving Self* makes sense and hopefully will change how mental health practitioners think about their work despite corporate pressures, which drive most graduate schools, medical schools, teaching hospitals, and institutes to train to the short-term.

With notable exceptions, such as *Harry Stack Sullivan: Interpersonal Theory and Psychotherapy* by F. Barton Evans III (1996), *Sullivan Revisited* by Marco Conci (2013), and the *Handbook of Interpersonal Psychoanalysis* (2015), much of the invaluable theories of earlier interpersonalists such as Sullivan, Fromm-Reichmann, and Pearce have been given perfunctory recognition or omitted altogether in new and popular psychotherapeutic volumes.[12] *Evolving Self* is not intended to replace the foundational works, but to make readable much of their somewhat dated and convoluted prose and to elaborate and expand their formulations into a modern, comprehensive theory. References to original conceptualizations are cited and readers are urged to study specific fundamental readings such as *The Interpersonal Theory of Psychiatry* (Sullivan, 1953), *The Psychiatric Interview* (Sullivan, 1954),

Principles of Intensive Psychotherapy (Fromm-Reichmann, 1960), and *The Conditions of Human Growth* (Pearce & Newton, 1963).

Most books and chapters in texts that reference the contribution of Sullivan have summarized his interpersonal theory but do not go into the depth his theory requires and deserves in its reinterpretation and modernization. These include *Psychology: Perspectives and Connections* (Feist & Rosenberg, 2014, 2021); the chapter on Sullivan in the nursing textbook *Psychiatry* (Tasman et al., 2015), which cogently summarizes his work; *The Interpersonal Perspective in Psychoanalysis, 1960s–1990s* (Stern, D. B., & Hirsch, 2017), composed of articles on Sullivan's interpersonal theory as applied to psychoanalysis, primarily for those not familiar with his work; *Relational Freedom: Emergent Properties of the Interpersonal Field* (Stern D. B., 2015), which covers comparative theories dealing primarily with the therapeutic interpersonal field, with many references to Sullivan; and M*aking a Difference in Patients' Lives* (Buechler, 2008), which integrates much of Sullivan's assumptions and is particularly useful for new psychotherapists.

The Purloined Self: Interpersonal Perspectives in Psychoanalysis (Levenson, 1991, updated 2016) is a series of essays from the interpersonal perspective of the author covering theoretical topics, Sullivan's theories, and analytic topics in psychoanalytic clinical work. Although more focused on transference and countertransference than advocated by Sullivan and the approach in *Evolving Self*, it is an interesting supplement to it, along with the *Handbook. Interpersonal Process in Therapy: An Integrative Model* (Teyber & Teyber, 2016) includes a brief mention of Sullivan but no mention of Pearce and Newton. Another very important supplement to this volume is *Interpersonal World of the Infant: A View from Psychoanalysis and Developmental Psychology* (Stern, D. N., 2000).

Using concrete examples within the contemporary social/economic/political milieu, *Evolving Self* delineates the internal conflicts and real-life opportunities and obstacles accompanying each human developmental era. Rather than just focusing on the individual, analyzing interpersonal interactions in a *developmental sequence* is crucial—in the context of the nuclear family or primary caretaker(s), the extended family, the community, and the larger world, especially in the era of social media.

As much as possible, the prose eschews technical terminology. However, some conceptualizations require the "shortcut" words and phrases defined in chapter one. The book strives to provide readers with an unencumbered experience.

LOGIC OF ORGANIZATION

After "Basic Concepts" lays the groundwork, the Developmental Eras section delineates how growth takes place involving interactive experiences with people. The next section covers aspects of personality structure, including cognitive development and learning. Although practical applications are discussed throughout, along with short "case" illustrations, the next section specifically addresses psychotherapy, including dream analysis. The last section, "Issues," brings the theory into the larger sociopolitical sphere, including how interpersonal theory relates to the development of society.

After "Basic Concepts," chapters can be read in any order. Nonetheless, the presented order is likely to offer the best understanding of interpersonal theory and practice. Because each subsequent chapter can stand on its own, there is some repetition. Since some issues can arouse discomfort, even for seasoned practitioners, repetition using different words and phrases can allow readers to "hear" better.

NOTES

1. Approximately the first 10.
2. First coined by Harry Stack Sullivan. See *The Interpersonal Theory of Psychiatry* (1953).
3. "Interpersonal" as a medical term is "being, relating to, or involving relations between persons" (*Merriam-Webster Dictionary*).
4. The Institute's theoretical contributions are published in *The Conditions of Human Growth* (Pearce & Newton, 1963) and comprehensively summarized in the *Handbook of Interpersonal Psychoanalysis* (Lionells et al., 2015). They are also contextualized in *Sullivan Revisited*, along with excerpts from Pearce's unpublished lecture on psychotherapy at the William Alanson White Institute in 1957 (Conci, 2013). Pearce was a student of Sullivan as well as interpersonalists Frieda Fromm-Reichmann and Clara Thompson.
5. This is not to suggest that medications that alleviate anxiety, depression, and psychotic symptoms should never be prescribed. However, if the work can be accomplished without long-term dependency on medications, a person has a better chance of gaining insight into the etiology of their debilitating issues, has a better chance of growing and changing, and is less likely to relapse. Because medications can feel like a "cure," a person may terminate insight-oriented therapy. Fearful that the symptoms will return, they deal with side effects over the long-term.
6. Just because physicians have ruled out physiological causes of a person's behavioral concerns, it does not necessarily mean that it is "all in the patient's head." The person needs to ensure that an underlying medical condition has not been missed.

7. This discussion refers to governmental and private insurance programs within the United States.

8. "Actual clinical benefit" is the lessening of symptoms that are troublesome because they are either unpleasant or socially "odd," for example, hallucinations, delusions, or powerful moods of despair or rage. The person is said to be cured if those symptoms disappear, regardless of what else is going on in their life. Stopping symptoms via medication and stating the cause to be some form of chemical imbalance is a simple, plausible explanation, but it leaves a lot to be explained.

9. At Sheppard and Enoch Pratt Hospital in Baltimore in the 1920s, Sullivan organized a closed, long-term, non-judgmental, and caring therapeutic community for inpatient schizophrenics that made use of his interpersonal approach. It is known for having approximately an 86 percent "cure" rate (Blechner, 2009, p. 110).

10. Damasio (2018), Malloch & Trevarthen (2018), and Trevarthen (2017), among many others.

11. "In the 1960s, partly because of the availability of television for micro-analysis of life in spontaneous communication with infants, there was a revolution in the scientific understanding of how the human mind grows. The inquisitive and responsive way a healthy baby moves shows that humans are born for intimate sharing of interests and feelings that are essential for acquiring cultural habits and understanding, including language" (Trevarthen, 2019a).

12. Earlier works did recognize their important contributions, including *Psychoanalysis and Interpersonal Psychiatry (Mullahy, 1980); The Contributions of Harry Stack Sullivan* by Patrick Mullahy (1952); and *A Study of Interpersonal Relations: New Contributions to Psychiatry*, edited with an introduction by Patrick Mullahy (1957). Mullahy reviewed *The Conditions of Human Growth* (Pearce & Newton, 1963) in *Psychiatry*: "This book is a major contribution to interpersonal theory. . . . [It] is the most ambitious work on the interpersonal theory of psychiatry since Sullivan lived and lectured" (1963).

Chapter One

Basic Concepts

"Interpersonal" is what goes on between people.

Human beings develop sequentially by living and learning in interaction with other human beings. Unless there are extraneous catastrophes, difficulties in human development are tied to interactions with significant people, particularly in the formative years (approximately the first 10). In addition to central significant relationships, broader social phenomena like racism, classism, religious oppression and anti-LGBTQIA+ oppression, and political and economic crises are also interpersonal and profoundly impact the growing person. However, people always have the capacity to change in an interpersonal environment.

Much of human functioning that we think of as purely physiological occurs in an interpersonal context. For example, defecating is a biological function, but its organization is determined by experience with the primary parenting figure(s). Many functions thought of as purely biological, like digestion, are impacted by the moods and actions of significant others as the functions are developing.

There is a developmental hierarchy of needs. Current need satisfaction is impacted by earlier need satisfaction. Infants have very basic survival needs like food, temperature maintenance, and cuddling.[1] People learn functions to satisfy those needs. Primary caretakers are needed to validate needs and functions required for each subsequent developmental era. Examples include encouraging the ability to crawl and walk in late infancy[2] and providing opportunity for interaction with other children during childhood.

Need satisfaction is required at all levels of human development. Sullivan also defines another kind of need, the "need for security," which a person organizes for the prevention of anxiety but not satisfaction (1953, pp. 42–43), such as the "need" to get blackout drunk. Getting blackout drunk delays or destroys learning how to satisfy an anxious-making need such as having an intimate conversation that moves from drinking companionship to deeper friendship.

THE INTERPERSONAL FRAMEWORK

In the interpersonal framework, human personality encompasses several components dynamically related to each other: the self-system,[3] the central paranoia,[4] the integral personality, and the dissociated.

The Self-system

The self-system is one's sense of self at any particular moment. It has productive and restrictive characteristics. It is available to grow from experience or to ward off growth from experience by omission or distortion. It is the part of the personality that organizes and focusses awareness. If it could be frozen in time, it would contain what a person has available to consciousness: the awareness of what one can do and who one believes oneself to be in relation to oneself, other people, and the world.

The self-system governs the ability to focus attention in order to do anything at all. This same capacity can be used restrictively using "selective inattention" to avoid awareness of anything that disrupts the historical emotional connection with the central parenting figure(s).

Some functions move in and out of the self-system's focal awareness, remaining much of the time in marginal awareness but available to be utilized in special situations. For example, a person might be quiet and unassuming, but in an emergency or crisis may assume a leadership position, provide direction to others, or speak out on an important issue when they had not previously done so or even thought they could. Basic physiological functions, like breathing or digesting, are also usually in marginal awareness and only come into focal awareness when there is a problem or a conscious decision to bring them into awareness, as in yoga.

The self-image, as opposed to the self-system, is mostly in *marginal* awareness, but periodically in focal awareness. It also appears in dreams. The self-image is a person's *symbolic* condensation of how one sees oneself: a symbolic encapsulation or representation of what the person believes is or isn't possible for oneself in life. Statements of self-image might be "I am a good teacher" or "I am a scaredy-cat."[5]

The Central Paranoia and Despair

The central paranoia is an organized, complex system of despair about what is possible, which forms the basis of a security system designed to ward off learning from new experiences that would threaten the tender connection with the original primary caretaker(s). At the beginning of life, the infant is dependent on the primary parenting figure(s) for its very survival. If a parenting figure is, for whatever reason, unavailable, the infant experiences discontinuity that results in instantaneous visceral distress because of the infant's fragility and dependence. The central paranoia is built upon those repeated threats to existence, functioning, and satisfaction that inevitably occur when an infant is most fragile and dependent.

In general, tenderness involves empathically sharing with another to satisfy any need at any time and in any era of development, but tenderness is most potent in the formative years, and particularly in infancy. All caretakers usually have out-of-awareness limitations based on their own upbringing. When the infant, in their newness and staggering potential, collides unknowingly with those limitations, they empathically experiences parental discomfort. For example, the infant explores putting their finger in their anus and takes pleasure in the sensation. If the caretaker finds that undesirable, continuity with the caretaker's tenderness is disrupted. Since the infant is dependent on the continuity of loving relatedness with the caretaker for survival, functioning, and tenderness, disconnection from that relatedness is experienced as a threat to all three needs.

Limitations are different for every caretaker, but the repetition of this dynamic forms the basis for the subsequent development of the person's central paranoid restrictions. For example, repeated parental disgust while changing diapers (whether because they are simply disgusted with feces or because they are generally disgusted with their baby) can ultimately become the basis for the child feeling like a disgusting person. This formulation applies to anyone who is the primary caretaker with continuity. Disgust by one babysitter, well-meaning friend, or relative who is no longer asked to do that task comprises only a short-time bad experience among many positive ones and won't form the basis for a person's self-disgust.

Despair is a compilation of one's worst fears. It includes the fear of death, the fear of disorganization, and the fear of loss of tenderness. It is usually a symbolic statement of why the project of learning something new can't work, or why one can't grow. Ironically, it is a formulation people experience most powerfully when they are in "danger" of growing beyond what was conceivable to the primary caretaker(s) during the person's infancy. To grow beyond the self-systems of those primary caretaker(s) would threaten very early continuity with them. For example, childhood and adult nightmares very often occur during periods of crisis and change in a person's life when they have reached a turning point toward growth beyond what was conceivable to those who originally validated their thriving during infancy. Nightmares are symbolic statements of despair, and they are useful therapeutic tools because they congeal or codify despairing assumptions a person continuously lives with, assumptions they are often unaware of.

A person most likely becomes conscious of despair when they are about to make a breakthrough into something new. It usually appears in the form of moods and dreams, including nightmares. Despair is most effective when it is formulated out of awareness but can also be quite powerful when it exists at the margins of consciousness: one lives by it uncritically. In situations when the self-system is not challenged, the despairing thought or perception is "it's just that way." The person doesn't think about what "that way" is, and is not critically aware of it. Once despair is exposed, it is open to criticism and available to change. Despair is like a distress signal that can marshal unspoken beliefs when the status quo is challenged. It can take the form of inner, unspoken beliefs that happiness, success, or any intense pleasure would be fatal, the "I'm about to die" feelings of an infant in distress from losing loving continuity with a primary relationship. "Despair is the watchdog of the self-system" (Pearce & Newton, 1963, p. 408).

Depression, usually a chronic state of a flattening or not noticing feeling,[6] is a state that occurs to keep out threats to the self-system that would imply forbidden opportunities for growth. Depression is different from despair because, in its apathetic shroud, there is no opportunity for the distress signal to occur. The alarm sounds when the apathy lifts with the intrusion of new experience and hope for change. That produces anxiety, with the attendant experience of the despairing assumptions. But therein lies the opportunity for a critical reassessment of those assumptions in a supportive interpersonal environment.

A person comes into therapy saying, "I can't make a friend, find interest in a project, enjoy anything in life. What am I living for?" The individual feels intensely discouraged because nothing feels satisfying and may even call this feeling "depression." To get past these pronouncements, the person would have to examine the original relationships that prompted the despair which, at the moment, would be too threatening to their self-system. However, it is an opportunity for the therapist to gently work toward bringing to light the underlying despair and the etiology of it by taking a history. Whatever words are used to describe problems in living, the therapeutic work is to finally push the self-system to grow and thus challenge despairing assumptions and discouragement that goes with them.

The Dissociated

The dissociated consists of all needs and perceptions, including memories and partially organized functions, that have been exiled from awareness because of the forbidding gestures[7] of early significant other(s). As discussed below, the dissociated is not a system; it is not organized in any way. It is a repository of forbidden needs and a "*chaotic constellation of amputated experiences*"

(Pearce & Newton, 1963, p. 21) that could not be validated. Dissociated needs and experiences are drawn upon by the integral personality (see below) in order of urgency of need and emerging opportunity for satisfaction.

Needs that are less dissociated may be partly available to consciousness: in marginal thoughts, fugue states (see below), or dreams. This partly dissociated material can be consciously considered because it is more accessible. Thinking about dissociated material consists of holding it up to scrutiny, perhaps in dreams, artistic work, discussions with friends, and/or in therapy. This work is done in awareness, in the self-system, usually with a supportive person, therapist, or friend; or it is worked on out of awareness, in the integral personality, in the form of dreams or fugue states, which may or may not be remembered, and, if remembered, can then be usefully interpreted by a therapist and/or helpful other. Then the person might begin to satisfy the heretofore partially dissociated need, which expands their self-system to include the new experience: to grow.

If a person experiences dissociated material when embarking on a forbidden expansion of experience, e.g., a relationship, a trip to another country or leaving their parental home, they will feel forbidden desire, disorganization, and subsequent despair. The security system, responding to the emergence of new vistas, may quickly marshal its big guns and resurrect old barriers. Paranoid convictions might be that life will never be any different, or even that it will be much worse, that they are on the path to destruction. The purpose of this maneuver is to repudiate and rebury the previously dissociated experience.

When a dissociated need moves into awareness, the productive aspect of the self-system has a chance to expand. If the emergent dissociated need is repudiated, the self-system's restrictive apparatus is strengthened. There is either growth or deterioration (see below). Much depends on the availability of other people who can validate the new experience.

Fugue States

Fugue states (Pearce & Newton, 1963, p. 347) are the intrusion of dissociated material into waking life, including both the forbidden functions and the forbidding thoughts that kept them dissociated. They are usually brief and not well remembered or rationalized away. Like a dream or nightmare, they are illustrative of the struggle between the integral personality and the security system, a person's push for satisfaction of dissociated needs versus their own restrictive, paranoid assumptions.

The Integral Personality

The integral personality is the total of all experience, conscious and unconscious. It is called integral because it integrates everything: the self-system, despair, central paranoia, and the dissociated, all relating to the integral personality.

Even those aspects of functioning that are forbidden by one's early experience, which one mostly dissociates, are contained in the integral personality. Because they are unmet needs, they continue to push for awareness. The degree to which they reach the borderline of one's awareness depends upon the intensity of need versus the strength of the security system.

For example, a child reaches the age of four or five having dissociated the need for relatedness to peers because of one or another unfortunate aspect of their upbringing. When it is time to go to school, the push to relate to other children by the new opportunity as well as by the ongoing need to play becomes more powerful than before. At that point, the need to relate to peers pushes for awareness. It may or may not succeed, depending upon what else is happening. When there is opportunity, and the more the need has gone unmet, the more the integral personality pushes to meet the need.

Sometimes functions forbidden in the conscious experience of the child are expressed in dreams or masked in fantasy and/or artistic expression, but not directly acknowledged. A person often plans and organizes how to get their dissociated needs met outside of awareness. They might know about it via dreams or creative work, such as writing, painting, music, or fantasy.

> As a kid, Jen was essentially isolated from other children. She had an ongoing fantasy of being with other children, building a log cabin, and getting more kids interested; together they build more cabins. Then they decide to build a wooden fence around the cabins, like the forts in cowboy movies. Now they're self-sufficient and no grownups are allowed. It has become a thriving cooperative community of kids. Jen didn't grow up in a community of kids, but in her fantasy life she was organizing a life consisting of a community of friendly people all working together to make something that excluded people they felt didn't love them. It was a very elaborate fantasy that went on for several years.

There is always pressure from the integral personality to admit dissociated needs to awareness. A simultaneous struggle occurs between the integral personality and the self-system's security operations, forged by the central paranoia, to keep them out. People sometimes take action, unwittingly pushed by dissociated needs, setting up situations to meet their needs, orchestrated by their integral personality. At the same time, people can set up structures to block themselves based on despair from the central paranoia. It is an internal dialectic that moves forward and backward to grow or restrict the self-system.

There's always pressure from the integral personality to admit needs into awareness, that is, into the self-system. In the dialectic process, there's always pressure from the security apparatus to keep those thoughts out.

OTHER EXPLANATORY CONCEPTS

Anxiety

"People who ride on roller coasters will pay money for being afraid. But no one will ever pay money for anxiety in its own right. No one wants to experience it" (Sullivan, 1954, p. 95).

Anxiety is the disruption of consciousness, organized according to the rules of the person's self-system. It is emotional, physiological, and perceptual—a confrontation with a forbidden desire previously dissociated, requiring reorganization to integrate into the new sense of self. The inner experience of disorientation and distress is on a continuum, depending on how much reorganization is needed and the relative strength of the person's security system.

It can be as mild as getting lost on the way to a class in reaction to discovering that one is mastering a new skill, or as severe as feeling the central paranoid fears of death, isolation, and insanity, such as hallucinating an attractive person as a demon when having sex with them. When the central paranoid system is involved, a person feels a threat to oneself—intense dread and despair. In short, anxiety is the emotional, perceptual, and physiological experience of disorganization and usually terror in the face of new self-awareness.

Anxiety is transitional, ending either with tightening self-system restrictions or self-system expansion, including previously dissociated experiences and needs.

Intruding needs may date from any time in a person's lifetime. But since they have been previously dissociated, their intrusion into the self-system can call up infantile terrors of the central paranoia.

It's said most people dislike change; they would prefer not to try. However, it's not change that is repugnant. If change were so scary, we'd never get past infancy. Throughout life every moment is potentially something new. What's problematic is challenging the assumptions of the original caretaker(s). Any change divergent from that can arouse anxiety, including disorientation and terror. It represents distancing from the original significant relationship(s). It particularly arises as the growing person becomes involved with environments psychically farther away from home. The occurrences of psychiatric crises and panic increase markedly in adolescents, coinciding with their increased potential for independence, mobility, and sexual desire.

In this context, "stress" is differentiated from "anxiety." Stress may be related to a realistically overwhelming situation, not necessarily from an expansion of the self-system. Anxiety occurs when one attempts to expand functioning, including previously inconceivable perceptions and functions. It is the difference between worrying about getting to a meeting on time (stress) and feelings of disorientation and dysphoria[8] when one is successful at organizing for the first time not to be late.

Security Operations

Security operations are perceptions and behaviors designed to avoid anxiety, functioning to limit experiences leading to anxiety-provoking expansion of the self-system.

They promote the status quo, how the self-system is organized, often functioning in anticipation of the point at which a person might experience anxiety.

Security operations are extremely varied. They could be anything and are very creative. For example, Frank works late, avoiding happy hour because, "My co-workers are just being nice and don't want me to join" and "I'll have nothing to say because I'm not very interesting," etc. Experience to expand his self-system has been successfully headed off.

Paradoxically, in some circumstances, productive capacities can be mustered to prevent expanding experience.

> A gregarious young woman decides to get her PhD. However, each time she plans to devote herself to her studies she finds herself embroiled in campus social activities: throwing a party for her friend's nephew, hosting old friends and showing them around town. These were productive activities, but now they are used to avoid needed study time. Obtaining her PhD would challenge her view of herself as a good-natured gal but somewhat intellectually limited. She's gregarious and organized enough to be accepted to graduate school, but God help her if she ever actually obtains a higher degree and realizes she's even more capable of using her productive skills.

Security operations can be behaviors, thoughts, perceptions, beliefs, and moods marshalled at crucial moments. Or they can be ongoing delimiting patterns running nonstop in the background of one's mind: "I'm always depressed. That's my personality, my diagnosis." Expressed dramatically, security operations can be a constant scowl.

While learning a new function, new security operations may develop as somewhat successful obstacles. For example, a young woman with low self-esteem finally forces herself to make it to a party but then acts like a wallflower once she gets there.

Or:

> A person needs to perform their latest song at an open mic, to share their creativity. However, on the evening of the event they decide they had better write a new song, so going public is delayed. Each time, on the evening of the weekly event, they decide they'd better write a better song.

This next example illustrates the expression of a need and its undoing:

> Bill, recently discharged from a mental hospital, finally decides to go to a party. In his subsequent session he describes a "horrible" time and that no one wanted to talk to him. The therapist asks him to start at the beginning: "I walked in, had a drink. A woman talked to me, asked me my name, and I said, 'My name is Bill and I have been in three mental hospitals.' I was being honest." He had successfully fulfilled his deeply embedded expectations of rejection.

Vague generalizations can also be used to maintain the status quo:

> An isolated boy tells his therapist that all the kids in school pick on him; they misbehave, and he gets blamed. The therapist says, "Okay, tell me about a particular time it happened." But the child wants to keep the generalization, keep this image that "nobody likes me." The devil is in the details. The generalization prevents him from being clear on what goes on between him and other children: their role in blaming him and his role in keeping other children at arm's length.[9]

All security operations operate via manipulation of consciousness defined as "selective inattention." Selective inattention is a major factor in the organization of consciousness necessary for a person to function (like not attending to ambient sounds during a lecture). As such, it is a vital ability without which a person cannot think. However, selective inattention can be used as a security operation to misdirect perceptions or dissociate them, thereby restricting awareness to avoid anxiety. For example, a person focuses on aspects they dislike about somebody, not noticing likeable traits. Or, in a different style, a person perseverates about a lost lover or a failed course, effectively blotting out constructive thought that might improve their life.

Validation

When learning a function, people need an audience, a significant person who responds to the process, consciously or unconsciously. The ability to function is dependent on the quality of that response and impacted accordingly. For example, in early infancy, the response by the parenting one(s), in muscle tone, mood, or voice pattern (to name a few), is validation for how the infant organizes digestion or skin integrity. If the parenting one(s) is comfortable and enjoys cuddling during feeding, digestion will probably go smoothly. If there is irritability or worry, that mood will be communicated to the infant,[10] with subsequent disruption of whatever function is being learned.

As discussed above, functions often seen as purely biological processes require validation, though learning must go on within the framework of the given physiological structure. Ribble, in *The Rights of Infants* (1965), and Spitz, in a series of studies (1945, 1946a, 1946b), describe how infants given adequate sustenance in the most sanitary conditions went into apathetic states and died unless they also received human contact, i.e., holding and cuddling. Survival rates improved with human touch, even if the holders and cuddlers were not the biological parents—a very clear example of the need for validation of basic physiologic functions at the beginning of life. As people age, their audience for various functions can be real or imaginary (fantasized), depending on their life experience. Some people experience substantial validation from fictional characters, TV personalities, athletes, or social media, to name a few.

Optimal validation occurs when one or more significant people take pleasure in a person's experience. Negative reaction is also a kind of validation. For example, a child has a close friend, but their mother constantly bad-mouths their friend or friendships. It is validation with a negative skew ("Friends are okay, but they always have ulterior motives"). Of importance is the acknowledgment of the friend's existence. If there is no response at all to the child's expression of need, there is even greater difficulty learning how to meet the need for friendship.

> Phil was an "army brat." His parents moved every year or two when his father was reassigned. They sent him to the local school wherever he was, but always with orders that whatever went on in the home stayed within the four walls. Phil's mother was an alcoholic, and his father was a severe disciplinarian. Phil was punished severely for small infractions such as not doing chores or talking back. He would either be beaten or grounded, sometimes not permitted to see anyone socially for months. His father encouraged school achievement and discipline, but both parents remained aloof from the local townspeople. They encouraged Phil to play sports and to win at any cost, but not to whine. Despite always being the new kid in school, Phil did well academically. He was also successful at sports, a star on whatever team he joined. He was able to engage in activities with other children and even work cooperatively in team sports, although he was extremely competitive and intolerant of teammates who were less skilled. But he was always a loner, never confiding in anyone. Completely forbidden was any kind of closeness or identification with his peers. No one specifically told

him intimacy with others was bad. However, his life was organized to avoid it. He remained aloof and did not experience loneliness. Occasionally kids made overtures to him, which he disdainfully perceived as some sort of weakness or seductiveness. When he reached puberty, he approached sex with the same competitive orientation he had toward any other activity.

There may be all kinds of limitations affecting the quality of available validation. It could be loaded with envy, disgust, competitiveness; it could be almost anything, but in some way or other if the validator at least recognizes the existence of the need with accompanying derogation, there is validation with accompanying limitations. To the degree that there are significant outside alternative validators, the person has an opportunity to learn, but with misgivings about the process.

Validation is rarely perfect. It usually comes freighted with the limits of the perceptual framework of the validator, along with whatever opportunities are available to the individual. As the person grows, there are more opportunities for experience and alternate validators. Sometimes a function moves from the dissociated to the conscious because of alternate validation.

A famous political writer was incarcerated as a teenager for stealing a bicycle. He was in prison for seven years and suddenly began to write, starting with a brilliant book that has since been published. The book is like a journal talking about his weekly life. It starts out monosyllabic. He's angry, he's depressed, he's barely talking, and one gets a sense of an extremely paranoid, closed, depressed person. Then he's visited by a lawyer who responds to his thinking with compassion and enthusiasm. He suddenly starts formulating theoretical concepts and writing long essays and poetry. Where did it come from? It is not that she taught him. She didn't. His capacities had been marginally developing inside him until someone responded to him enthusiastically and it came flooding out of him. It is evident in his book.

Sometimes that movement happens when a student has been sitting on a lot of potential until a teacher recognizes it and simply comments about it.

The degree of responsiveness to validation is based on a person's readiness to respond to it, depending on previous experience. If validation in later life is effective, it has the potential to increase the momentum for change in wider and wider areas of living. No matter how old, a person can change with validation.

Envy

Envy is rooted in the unsatisfied, dissociated needs of the envious person. It's not possible to validate a person's need if it is inconceivable to the other person. While the envious person is not conscious of their own unsatisfied need, they feel and express rejection toward the articulated need of the other by ignoring or disparaging it in some form. In its most subtle and thorough form, envy may be manifested by not noticing the other's need or by responding unwittingly but accurately aimed in a way that is antagonistic to it. In all cases the unconscious message communicated is: "If I can't have it, think it, or feel it, neither can you."

> Henry won a coveted award in the movie industry along with two friends. After he and his co-editors received an Oscar, he called his mother. "Me and Hannah and Jack got an Oscar!" His mother responded, "Hannah, Jack, and I!" Henry finally understood what he had been hearing in therapy about parental envy.

When it occurs, envy is a powerful disruptive force; it moves to stunt personality growth by restricting satisfaction of a need in the envious person as well as the person who is the object of it. Parental envy of the developing infant or child is particularly damaging because it takes place in the earliest stages of growth and learning, fundamentally limiting the child's experience. A depressed, envious primary caretaker, for example, whose restrictive self-system will not allow curiosity in themself will not be able enjoy the child's investigation of the world. Instead, they either will not respond to the child's actions at all or will prohibit, for example, the child's exploration of their body or their friendliness toward strangers or their pleasure in the mastery of a project because the caretaker's perception—a consequence of envy—is that such behaviors are somehow bad. These perceptions had been developed in the caretaker's own early experience with significant others and were not challenged later with alternate validation.

To prevent a rupture in connectedness to the parenting one(s), the developing, dependent child experiencing their envy must view the forbidden need with the caretaker's perception. They would experience a rupture in this life-sustaining relationship as chaotic and terrifying. There is no other option but to preserve the relationship with their most important human contact.

Needs colliding with parental envy will continue to push for recognition. The integral personality's push to get the dissociated need (and its functions) into awareness and belatedly satisfied is a struggle, no matter when it occurs later in life. The degree of struggle, with accompanying anxiety, is consistent with the magnitude of the threat of disconnectedness from the early envious caretaker the person reexperiences. Along with making use of alternate validation, it makes a huge difference when they understand the historical effects of early parental envy on continued growth throughout life.

In interpersonal theory, envy is different from jealousy, when a person consciously wants something the other person has that they do not have. In jealousy, the person may go after it too, as if inspired, or, on the other hand, might be angry at the other for having what they want and use it to feed their own low self-esteem or even *consciously* go after the other person for having it. Jealousy can actually be inspirational and useful to the jealous person. It's then possible to organize to have something they didn't, up until then, think they could have. In contrast, envy is *out of awareness* on the part of the envious one; if confronted with it, the envious person would, understandably, strenuously deny it or attempt to use a cover story, such as, "That person's behavior is disgusting!" The goal is to stop satisfaction in the other, not organize satisfaction for oneself.

> Abe is jealous because their friend, Clyde, has enrolled in a theater group at school and is appearing in class plays. Abe feels left behind and inadequate. They can't be popular and talented like Clyde. Somebody friendly tells them that if they want to do something that shows off their talents, they can join the school band since they play a mean trumpet. It had never occurred to them, but they timidly audition for the school band and get in. They stop being jealous of their friend.
>
> On the other hand, if Abe were envious of Clyde, having dissociated the possibility of belonging to anything, they might not welcome the suggestion to audition, but they continue to mock Clyde for being a show-off, a phony, etc., without realizing that they were unconsciously, out of envy, trying to destroy the other's enthusiasm for belonging to the theater group.

Point of Fixation

Development occurs in an orderly sequence, one function building upon another (Pearce & Newton, 1963, pp. 56–57), based on previous learning and maturation. You can't learn if there is no basis for learning—without the required antecedent-validated consolidated experience. For example, the ability to grasp objects comes before scribbling with a crayon. In development, there is always a zone of experience not yet consolidated which would be the individual's expected next area of development. So it is just these experiences that should be incorporated into the self-system with a minimum of anxiety. This zone is the focus of the integral personality in its push to growth. The integral personality is focused on this zone of developing functions in the individual in whom growth is proceeding optimally in sequence and timing. The term "fixation" is not ordinarily used to delineate where the focus of attention is. The concept of fixation applies when the situation is not ideal, when some necessary functions are forbidden and thus blocked by the self-system's restrictions, when progress in the ability to relate stops expanding because of earlier prohibitions. As a person continues to grow in other areas, there may be learning that also occurs in the forbidden area, and so the point of fixation may advance but with a skew, like a stream flowing around rocks in its path but continuing to flow forward, propelled by the force of a person's needs (Pearce & Newton, 1963, p. 58).

The point of fixation moves along as the person manages to accumulate more learning. Insofar as someone is continuing to grow, the point of fixation moves up the hierarchy of functioning toward greater complexity. The integral personality, which operates based on the pressure of the most urgent need, provides the pressure to move past early prohibitions. It is the push toward growth, which may or may not be strong enough to overcome the security system. So in determining the point of fixation, one needs to look at what a person has *next* to master in the developmental sequence (Pearce & Newton, 1963, p. 58).

For example, a person reaches the age at which they are called upon to be a functioning member of a team—the juvenile era. The person now must cooperate, compromise, and compete for the sake of the team. However, while learning some of the political aspects of group dynamics, the individual might still be focused on the childhood goal of getting parental approval more than meeting team goals or is maybe focused on being the star. They are still operating within the childhood era, which is more self-centered, as opposed to focusing on the goals of the team as a whole. The individual is uncomfortable about actually belonging as a member. Their point of fixation is at the beginning of the juvenile era, with some aspects of it continuing to develop but blocked at the forbidden function of belonging (Pearce & Newton, 1963, p. 58), not yet feeling membership in a cooperative group. Whatever political success the child has achieved using some juvenile functions has not become the basis for the next stage of development after the juvenile, which is the development of "warm personal relationships within the group" (Pearce & Newton, 1963, p. 58), the move toward interpersonal intimacy with a best friend in preadolescence. If the person does not feel like a member, further growth beyond the juvenile is much more difficult because whatever functions are learned in the group, such as the political arts of cooperation, compromise, and competition, are already skewed. It is a large barrier in the flow of the person's life.

All new functions are based on the degree of consolidation of previous ones. The close preadolescent relationship with a best friend is limited if a person has not yet learned how to comfortably feel like a member of the group (Pearce & Newton, 1963, p. 58).

Residuals

Residuals are functions not adequately consolidated in a particular developmental era that affect how one functions in later life.[11] Residual deficits skew later learning until those aspects of functioning are integrated. For example, during the juvenile era, a person develops and consolidates the experience of group membership. If they cannot make up for poorly consolidated juvenile functions later in life, they are, to varying degrees, self-centered and childish in their interactions with other people.

Regression/Growth/Deterioration

Regression is a disruption of functioning back to earlier functioning in the face of anxiety. The point of fixation is what one hasn't yet learned. The latest learned function falls apart with anxiety. A fixation is a point, and regression is a process backward to that point.

Growth and deterioration depend on the processes of hope and despair. On the hopeful side is the integral personality, the repository of all experience, conscious and dissociated. It operates on the pressure of need, constantly pushing for more satisfaction, responding to any potential validation of one's need to grow, always searching for new validation of the continuous pressure of need pressing against the limiting warnings of the security system.

Adult growth, while still dependent on tenderness and validation, is different from growth in childhood because societal expectations of adult behaviors are different. To continue to learn how to relate past one's point of fixation as an adult, one needs to explore solutions that may seem unusual or unconventional (Pearce & Newton, 1963, p. 61).

> Joe was so phobic about touch that he experienced only pain during attempts at sex. He began exploring ways to learn about cuddling. Drawing on the early positive experience of owning a cat, and only after a great deal of effort, he adopted a kitten that reminded him of the one he had as a child. While cuddling with his kitten, he was finally able to experience pleasure and comfort. Many of his friends thought his desire to rush home to be with his cat extreme and inappropriate for a man in his 30s.

The adult has more opportunities for growth and to make changes than the child because they are mobile and less dependent upon their original caretaker(s). However, because of the increasingly complex web of social relationships, functionality, and responsibilities as one moves throughout life, the self-system becomes a more rigid adversary to the push for new growth experiences (Pearce & Newton, 1963, p. 62). So much more has to be shifted.

The adult needs the experience of affectionate, validating relationships to make it easier to tolerate anxiety when the self-system is reorganizing. Tender validation reduces anxiety and the fear of isolation from the original caretaker(s) and, therefore, from the world one has known up until then (Pearce & Newton, 1963, p. 62).

That is, if there are more friendly people in one's life than there had been in their childhood, anxiety is more tolerable.

In adult experience, the integral personality and the self-system are in constant struggle. The integral personality uses the accumulated new experiences in living to build for new learning; the self-system's security apparatus twists or dissociates the new experience to justify maintaining old restrictions. The opposing forces push each other in a hopeful or despairing direction, depending on how much validation for change exists in the adult's life. The point of fixation, therefore, is constantly fluctuating.

There is also momentum. One thing leads to another. When a person incorporates a new function, expanding one's self-system, the next attempt to grow is easier, based on previous success. On the other hand, if the new experience is repudiated in some fashion, the next opportunity for growth will be more difficult and fraught with even more anxiety (Pearce & Newton, 1963, p. 62). That is the beginning of deterioration.

Awareness of one's setbacks is on a continuum. A person may be aware of trying to make a friend but fails to do so. In such an instance the person might say, "You see? I could never make a friend. I'm unlovable." Or a person might repudiate a friendly gesture, but not be aware that more despair has been created by this casual rejection. If pushed, say, by a therapist, the person might retort with bitterness, "Don't be naive. It's a hostile world. You can't trust anybody." The person has moved from making timid attempts at closeness to a more entrenched position that rationalizes the distance already existing between them and others.

The process of deterioration, like the process of growth, is cumulative. If needs are not satisfied, the person deteriorates. Absence of or the inability to accept tenderness is the primary condition for deterioration, first for the erosion of interpersonal and then for intellectual capacities. When people start denying and rejecting experience, they also deny and reject their own perceptions; they begin thinking less clearly and in a more paranoid, restrictive way.

Regression, as opposed to deterioration, is the process of *temporary* disorganization of the latest learned functions under the impact of anxiety and the return to earlier modes of functioning (Pearce & Newton, 1963, pp. 63–64).

> James, infantilized by their parents well into adulthood, lives at home even though they can afford to get their own place. Because their job requires relocation, they very reluctantly move to a new city, and for the first time must learn to organize their own household, cook their own meals, meet strangers, and explore a new environment. They suddenly discover they have difficulty driving and need much more help navigating the new transportation system, although

they once prided themself for being very well-oriented and mobile when traveling for work or as a tourist. They are temporarily disorganized because of the anxiety of leaving their parents. As they begin to integrate the expansion of their world of new people, places, and situations, the ability to navigate and orient themself improves. Once the new experience is integrated, they begin driving and orienting to their surroundings with more confidence.

Regression and deterioration consist of disruption of functioning, but deterioration is about decay, the repudiation of function. The person is not learning anything new and discarding what has already been learned. If it keeps going, they discard more and more, becoming increasingly limited in intellectual, perceptual, and emotional capacity. The process involves repeated paranoid formulations that increasingly restrict functioning. The pull to paranoid reformulation destroys their capacity to organize perceptions in relation to direct experience. The attack, then, is aimed at not only one's closeness with other people but also their perceptual-cognitive functioning.

Mary, an only child of very reclusive parents, dropped out of high school and joined the Peace Corps. She was forced to live with large numbers of strangers her age, and became agitated and delusional, asserting that her dreams foretold the future and that she was destined to be a prophet who predicted disaster. She was hospitalized. She calmed down and was soon placed in a residence and given a job in a sheltered workshop. She seemed to enjoy her job, but in therapy she complained she was better than her co-workers and underestimated by her supervisors, who lorded it over her because of her "patient" status. In her estimation, she would reach her true potential once she was discharged to her parents. In sessions after discharge, she expressed increasingly negative feelings about people outside the home: job interviewers, strangers in the street. She no longer had a good word to say about anyone she met and was increasingly discouraged about finding work or any kind of social interaction. She was also increasingly silent about interactions with her parents, declining to discuss her parents' and her own isolation and phobia about the outside world. She began focusing more insistently on her belief that she was a prophet whose dreams predicted the future. Her belief in her prophetic abilities focused more and more on how special, important, and unappreciated she was. In her increasingly grandiose mood, she was unable to negotiate job interviews or simple social interactions. She was eventually rehospitalized.

Mary's deterioration started with the derogation of her peers, but because of the pull to justify her alienation from people, her judgment and ability to think began to deteriorate as well. Her curiosity withered as her interest in learning new things about the world around her diminished. She was at the same time less able to communicate with others. The loss of function became cognitive as well as social.

Empathy

Empathy is the ability to feel what another is feeling. In the words of Trevarthen (2006), a clinical researcher of communication in infancy, "the core of human consciousness is the potential for rapport of the self with another's mind. This potential is immediate, irrational, unverbalized, conceptless, and atheoretical: A delicate and immediate [being] with-the-other" (p. 121). He is talking about empathy. For Sullivan (1953) and Pearce and Newton (1963), empathy is the main means of communication between the infant and mothering figure(s). They describe it as crucial to the infant's survival and cite studies by Ribble (1965) and Spitz (1946a) to show that without that empathy or empathic identification, the infant will die, even with the provision of basic food and shelter. Trevarthen's (1979, 1993a, 1993b) research provides even more empirical evidence of the ongoing responsiveness of the infant to available human beings.

The capacity for empathy exists throughout life. It is a significant method of communication between people who are close to each other.

The infant relies almost completely on empathy for all communication. As they grow into late infancy and childhood, when the child depends more on dramatic gestures and language for communication, the reliance on empathy recedes but does not completely go away.

Throughout life, empathy, as the underlying method of communication, emerges as random thoughts, disconnected associations, memories, and intuition. People experience it, for example, in concerts and rallies and when stuck together in an airport; it becomes intense during states of personal and communal crisis as well as in day-to-day adult interactions. It forms the basis for communication in the myriad ways that occur when people are relating (Pearce & Newton, 1963, pp. 52–53).

Primary Relationships, Productive and Restrictive

Human beings develop within an interpersonal context. In other words, we become human by "being raised by people" (Pearce & Newton, 1963, p. 13). In the beginning, the parenting figure(s) are the preeminent relationships, the first audience for any action or thought. People continue to think to that particular audience, present or imagined, although their importance may diminish over time. It isn't possible for perception and thought to exist without interaction with another person, current or remembered.

Throughout the early years, there can be primary relationships with other people besides the parent(s), who become alternate validators if they are acceptable to the parent(s), such as extended family members, close family friends and teachers. If all goes well, the person becomes emotionally intimate with a best friend peer in the preadolescent chumship, and hopefully goes on to establish important relationships with an expanding number of people. The audience for thought continues to be expanded. These are primary relationships, the primary audience in thoughts and actions, the ones who make life meaningful to a person (Pearce & Newton, 1963, p. 191).

Primary relationships govern all patterns of interaction, whether they are with the early primary figures or not. A person's way of relating to the rest of the world is limited by the need to maintain continuity with the primary relationships. As with a parenting one and child, any new experience that would expand the self-system in ways that threaten the connection between the person and their primary relationships will be met with inner resistance and anxiety (Pearce & Newton, 1963, p. 191). Since there are always primary relationships by necessity, if a person is unable to form significant relationships with anyone beyond the parenting figure(s), they remain the primary relationship(s), whether or not their parenting one(s) are currently present in their life. When a person can go beyond inner restrictions, new primary relationships are possible. New relationships are easier to integrate if they bear some similarities to the relationship with the parenting one(s). The issue becomes: Are the new relationships merely repetitions of what went on with the original parenting figure(s), or are they expansions beyond what a person is used to? As a person continues to have new experiences—in school, the workplace, social groupings—and develops new relationships, expansion beyond the original, parental, primary relationship(s) can increase indefinitely. In other words, a person can expand indefinitely in one's range and depth of functioning in the world depending on the range and depth of their relationships. This is true no matter how productive or restrictive the original parenting relationships have been. There is always room for expansion.

However, if establishing relationships with others is deficient or non-existent, there is an intensification of resistance to new experiences in the service of maintaining parental continuity, with an increasingly limited ability to relate to the rest of the world. Depending on a person's opportunities for interpersonal interaction, this can have a crippling effect on a person's satisfaction in life.

A primary relationship functions to validate perceptions and provide tenderness, cherishing, and respect of the other—or their opposite.

Tenderness involves empathic relatedness to the other's need to expand their self-system; if tenderness isn't present, the other has a much harder time and feels isolated and in pain. They might give up trying.

Cherishing has to do with relatedness to the other's physical survival and can range from great pleasure in the existence of the other to slight interest in the other's survival (Pearce & Newton, 1963, p. 192).

Respect involves loving feelings toward the other's integral personality (their potential) with tender disregard for the other's security operations, or those aspects of the other person that limit that potential (Pearce & Newton, 1963, p. 193).

A loving, or productive, relationship is distinguished by a high degree of mutual validation, tenderness, cherishing, and respect; all push for growth. It involves an intermingling of integral personalities, which mutually force into awareness heretofore thwarted areas of growth into their self-systems (Pearce & Newton, 1963, p. 193).

A restrictive relationship is characterized by the opposite and the dominant integration is between the two central paranoias.

The relative stability of these relationships, productive or restrictive, is dependent on the strength of the meshing of either the integral personalities or the central paranoias (Pearce & Newton, 1963, p. 194).

Most primary relationships start with a mix of growth and restrictiveness, but as the interaction progresses, a dominant pattern emerges which is either productive or restrictive. Loving integrations can grow, dissolve, or deteriorate into restrictive ones. Restrictive relationships can become increasingly entrenched, dissolve, or even shift for the better with a change in circumstances, usually when the partners reevaluate their situation (deciding to move from a studio apartment to a larger space, deciding to live separately, or encouraging each other to have more friends). The value of a relationship is not determined by its longevity, but by the degree to which it promotes growth in the partners. Unfortunately, a relationship may last long after the merging of central paranoias, long after the relationship has outlived its usefulness. Just because two people live together for a long time doesn't mean the relationship is satisfying to either person. They could be deteriorating together, convincing each other that the world is a dangerous place and becoming more entrenched in an isolated way of life. On the other hand, if both people continue to expand in their relatedness to other people and increase their creativity and productive work, the relationship might be mutually validating over a long period. Either is possible.

SUMMARY

Human growth involves a complex and ever-changing interaction between people in a developmental sequence from infancy onward. This chapter briefly introduced the basic concepts of interpersonal theory as elucidated in this volume, including the self-system, integral personality, the dissociated, and the central paranoia. Other concepts discussed include depression, despair, tenderness, anxiety, security operations, validation, deterioration, envy, point of fixation, empathy, cherishing, and respect. Personality is the interaction between the self-system, the integral personality, the central paranoia, and the dissociated, utilizing the described mental phenomena in repetitive patterns.

NOTES

1. See discussion of life-threatening infantile apathetic states below.

2. As discussed in the introduction to Developmental Eras, differently abled people require empathic relatedness to their needs. Someone who does not have the physiological ability to crawl and then walk because of cerebral palsy requires tender and proactive relatedness to their need to learn alternate methods of ambulating, including providing people and devices to facilitate mobility.

3. Sullivan (1953) coined the term "self-system." Pearce and Newton (1963) coined the terms "integral personality, "central paranoia," and "the dissociated." All are discussed and elaborated upon in this volume.

4. The use of the word "paranoid" in this context is not what is commonly accepted as a diagnosis in the *DSM* (*Diagnostic and Statistical Manual*, 2013). It defines a despairing conviction that is a departure from what is true in reality on a continuum from a false assumption that regulates one's life (like, "I'm a loser") to the florid paranoid psychotic belief that aliens are in control of one's mind (as described in the *DSM*).

5. See chapters 9 and 11 for full discussions of the self-system, self-image, and perception.

6. Depression, a lack of feeling, is very different from grief, which is an intensely felt emotion in response to an actual loss of some kind.

7. A forbidding gesture is a non-verbal mode of communication that expresses dissatisfaction or disgust with what another is doing or saying. For example, a significant parenting one signals dissatisfaction by stiffening when their toddler tries to climb on their lap, or grimaces and walks away when the child tries to show them something they drew. Often the gestures are spontaneous, and although keenly felt by the child, they are not in the adult's awareness. In early infancy, when empathy is the mode of communication, a forbidding gesture might be the adult's rough and hurried handling of diaper change. A person cannot remember the actual gestured message of disgust from infancy, but now, as an adult, they might be able to get in touch with the mood-memory of self-disgust and be able to connect that mood-memory to stories about their infancy.

8. An overwhelming uneasy feeling accompanied by strenuous dissatisfaction with one's life.

9. There are also situations in which the child is accurate. For example, they attend a racist school, or others are demeaning their emerging gender expression. Adult actions may be necessary to change the environment, such as official interventions, a school transfer, if possible, or guidance on how to deal with the situation.

10. See discussion of empathy below.

11. The term "residuals" as defined here was coined by Pearce and Newton (1963, pp. 83, 89, 94, 102, 107, 113).

PART I

Developmental Eras

From the moment of conception, the human organism builds upon itself, each cluster of cells growing out of earlier ones. Starting with the fetus, each integration of a capacity relies on earlier integrations of capacities, the way a blastula doubles and then doubles again in the womb. "It spreads out over the course of a lifetime in a fanlike direction, to include more specific and more elaborate functions" (Pearce & Newton, 1963, p. 29). As discussed in chapter two, interpersonal validation from the person or people most intimately responsible for the neonate's very survival is essential for the integration of functions, including digestion and skin integrity. The integration of new functions from developmental era to developmental era is also based on validation from those who matter. What happens next depends upon the quality of essential intimate communication. Interpersonal theory posits that all functioning, starting in utero, depends upon the quality of the two-way communication between the primary caretaker and the growing individual.

In the beginning, communication is purely empathic. Babies "in the first hours after birth wish to imitate, and with astonishing discrimination and skill. Indeed they are happy to negotiate exchanges of imitation, taking their turn and inventing new messages" (Trevarthen, 2019b, p. 1, summarizing Nagy and Molnár [2004]).

> This attentive aiming of the baby's sense organs is imaginative and creative using the wisdom of a body feeling its movements intentionally. It is not reflexive, triggered and "conditioned" by stimuli. Thus a blind baby can look, a deaf baby can listen, making the required movements "as if" they had sight or hearing, expecting new experience. Books for parents with powerful photographs show how rich infant sociability normally is in intimate communication. (Trevarthen, 2019b, p. 2, summarizing Nagy and Molnár [2004]; Nugent and Morell [2011])

As the individual grows from era to era, so does the mode of communication, from idiosyncratic—between the infant and the mothering one(s)—to articulation in childhood that is understandable by an ever-expanding interpersonal milieu. Likewise, as the child develops motility and other capacities, understanding the world beyond the bassinet widens exponentially, to varying degrees of satisfaction, depending upon the quality and quantity of interpersonal validation.

Basic assumptions underlying this process are the universality of human needs and the resilience and adaptability of human beings.

In discussing how one function is a prerequisite for the next, such as crawling is essential before walking, it is necessary, as it is with any child, to keep in mind how their needs are met and the extent to which they are met. A caretaker with a deaf child or a child born with cerebral palsy benefits from an understanding of what all children need. Figuring out how to provide appropriate opportunities to satisfy the needs of a differently abled child or one born under the most unfortunate conditions, in most instances, depends mainly on who the caretakers are and what opportunities are or could be made available in a particular community or society. Here are some examples.

Some human needs are more complex than others. Consider the need to communicate with others. If an infant is born deaf, for example, a major adaptation is required on the part of the parents and others, as well as on the part of the infant (the physiology of the infant may be able to compensate for the deficit), in order to meet that infant's need to communicate and feel emotionally connected to others—a vital need across the life span that is intertwined with the need to communicate. Under the most fortunate circumstances, throughout this adaptive process, the caregiver(s) and others never lose sight of the fact that a deaf child is, most importantly, a child with the same needs that every other human being has.

Likewise, when discussing the necessity for "articulate" speech to develop in childhood as a prerequisite to mutually satisfying relatedness with the wider world, the concept of "articulate" must include all modes of communication, such as sign language or, for people like Helen Keller, a reliably different way to communicate. It all depends upon how related the particular caretaker(s) is to the need for the child to develop the capacity to interact with mutual satisfaction with the wider world.

In a sense, then, all humans are differently abled as soon as they have been placed in the arms of their significant, yet imperfect, parenting one(s). The degree and kind of differently abled matters, but "we are all more simply human than otherwise" (Sullivan, 1953, p. 32).[1]

NOTE

1. With this principle, radical for his time, Sullivan was emphasizing that "homosexuals" and people diagnosed schizophrenic must be not be placed in a category of "other" and treated as such. In the current social climate, not only must his one-genus postulate be reasserted, it must particularly call attention to "recently acknowledged complexities in gender identity, development, and both the vulnerability and resilience of transgender communities; in other words, a greater understanding of the diversity in the human condition" (Taffel, 2020, p. 17). This applies to all peoples who are oppressed and whose common humanity must be emphasized.

Chapter Two

Early Infancy

The Development of Initial Blueprints for Later Experience

Early infancy describes the initial stage of a person's development from pre-birth (Goodrich, 2010) to approximately eight months, when the infant is more able to relate to the object world and to issues of mobility (Stern, D. N., 2018).

Repetitive interaction with the infant's primary caretaker(s) organizes the infant's physiological, perceptual-cognitive, and motor functioning (Sullivan, 1953) via the process of validation from this initial audience (Pearce & Newton, 1963). This relationship between infant and mothering figure(s) is the primary force for development of the self-system.

This chapter integrates recent findings that infants demonstrate a high level of responsiveness to their interpersonal environment from even before birth, and how empathy[1] and mood operate in interactions between infant and primary caretaker(s). It briefly covers the development of physiological functioning during early infancy, how deficits during this developmental period might show up in later malfunctioning (residuals[2]), and how to address them. It also discusses the potentially debilitating experience of anxiety that occurs when the person responsible for care is unresponsive in some way to the infant's needs. Even before birth, the caretaker's validating and forbidding moods empathically initiate the formation of the person's self-system. Finally, this chapter studies the impact of these interactions on later functioning.

Because the human being develops through relationships with human beings, the infant develops in relation to what those people are available for.[3] When Sullivan (1953) and Pearce and Newton (1963) developed their theories, the quality of infantile consciousness could only be inferred. Subsequent observational research of psychobiologists who study or cite the normal development of physiological actions and response, along with many earlier psychobiological and ethological researchers in the latter half of the 20th century and early 21st century, empirically confirm the developmental importance of early interpersonal relationships in infancy.[4] Even from before birth the infant actively engages in relating to whatever interpersonal environment is available to meet their psychobiological needs (Goodrich, 2010).

Trevarthen (2006) concludes from his observations that "an infant who is only a few months old has a remarkable range of perceptual capacities that allows for imitative identification, emotional empathy and reciprocal communication that all humans possess" (pp. 127–128). He goes on to say that "the core of human consciousness is the potential for rapport of the self with an other's mind." This potential is "immediate, unrational, unverbalized, conceptless, and atheoretical: A delicate and immediate [being] with-the-other" (p. 121). In interpersonal theory terminology, as discussed by Sullivan (1953) and Pearce and Newton (1963), Trevarthan (personal communication, 2018) is talking about empathy. He uses the term *intersubjective sympathy*.

The infant gradually organizes experiences into a pattern of expectations from its point of view, depending on its needs in that moment (Stern, D. N., 2004). Interpersonal theory infers that initially anyone who creates satisfaction and provides social responsiveness, nutrition, cuddling, rocking, and physical comfort is part of the infant's experience of the "good mother" (Sullivan, 1953, pp. 161–165).[5] By the same token, the infant experiences the "bad mother" with deprivation of need. In fact, Sullivan says, an infant may experience two different "mothers," good and bad, in the same person, or the same "mother" in two different people based on the mood or level of care perceived by the infant. The difference between "good mother" and "bad mother" resides in the infant's experience, which may not resemble the caretaker's or observer's experience.[6]

The infant begins to experience expectations of good and bad in one person in gradually developing foresight and awareness that many of the same characteristics are in the skin of that person, the primary caretaker. If there is more than one important caretaker, the infant gradually develops expectations about each. Although research with newborns reveals that they may identify their mother by their voice (DeCasper & Fifer, 1980), they will learn to get satisfaction from each important person and how to avoid the "bad mother" in each. The process can become rather complex but is important, considering that the infant is growing within a larger cultural context requiring interaction with many significant people (Trevarthen et al., 2014).

PHYSIOLOGICAL DEVELOPMENT IN THE INTERPERSONAL MILIEU

Early infancy is the busiest era of anyone's life and the first 24 hours after a full-term birth involve the most massive reorganization (Pearce & Newton, 1963, p. 78).[7] Most dramatically, the infant transforms from water animal to land animal, requiring changes in skin functioning, breathing, digestion, and temperature control. Oxygen exchange shifts from placental to pulmonary. These changes and many more must be mediated via interaction with a significant person or persons, the primary caretaker(s).

In the last half of the 20th century, researchers[8] began to study interactions between infants and their caretakers via videotape and other means. Citing repeated patterns of preverbal behavior, they attempted to describe hypothetically the subjective experience of the early infant.[9] While they came to many different conclusions, they seemed to agree that the infant begins to interact preverbally with the caretaker much earlier than had been previously thought. For instance, Stern (2018) sees a marked shift at nine months to a symbolic way of thinking. They also observed that crucial information is transmitted between infant and caretaker via a multitude of means, including motor, visual, smell, and proprioception, all of which constitute empathic communication. The infant can also immediately perceive the same message via proprioception, smell, vision, etc.

The human animal is social from the start. In the literature, there much discussion about the role of heredity in infantile development and the relative importance of heredity versus environment (nature versus nurture) in determining a person's future outcome regarding intelligence, the ability or proclivity for particular skills, and the tendency for various forms of mental illness or temperament. Therapists often meet people preoccupied with fears that they have inherited parental life patterns and will inevitably make the same mistakes, often the basis for an unfortunate decision to avoid many major life projects.

While certain effects of genes in determining human development are incontrovertible, how the mothering one(s) relates to emerging functions and needs of the infant are also crucial. "A kitten will grow up to be a cat no manner how much one cuddles with it or talks to it. It will never be a person. How one treats that cat will significantly influence its temperament, health, activity level and relatedness to people, but the cat will still develop within a specific, feline autopoietic structure" (Maturana & Varela, 1980).

Many studies attempt to prove genetic differences between human infants that lead to various forms of mental disorders,[10] but they fail to provide a specific, detailed understanding of how this happens (except perhaps to suggest that certain genetic traits are activated or remain dormant in the brain depending upon experience). There is also a tendency to tie such studies to the clinical use of medication based on the assumption that particular behavioral traits are genetically determined and therefore unchangeable except by use of physiological agents such as psychotropic medication or electric shock therapy.

The interpersonal orientation to human development and infant potential examines the interaction between physiological and social phenomena affecting human development. It assumes that human potential and behavioral traits can be profoundly and effectively influenced by interactions with others and the feelings of joy and pride, sadness, fear, and shame that are produced by those interactions (Damasio, 2018; Jaswal & Akhtar, 2019; Pearce & Newton, 1963; Sullivan, 1953).[11]

PERCEPTUAL DEVELOPMENT

From birth or before, the infant responds to surrounding people. Researchers have described the remarkable capacity of babies within the first minutes of birth to respond to visual and auditory cues such as tone of voice and facial gestures (Trevarthen, 2006, p. 151).

From this it is inferred that to meet their needs, the infant learns the caretaker's response patterns. The infant is all about survival, learning to cope with parental emotional patterns, including disjunctive, repeated patterns of anger and unrelatedness.

Notably, parental dysfunctional moods must be repeated often before permanently affecting the infant. Occasional vicissitudes in mood do not constitute ongoing patterns. Parenting ones don't need to monitor every mood, fearing to inflict permanent damage.

Repeated disruption of response to the infant's needs for tenderness can come from many sources, such as economic instability, war, environmental crisis, or parental unavailability. The infant doesn't know the reason for deprivation. They just need to get their needs met.

During early infancy there is only rudimentary development of foresight, the ability to form expectations based on experience. This ability becomes more complex over time.

Nevertheless, caretakers often ascribe complicated motivations to babies, such as seduction, malevolence, or willfulness, but these are adult expectations. The infant is simply crying when hungry, cold, irritated by a wet or soiled diaper, colicky, or experiencing parental anxiety and disapproval, etc. Motivated to relieve the tensions of hunger and pain, to satisfy the need for tenderness and to avoid anxiety, the infant is incapable of manipulation, seduction, or domineering. "The baby won't let me rest" is a commentary on the adult's state of mind. Such characterizations can become an accepted part of the infant's developing self-image, if it goes on long enough, because they learn to accommodate to the caretaker's expectations.

> Elaine's mother experienced her as an annoyance from birth. Elaine was her first child and she felt unprepared to take care of a baby who not only cried but also defecated, spit up, and wiggled. Throughout Elaine's childhood she continued to attribute her emerging needs as repeated offenses cooked up to irritate her. Elaine gradually accommodated to the accusation that her needs were a deliberate provocation. She learned to express her needs provocatively because it was the only way that she was able to get recognition of them. As an adult she became a bully, picking fights with strangers and associates and unable to accommodate others' needs. This pattern developed through the preverbal empathic communication between mother and infant long before memory was established. Elaine accepted her mother's perception of her as reality and acted accordingly into adulthood.

EMPATHY

Empathy, communication by resonance with the caretaker(s)' mood, is the primary mode of communication in infancy. All available senses are involved (Trevarthen, 2011a, 2011b), including voice and other sounds, gestures, and facial expressions, as well as the quality of touch, texture, temperature, and pressure. Smell, the most primitive of senses, is also likely involved.

Sullivan (1953) and Pearce and Newton (1963) posit that empathy is most intensely experienced in infancy. Empathic cues that adults assume they are concealing from the infant, or don't notice themselves, may be transmitted via muscle tension, proprioception, smell, temperature, and sound. The baby responds to these cues. Some say that empathic communication can be felt through walls, an experience that can go on well past infancy.

Margaret Ribble (1938) and René Spitz (1945, 1946a, 1946b) solidly established the importance of some kind of an empathic bond between an infant and a caretaker. Without an empathic bond, the interpersonal interaction with the caretaker(s) involving physical contact, the infant cannot survive (Cytryn & McKnew, 1996; Emde et al., 1965; Ribble, 1965). Substitutes, such as always propping a bottle up for the baby to drink alone, produce, at best, severe malfunction. When Spitz studied infants who were efficiently cared for but rarely handled in a pristine foundling home, he observed that they became increasingly listless, unresponsive, and prone to infection. They were suffering from "anaclitic depression."[12] Many died, and those who survived were hardly able to function. Infants who received consistent tender contact with their primary caretaker(s)—including rocking, cooing, talking, or singing to them while giving them their bottles—did not suffer from anaclitic depression, even in an institutional setting.

Participant-observation of empathic communication from birth to 16 hours of life has provided very valuable, empirically demonstrable evidence of this crucial developmental period (Beebe et al., 1965; Trevarthen, 2011a, 2011b).

Every caretaker has limited capacity to relate tenderly to *all* the infant's needs. To the extent that primary caretaker(s) cannot respond appropriately to an infant's need, that function is denied validation and poorly consolidated. The infant, totally dependent on mood and relatedness of the caretaker, mirrors the limitations of the caretaker, even for physiological functioning. For example, a caretaker who is uncomfortable with touch communicates that discomfort to the infant, whose skin integrity and muscle tone are developing and susceptible. Eczema, hypersensitivity, insensitivity, and poor muscle tone are ways skin and musculature falter in functioning as a result.

When a caretaker responds, the infant resonates with the response. If a caretaker is unresponsive to the surrounding world, so is the infant. If a caretaker perceives the infant's behavior to be in a particular mood, e.g., demanding, petulant, imperious, playful, charming, or cute, the infant's behavior will mold itself to parental expectations, "mirroring" the caretaker's perception more and more as the interaction between the two develops over time.

BEGINNING THE DEVELOPMENT OF FORESIGHT

Sullivan, theorizing before the emergence of much of the neurological research, posited that infantile consciousness consists of an unorganized flood of sensation without a sense of time or sequence (Mullahy, 1948, pp. 286–291). He called it *prototaxic* consciousness. According to psychobiological and neurological research published beginning in the last half of the 20th century up until the present, perception and foresight begin developing in the human embryo proprioceptively[13] via interaction with the embryo's surroundings in utero (Goodrich, 2010). The infant at birth is already attuned to communicating with its environment. These later findings place the beginnings of awareness at a much earlier time in human development, in utero, and stress the importance of sensory interaction via the whole body.

From birth, the experience of need and the satisfaction of need provide the structure for the development of infantile perception. The infant experiences the tension of a very basic need, such as food or cuddling. They cry and hear and feel their own cry. They feel the repeated experience of need satisfaction through the tender presence of the caretaker, preceded and accompanied by cues such as smell, touch, and tone of voice. A particular expectation develops, *crying with the expectation of satisfaction.*

Foresight also develops as the infant grasps what Sullivan (1953) calls "forbidding gestures" (pp. 86–91, 121n, 166) in the parent-while-anxious: a shift in parental mood from playful to angry or withdrawn, or a shift in muscle tension from cuddly to stiff. As they move into more complex levels of perceptual capacity, they learn to tailor their responses toward satisfaction and anxiety avoidance. For example, the infant may begin to refrain from touching their genital and anal areas if parental anxiety increases when observing such behavior. The infant starts "testing the limits," gauging their responses to the parental anxiety level. Sullivan (1953) calls this an "anxiety gradient" (pp. 151–153), which can go on long after early infancy.

Early infancy is fraught with breakdowns in functioning; infants are primarily focused on learning to accommodate to parental expectations (and vice versa). The functions they need to learn are urgent but dependent on the comfort level of the primary caretaker and, empathically, the infant.

ANXIETY

When the infant's need makes the caretaker anxious, the caretaker makes a forbidding gesture, often outside awareness. The infant tailors their response to the caretaker's limitations. This repeated interaction between them generates the formation of the self-system.[14] The level of anxiety in the caretaker(s)' response to the infant's need determines how much the infant can relate to that need. If there is relatively little anxiety, the learning of the function to satisfy the need becomes part of the "Good-Me" personification of the self-system (Sullivan, 1953, pp. 162–163). If the response is somewhat negative but only moderately anxious, the need and the function to satisfy it become part of the "Bad-Me." Severe anxiety about the infant's need feels much like a "blow on the head" (Sullivan, 1953, p. 160), obliterating awareness of the need, relegating it to the "Not-Me." Such experience can only be brought into awareness with severe, uncanny emotions, like dread, loathing, or horror.

When severe parental anxiety continues, crying to stop that disjunctive mood doesn't work. However, the infant has no other means to bring relief; crying continues, possibly leading to a physiological crisis, such as convulsions and difficulty breathing. Mechanisms such as somnolent detachment, a retreat to sleep, bring relief but can also result in an attenuation of functioning. If the caretaker is still anxious when the infant awakes, crying begins again. The cycle of caretaker and infant anxiety spirals because continued crying creates more adult anxiety, exacerbating the situation.

If possible, a solution is for the caretaker to find an alternate adult who can tenderly relate to the infant until the primary caretaker can relate more comfortably. Another solution may be for the caretaker to locate a more comfortable setting to relate to the baby. Ability to help the baby stop crying is often viewed competitively or morally, not pragmatically, so parenting ones, particularly new ones, often feel watched and judged if their baby doesn't stop crying right away; they need to feel less judged.

The scenario of the incessantly crying baby is common. Child-rearing literature and common lore offer many solutions that are often morally tinged. People may grow up with stories about being an "angry baby" because they wouldn't stop crying. The concept of "spoiling," giving in to infant's "imperious" demands by providing food or cuddling, is a belief that the infant is motivated by something other than simple infantile needs. The solution is to determine how to relieve the tension of need, whatever it may be. If the caretaker is unsuccessful, it is not a moral issue; it is a practical one.

Additional helpers, a spouse, partner, friend, relative, nanny, or nurse can bring relief. In traditional households of previous centuries, and in some cultures today, a wider range of people would assist with caring for the newborn. The baby might be passed along to adults who are more available, experienced, and effective in helping the baby stop crying. A solution is rarely perfect, but the projection of complicated adult motivations onto the infant never helps.

A frequently recommended way to cope is to "let the baby cry it out," or to muffle the crying by putting the infant in the basement or a soundproof nursery. Non-response to the baby's only mode of expression of urgent need may provide relief for the harried parenting one, but it also disrupts the intimate relationship between the parenting one and newborn and provides a particularly dismal lesson in the early development of foresight, which in adulthood can be deficient or distorted, starting from the lowered infantile expectation of need satisfaction. Depending on the amount of isolation, the solution of letting the infant cry it out can have serious consequences, as discussed above.

> A woman described being placed on the back porch out of earshot as an infant to "cry it out." As an adult she exhibited marked anesthesia regarding her current needs. She was depressed and phlegmatic with peers. She was severely obese and did not notice hunger or discomfort from overeating.

VALIDATION AND THE DIFFERENCE BETWEEN BAD-ME AND NOT-ME

Lack of validation is not purposeful. The parenting one(s) who has dissociated a particular need is unrelated to the need the infant expresses. If the infant blatantly expresses their need and a parenting one's avoidance operations fail, the parenting one's reaction is severe anxiety accompanied by "uncanny emotions," such as dread, horror, or loathing. It is so severe, it is like that "blow on the head" which usually wipes out the infant's conscious memory of the impulse or need. It is communicated empathically via mood or other forbidding gestures.

Not-me: During diaper change, a four-month-old touches their genitalia in obvious pleasure, which the parenting one finds very anxiety provoking. The parenting one has long ago completely dissociated their own experience of masturbation. In response, they might abruptly break off diapering, frantically remembering an "extremely urgent" household task that must be done immediately or something terrible will happen. They hurriedly leave the undiapered baby, possibly covering the offending parts, to do the household task. A little while later, they calm down, hear the baby crying, and remember the baby needs a diaper. Now, during diapering, the baby does not resume offensive touching. To complete their dissociation of this pleasure, the experience must be repeated several times. Starting in adolescence, they might experience sexual feelings and urges to masturbate with severe anxiety, dread, and confusion.

Bad-me: If the same behavior is not totally dissociated by the parenting one, but they consider it "bad" or undesirable, they may relate negatively, perhaps thinking, "My baby is a sex fiend!" or exclaiming, "How can I keep you clean?!" They might become preoccupied with "catching" the odious behavior. In this case, the need and the function are conscious in the infant, but experienced as bad or dirty, certainly offensive. Starting in adolescence, they might satisfy sexual needs, but with some misgivings, perhaps including shame and revulsion.

RESIDUALS AND TREATMENT

Residuals are difficulties in living manifested in later life that originate from dissociation in a developmental era. An adult starting psychotherapy may have deficits beginning in infancy. The relationship between the infant and the primary caretaker(s) forms the basis for skewed emotional patterning, unique to each individual and persisting throughout life. Vivid infantile mood-memories[15] persist and become more noticeable at moments in adult life, particularly when they are faced with the emergence of the dissociated need.

Human consciousness develops in the context of other human beings, that is, in relationship to one or more significant persons: the *audience*. From the beginning, all experience is developed in relationship to other significant persons and tailored to what is conceivable to that audience. This includes mood. The emotional patterning that begins in infancy remains a kind of bedrock upon which other, broader experiences are built, based on interactions with new people who become significant. All people carry with them a characteristic way they view the world and a characteristic mood in which they experience events. To the extent that they have been taught to be comfortable with people beyond the first significant caretaker(s), they can become broader and more flexible with the expansion of significant relationships (or new audiences) in their lives.

Encouraging development of new audiences is therapeutic. If a person's early experience has been with parenting figure(s) whose capacity for tenderness is limited and whose mood is disjunctive, i.e., paranoid, rageful, depressed, or fearful, the person's attempt to push the boundaries of their parental acceptability will powerfully thrust that mood into awareness as they, in the present, begin to again challenge the limitations of their earlier experience.

A very useful therapeutic intervention can be: "You are talking as if you are still living by your mother's rules." The rejoinder, understandably, may be, "My mother has been dead for 15 years. This has nothing to do with her!" It is important to establish that the first years are the most formative. Through exploring their history and connecting current intense moods with earlier memories, particularly mood-memories, they learn that interactions with primary caretaker(s) during early years are wittingly or unwittingly still living with them. Forming the basic patterning of personality, the formative primary audience can still promote or limit growth. When an area of functioning is limited, a change in the current audience for it is crucial, even though the person may have expanded their functioning in other areas and moved on. Teachers, mentors, friends, and partners are profoundly influential audiences for functions forbidden by the original audience.

> James's mother was fairly unresponsive to her infant's curiosity and enthusiasm. He grew up somewhat subdued in mood, avoiding exploration beyond certain limits. His seventh grade teacher, excited about learning, involves the class in simple experiments. The students work in pairs and the timid preadolescent starts a project with a particularly enthusiastic partner. James begins looking forward to science class, the highlight of his day. He may not talk about it at home, but now he even considers majoring in physics in college.

Making up deficits isn't an intellectual process. It involves, usually through therapeutic inquiry into a person's history, reliving experiences, remembering, noticing, and feeling what has been unattended or poorly attended to. That process is particularly difficult when deficits originate in infancy, when there are no describable memories except for mood-memories, those moods that seem to pop up mysteriously out of nowhere. The therapist attempts to obtain the person's history from birth through early infancy from remembered stories told by parenting one(s), relatives, and family friends; baby books, photos, and videos also help. Useful questions include: What were you told about people's first reactions to you when you were born? What kind of an infant were you (did you sleep through the night; did you cry a lot)? Were you considered a good baby, bad baby, spoiled, colicky, sickly, fussy? What was going on in the household when you were an infant? Did they say you "took after" someone? Who was that?" What stories did they tell about that person? These early pieces of information can provide a framework for exploration and an intellectual understanding of current problems. It can sometimes provoke an emotional reliving of an earlier mood. However, that kind of reliving requires detailed exploration that reevokes infantile experience of need.

> In working with a man severely uncomfortable with physical contact, who experienced another's touch with numbness or pain, the therapist was looking for experiences that involved touch and caretaking that were more accessible to consciousness. His brother was born when he was three. He remembered how protective he felt of the tiny baby and his subsequent delight when he could make them smile. He got in touch with powerful emotions he had buried from the age of three in the service of maintaining an aloof, complaining, and distant persona. Recalling the intensity of his feeling with his brother seemed to open availability to similar experiences in the current. While not directly accessing his negative, infantile experiences with the anxiety-laden touch, the person was able to make up for unfinished business by remembering later pleasure with that function in the experience as a three-year-old.

PSYCHOSOMATIC SYMPTOMS

Basic, physiological functions[16] *cannot develop without* the tender, loving care of at least one other human being. With little validation, physiology will develop with a skew.[17] This includes physiological functions that may or may not have direct interaction with the primary caretaker(s) but are affected because they are impacted by the caretaker's anxiety or lack of relatedness to the infant's well-being during the crucial period of their emergence. For example, though not directly affected by the early caretaker(s), the organs of the digestive tract may be affected by disruptive moods the infant experiences while feeding or afterward.

Symptoms commonly thought of as psychosomatic may have developed in part because of this disturbance (Pearce & Newton, 1963, p. 86).[18] The therapist needs to employ a two-pronged approach to psychosomatic symptoms: Their analysand needs to obtain appropriate medical attention for structural damage already affecting the body. Simultaneously, the analysand needs to address the ongoing lack of awareness or distortion of certain vital infantile functions and its effect on adult functioning. Increased awareness of the origins of the problem and the behaviors that exacerbate it can, little by little, prevent the same dysfunction from recurring or diminish its frequency, severity, and/or duration. They also learn to notice the timing of symptoms. While treating them medically the person also strives to understand the emotional triggers and recognize them as reactions from very early infantile experience.

For example, in the case of a person with chronic digestive problems, in addition to a medical referral, the therapist and analysand investigate the context in which indigestion occurs and identify accompanying moods. Broadening awareness of one's moods allows them to be more in touch with disjunctive and/or angry emotional states affecting the gastrointestinal tract. It is also important to explore the analysand's early interpersonal experience around food intake, including stories of nursing, incidents of colic and/or other digestive problems, memories of what it was like at meals (to perhaps infer earlier parental moods around food), and the range and depth of their freedom to explore and choose food as an infant and young child. As awareness increases, the person's mood around eating can change, including expansion of food choices and sensations and making more educated food selections to give the digestive system a break.

The issue of psychosomatic symptoms is important because all physiological systems, including the neonate's skin, digestive, respiratory, sympathetic, parasympathetic, and circulatory systems, are in very immature states. Their development becomes skewed when the infant is anxious.[19] Later in life, under the impact of anxiety, organs that developed with a skew may break down, causing a range of dysfunction severity from minor, such as hives or contact dermatitis, to severe, such as proneness to infection or ulcers.

The emotional climate during early infancy also affects the immune system. For example, one might become ill at particular times of crisis or change. Since anxiety disrupts functioning in general, if a particular organ is already weakened by prior infection or damage, it can be further compromised during a period of crisis or anxiety.

At three months, Catherine had a severe life-threatening strep throat infection, which was successfully treated with antibiotics. The infection reoccurred at key moments of crisis during her childhood and adolescence.

Catherine's parents were not comfortable with strangers. They were extremely paranoid about allowing her intimate social contact with other kids. However, because of their need to work, it was convenient to send her to sleep-away camp every summer from the age of 10 to 17. Given her parents' discomfort with people, Catherine was shy in the informal peer setting of camp. Despite enjoying the camp experience, she would spend at least one week in camp infirmary with a strep infection.

At 18, anxious about moving out of her parents' home, Catherine fell ill with her most severe strep infection, which then reoccurred more frequently. In therapy, she achieved insight about the connection between that susceptibility—her poorly developed immune system in early infancy—and strep throat during an anxious time. It required insight before she would agree to a tonsillectomy to reduce bouts of upper respiratory infections during periods of anxiety-producing change.

SUMMARY

Development takes place in the context of interpersonal interactions. The primary caretaker(s) has a profound influence upon functions developing in infancy, even upon physiological functions not ordinarily considered susceptible to human interaction. To the extent then primary caretaker(s) is not available to tenderly relate to the infant's needs, there is a gradient of disruption to physiological functioning that, in the extreme, can lead to death. In less extreme situations, residuals often take the form of chronic physiological disorders, difficulty with physical contact, and disjunctive moods.

Strenuous and disruptive moods and psychosomatic symptoms rising out of current experiences can be, through therapeutic inquiry, traced to early infancy. They occur whenever the person wittingly or unwittingly has an experience that challenges their original infantile audience, threatening to expand current personality.

In treatment the person gradually learns to connect such moods to repeated historical events and to understand their function in the maintenance of old dysfunctional patterns. When the person uses such reactions to retreat to those old, dysfunctional patterns, such as avoiding physical tenderness as an adult, the person is actually exploiting the unwanted mood or physiological symptom to maintain connection with the original primary caretaker(s), the original audience.

Maintaining the original audience in these situations prevents growth. The person learns in therapy to understand where the uncomfortable and undesirable reactions come from and to change their original audience to appropriate validating peers in the current. They also understand that anxiety comes with the territory of change and that they need a positive audience to help them weather the storm.

Physiological symptoms must also be addressed medically. There is no such thing as "it's just emotional." It is necessary to treat such symptoms on both fronts.

However, one of the most significant lessons a person can learn and retain is that weathering the anxiety storm can result in positive growth. One works through it like a "charley horse" of the brain. The emotional muscle will emerge stronger and ready to take on even more growth.

NOTES

1. Empathy, as described by Sullivan (1968) and used interpersonally, involves communication of feeling by mood and gesture or via means not yet understood. Trevarthen and his associates use the term "intersubjective sympathy" in reference to the communication between the infant and its caretaker(s). There has been much empirical research over the past 50 years on the physiology of modes of response in infancy, for example, Cytryn & McKnew (1996), Damasio (2018), DeCasper & Fifer (1980), Goodrich (2010), Maturana & Varela (1980), Trevarthen (1989, 1993a, 2011a, 2011b), and Trevarthen et al. (2014).

2. Residuals are functions not adequately consolidated in a particular developmental era that affect how one functions in later life. The term as defined here was coined by Pearce and Newton (1963, pp. 83, 89, 94, 102, 107, 113).

3. Bowlby (1982) states that to understand attachment in an infant, it is necessary to know what the mother's condition is because "only when this has been done can the pattern of interaction between them be seen and the child's part in it understood" (p. 334).

4. For example, Bowlby (1982), Damasio (2018), Goodrich (2010), Stern, D. N. (2018), Trevarthen (1989, 1993a, 2011a), and Trevarthen et al. (2014) .

5. Sullivan employs the word "personification" in relation to good and bad mother. He takes pains to emphasize that the infant formulates its own expectations based on experience with satisfaction and dissatisfaction. There is no good mother or bad mother out there in the real world.

6. For a more detailed discussion of the concept of personification in infancy plus a comparison with Freudian theory, see Sullivan (1968, pp. 166–167). Also, for further elaboration of the concept, see Pearce and Newton (1963, pp. 184–189) in the chapter called "The Personifications of Infancy." For more detailed observational research on the ability of the infant to engage in responsive interaction with people, see Trevarthen (2011a, 2011b).

7. For a more detailed discussion of the development of physiological functioning in infancy, see Pearce and Newton (1963, pp. 77–83).

8. For example, Beebe (1973), Beebe & Gerstman (1980), Beebe & Sloate (1982), Beebe et al. (2003), Brazelton (1982), Brazelton et al. (1974), Butterwoth & Castello (1976), Meltzoff & Moore (1983), Stern, D. N. (1971, 1974, 1977), and Trevarthen (1977, 1979, 1980).

9. Bowlby (1982) concludes that the child's ability to relate or not to others stems from the interaction with the mothering figure and that to understand the nature of the dyad, it is necessary to study the interaction between them (p. 361).

10. For example, Faraone et al. (1999), Hyman (2000), Insel & Wang (2010), and McGuffin & Murray (2013).

11. Also see commentary on the article by Jaswal and Akhtar (Delafield-Butt et al., 2019).

12. A term coined by Spitz (1946a) to refer to the immediate effect on a newborn when it is deprived of affectionate contact from another human being.

13. Awareness of the position of one's body mediated by sensory neurons in the inner ear, muscles, and ligaments.

14. In interpersonal theory, the term "self-system," coined by H. S. Sullivan (1953), is one's sense of self at any particular moment. It has both productive and restrictive characteristics. It can grow from experience or ward off growth from experience by omission or distortion. The self-system organizes awareness. If the self-system could be frozen in time, it would consist of what a person has available to consciousness, that is, awareness of what one can do and who one believes oneself to be in relation to self, other people, and the world.

15. As discussed in chapter eight, in adulthood, the memory of infantile experience such as pleasure, satisfaction, euphoria, terror, and anxiety are intensely felt and can reappear later in life as if from nowhere and in powerful form as mood-memory. The mood-memory can be negative or positive, reflecting the actual experience in infancy. They can also be dredged up from slightly later experiences (past the age of four or five months) in the parataxic, when there is still very limited capacity to verbalize and limited ability to orient oneself enough to have conscious memory.

16. Functions are the operations an individual learns to satisfy needs.

17. Empirical evidence indicates that early negative experiences produce pro-inflammatory phenotype cells in the immune system, which are directly related to cardiovascular disease, autoimmune diseases, and certain types of cancer (Chung et al., 2009).

18. Although children vary genetically and every individual requires different attachment relationships, there is consistent evidence that maternal warmth during infancy and childhood creates a safe haven for individuals resulting in superior immune system functioning (Chen et al., 2011).

19. The quality of caregiving received at infancy and childhood directly affects the individual's neurological systems, which controls stress regulation (Fox & Hane, 2008).

Chapter Three

Late Infancy

Exploring Beyond the Self

Late infancy begins as the infant moves from total dependency on primary caretaker(s) to involvement with the wider world, including alternate validators.[1] Major areas of functioning that begin to develop include relatedness to the object world, increased mobility, and increased communication, each developing sequentially. The infant also begins learning to relate to a wider world of people. Pearce and Newton (1963) define late infancy as the time the child is learning to walk until they achieve some ability to form phrases (about one to two-and-a-half).[2]

The infant continues developing rudimentary foresight and learns to identify who is coming in response to their crying. Not only can they begin to distinguish between adequate or inadequate responders, they also learn to distinguish between moods that tend to be helpful and those that will just make things worse within *one* caretaker. Through ever-sharpening perceptions of who's who, they continue developing methods to get a "good mother"[3] response for a need to be met and to avoid anxiety in those responsible for their well-being. They are expanding upon the earliest forms of learning, the "organization of experience" (Sullivan, 1953, p. 150).

In so many ways the toddler is no longer completely helpless and dependent, which the primary caretaker(s) may perceive as positive or negative. In either case, the parenting one(s) must adjust to the change in a variety of ways because of the infant's now highly energetic relating to the world beyond itself. Simultaneously, the primary caretaker(s) must learn to provide the support and tenderness the toddler continues to need despite their increased mobility.

Because they are sharpening differentiations between people and how to relate to them, they are developing preferences for particular people, a sense of attachment,[4] upset by separation from select people and very in tune to the primary caretaker(s)' approval or disapproval. Who else matters (siblings, grandparents, babysitters, daycare teachers and godparents, etc.) depends upon that assessment. Empathically responsive to the primary caretaker(s)' approving and disapproving moods, they mirror those responses in relating to alternate validators.

As other people emerge as desirable and significant, they are nevertheless not as important as the primary caretaker(s) but still "rank" as potentially available. With these additional interactions, their perceptions of the world expand. Household pets are interesting toys and potential alternate validators; the toddler learns how to relate to them as well.

EXPLORATION OF THE OBJECT WORLD

Development of increased visual-motor coordination, coupled with curiosity and increased mobility, makes it possible for them to explore objects within reach using all receptive modes, including the mouth. This exploration, which benefits the toddler by enhancing visual-motor coordination and mobility, happens regardless of adult assumptions about what is appropriate for them to play with—whether it be a speck on the floor or a dangling electric cord. The adult(s) must adapt the home to safely accommodate this curious, mobile explorer. "Babyproofing" the house or the baby's area is crucial so the toddler can comfortably explore without getting reprimanded at every turn. Even with babyproofing, the caretaker(s) must remain vigilant.

They begin to cherish particular objects, maybe a favorite cuddle toy or a baby blanket that absolutely must go wherever they go. There can also be temporary "crushes" on particular objects that change unpredictably. The primary caretaker(s)' respect for the toddler's designation of favorite objects is important and goes a long way in teaching the budding personality comfort with cherishing.

MOBILITY

The process of mobility, a major milestone in late infancy, has stages, as with any other function. It starts with motility, then the ability to roll over in early infancy, then crawling, which may start as crawling backward. This takes a while, perhaps producing initial frustration in an impatient parenting one. Crawling is very important, linked with interest in exploration of the object world and, most critically, increasing autonomy. The ability to stand and then toddle occurs toward the end of the process.[5]

Parental attitude is important. Learning to walk can be accomplished in an enthusiastic atmosphere, one of apprehension, or anywhere in between.

Unfortunate parental attitudes include insistence on rushing things (trying to skip the crawling phase or irritability at the baby's pace) or apprehension about falling. Learning to fall is part of the process.

Accomplishments develop in logical sequence. For example, if a baby crawls comfortably, chances are they'll start walking easily. If the primary caretaker(s) rushes the process, pushing them to walk before they're ready, they may have an unfortunate beginning in learning to walk that can manifest later as poor balance, disorientation, or uncertainty. As with any function, adult mood influences how they learn to walk, maybe conveying the assumption that the physical world is dangerous and the infant should be fearful ("Uh oh, be careful!") or that falling is tragic instead of a learning experience. On the other hand, with a sufficiently energetic and alert caretaker(s) who babyproofs the environment, exploration can be a game; the adult(s) is a reliable backstop, encouraging them to try again.

OTHER SKILLS

During this time, other behaviors emerge, depending upon opportunities the primary caretaker(s) provides, often within the widening circle of parentally approved validators. In the development of perceptual-motor skills, artistic skills can burgeon.[6] The toddler can develop musical skills by singing along with the adults or the music they play for them. They also can develop rudimentary art skills, such as scribbling with a crayon, or rudimentary problem-solving by taking pleasure in solving simple puzzles. Exploring textures and tactile experiences involving paints, food, or mud is fun, depending on parental tolerance of the experience.

TRAINING AND "SOCIALIZING" THE TODDLER

Socialization training intensifies depending upon the frequency and consistency in which it takes place (Sullivan, 1953, p. 173). In addition to toilet training and learning how to self-feed, the infant is now being trained to walk, talk, and identify objects (even if they can't name them), among the most obvious socialization lessons. The infant has more control over bladder and bowels and is learning how to use the potty. This process is long and very dependent on the caregiver(s)'s sensitivity to the infant's actual muscular ability to maintain control, along with the nature of their response to the infant's efforts. Potty training is usually not fully integrated until after late infancy.

Useful conscious and unconscious training via mood, gestures, and other overt reactions occurs as a part of teaching the toddler how to behave in the world of humans. Teaching comes out of tender parental feelings toward the growing baby: The caretaker(s) is thrilled when the baby pushes up from crawling or they take that first step. When the baby points at an object of curiosity, the parenting one(s) hands it to them (assuming it's safe) or tenderly redirects them to another more appropriate item. When they point to a colorful poster of a clown, trying to get the parenting one(s) to look too, the adult(s) pays attention, is enthusiastic, and might even name it. When they start imitating a musical phrase, the parenting one(s) claps, sings along, and may enthusiastically comment about their good ear, just like Aunt So-And-So.

Significant adults can interfere with comfortable learning of functions in several ways. One interference is demanding that the baby learn things before they're ready. For example, a parent may insist the toddler be completely toilet trained by 15 months, generally too young. These kinds of demands can make a toddler feel bad or disgusting, creating terrible anxiety around a process that should be simply practical and useful information (Sullivan, 1953, p. 174).

Adult moods during training interact with the particular functions being taught at the time. They can affect how people ultimately see themselves and how they experience learning. These late infancy experiences can become the bases for lifelong patterns of behavior and self-image.

> As a social worker Kitty's supervisors often praised her for excellent services to her caseload. Nevertheless, she always felt guilty and ashamed because she had trouble finishing required paperwork, understandable given her large caseload. She chose social work against her parents' wishes. Finance was much more prestigious. Kitty felt guilty about disappointing them but loved her work. Her career choice was among the many ways Kitty experienced herself as shameful: she failed to fulfill her responsibilities and didn't live up to parental expectations.
>
> Therapeutic historical inquiry provided clues to the possible genesis of her deep feelings of shame and guilt. A key memory was from late infancy. Her mother was scrubbing her in the bathtub, punctuating her words with every scrub: "When will you learn to use the potty?" When she was seven, her aunt told her a story about when she was two. She had asked Kitty why she was sitting under the table during a family get-together. Her mom answered, "Kitty probably wet her pants." Her impatient and critical moods around toilet training and learning how to hold a cup without spilling, for example, established a framework for future learning experiences. Kitty was supposed to learn immediately and her "slowness" was disparaged. Shame was the "normal" way to react to a mistake; she was not taught to understand learning as a process with predictable errors. Later, her parents' impatient and critical reaction to her school

performance ("Why didn't you get 100?"), success at sports, skill at parking the car, etc., reinforced her early experiences with learning.

The early infant's innocent incessant demand that needs be met is in essence "teaching" the caretaker(s) about how to respond to their needs, satisfactorily or not, with whatever amount of empathic connection exists at a given moment and with whatever gradient of anxiety (see below). The mothering one(s), particularly a new one(s), learns how to respond as the baby makes their needs known. Their early infant's need for tenderness stimulates or evokes to varying degrees the experience of tenderness in the mothering one(s). But as the baby grows into late infancy, the parenting one(s) may expect them to respond to *their* training and be more obedient in communication and behaviors that go along with that training. They might also assume that the baby now has a *will* to defy.

In early infancy, when the baby defecates, they get a nice clean diaper. In crying, the baby has "asked" for things to be removed so they can feel good again. In later infancy the infant is rewarded twice for telling mommy in a better way, "Potty!" When mommy brings them to the potty, the baby receives two rewards: no messy diaper and warm satisfaction that mommy is happy with their behavior. Acculturation takes place: now the baby is more trainable. Regarding defecation, many adults (maybe because of how their own infancy went) may be so phobic, controlling, or insensitive about how to relate to this piece of acculturation that the whole issue of toilet training might be full of contradictions.

Recall that there are many unfortunate situations in which parenting figures see themselves as training the baby, even from birth. In fact, they *are*, outside of awareness, training the baby around needs by their moods and unconscious forbidding gestures. Even in early infancy, a mothering one who is disgusted while changing diapers is, through mood and forbidding gestures, conveying to the infant that they're disgusting. But it's another story if a mothering one is also consciously determined to train the early infant as if they are already trainable. For example, if the infant is shaking a rattle, and in their enthusiasm bops an older sibling's head, they cannot be trained not to hit as if they are already bad. Sometimes the story about how the infant was "a bully from the very beginning" gets repeated and may even become a prophecy the child fulfills—as early as late infancy—having accepted the mantra as the "reality" of who they are.

COMMUNICATION

While the baby's first words are generally uttered before 12 months, the mode of communication is increasingly dramatic. Vocabulary is largely developed with the primary validator(s) as the audience. When cooing and babbling are met with delight and encouragement, when the primary caretaker(s) talks comfortably with the baby, first words come naturally but are still used dramatically—part of private communication with the caretaker(s). Words have private meaning known mostly to the parenting one(s) and people close to the home environment. In fact, those people are often asked to "translate" for those who are not in the charmed circle. Words, still private between the primary caretaker(s) and the late infant, are part of dramatic communication even when others can understand them.

Verbal communication is primarily dramatic, such as the use of simple words or phrases, like, "No!" "More!" and "Bye-bye." "No," easily learned because adults repeat it as the toddler tries exploring forbidden or unsafe objects, is often an attempt to establish some autonomy, not necessarily simply defiance. When a toddler has their heart set on something, it can be very difficult to change their mind. Even redirection doesn't help. But the temper tantum is not willful defiance. It's toddler inability to understand adult reasoning. These behaviors, often extending into early childhood, are often called the "terrible twos." How caretaker(s) handle them significantly influences how to relate to any authority and the development of independence.

DEVELOPMENT OF OBJECT CONSTANCY

Playing games becomes gradually more sophisticated, perhaps starting with mimicking adults in "peekaboo," which goes a long way in developing "Object Constancy" (Piaget & Inhelder, 1969). If the younger infant's crying for a need gets met in a timely fashion, it is more or less oblivious about whether mommy is in the room at all times. However, as the older infant develops distinct preferences for who will satisfactorily fulfill their needs, they become upset if that particular person(s) is not in plain view. Once they achieve object permanency, they understand that when the object disappears it may still exist, just hidden. The infant may vociferously demand mommy come back, but mommy-out-of-sight no longer means mommy-out-of-existence. Leach (2010, loc. 4763) provides a marvelous explanation of how the development of object permanency helps an exhausted mother cope with her ever-demanding, be-with-me-all-the-time infant.

MODES OF LEARNING

Unlike in early infancy, the baby begins to organize experience along a "gradient of anxiety" (Sullivan, 1953, p. 153). There is never really a true all-or-nothing anxiety/euphoria phenomenon, even in early infancy, but people primarily learn behaviors in their society based on the gradient (Sullivan, 1953, p. 153).

Withdrawal of tenderness in the form of forbidding moods and gestures by the primary caretaker(s)—for example, if a caretaker is disgusted while the toddler explores finger foods on the highchair tray—is devastating and tied to forbidding moods. Adults can perhaps better understand it in its later manifestation, during the juvenile era, when they have clear memories of how they adjusted behavior to fit with peers for fear of ostracism. The experience of adjusting based on forbidding gestures in late infancy is less available to memory, but much more potent than what happens in the juvenile. But the degree of intensity from the earlier experience of estrangement from the mothering figure(s) in infancy, early and late, can fuel the intensity of the juvenile's fear of ostracism. *How* vulnerable the juvenile is has been determined by earlier experiences.

Another example is the attempt to satisfy the need to explore the environment without getting in trouble. The baby picks something off the floor and puts it in their mouth; mommy reacts negatively. But if they pick something up from the table, mommy *doesn't* say, "No!" or is less discouraging. It has to do with what is tolerable and what is beginning to be not so tolerable. The baby may test things out as if saying, "Can I pick this up?" while looking at mommy to check.

If there's massive anxiety on the part of the parenting one(s), learning can't take place; it feels like a "blow on the head" (Sullivan, 1953, p. 160). The growing infant may figure out how to get their needs met by finding less anxiety-provoking ways to satisfy them, perhaps when the adult isn't around. They're still pursuing what is forbidden with some degree of anxiety, but without the all-or-nothing "knock on the head" feeling that makes them forget about it altogether. While they might still feel taboo, they have unwittingly found ways to avoid or diminish the parenting figure(s)' anxiety level, and in the process are learning behavior acceptable to where they live (Sullivan, 1953, p. 154).

The baby also begins looking for approval and eschewing disapproval from all-important caretaker(s). If a primary caretaker disapproves of a behavior, they experience an anxiety-producing withdrawal of tenderness. The baby figures out how to modify their behavior, particularly when learning actions not acceptable to the parenting one(s). They begin to discriminate when euphoria is beginning to diminish, when they are getting more anxious, which is the "discrimination of a gradient" (Sullivan, 1953, p. 153).

An example is the process of "testing the limits." There is just so much of a certain thing, such as loud screaming or playing with food or touching one's genitals, before there is a sharp drop in euphoria. This is not thought out consciously or verbally in the infant, but in an adult's words it could be, "How much can I get away with before Mommy blows up?" It's an important tool in learning the limits to one's behavior in relation to one's significant others.

Learning also occurs through reward and punishment. The need for human approval exists practically from the get-go. As explained in the "Early Infancy" chapter, the caretaker's indifference to a need produces indifference to that need to the same degree in the infant. Attempts to satisfy the need diminish. In late infancy, what the infant pursues and tends to ignore becomes very obviously connected to the need for approval from those who matter. Withdrawal of tenderness by the primary caretaker(s) in the form of forbidding gestures is devastating, but much more subtle than conscious adult forbidding. Much goes on outside the awareness of the adult(s) and infant, in a thousand tiny forbidding gestures. To be sure, parental conscious or unconscious opposition has its effect, but it's much more powerful if repeated many times, such as continual opposition to the infant's exploration of their genitals. There is also the issue of how the genitals are touched, handled, etc., during diapering.

Larry's anesthesia for sexual feeling is striking. Even after a long process of successfully establishing an honest and comfortable therapeutic relationship, starting to talk about sexual interaction causes the same uneasiness. It's almost impossible to talk about. Anxiety around physical contact, including around touching oneself, was so severe, so prohibited, that not only is sexual desire dissociated, but the rage and all the attendant emotions with the initial experience have been dissociated. He cannot even begin to think about it, his anxiety is so acute. It seems as if this phobia about physical contact—the badness and horror of it—was inculcated with so much rage and terrorization that the therapist can't even approach it without throwing Larry into a total panic. The stated experience in this young adult is: "Everybody else has some preoccupation with sex. Everybody else has an interest in the opposite sex, or in the same sex, and feels desire. I don't feel anything, and I never have."

Larry's experience is total anesthesia regarding another person. There is, in addition, dissociation of not only desire but also rage and anything attending that earlier experience.

James has a similar but less acutely dysfunctional history. When cuddling, he suddenly has an itch and becomes fidgety. If he tries to ignore the itch, it becomes unbearable. When he finally scratches it, there is momentary relief until the next itch starts.

Late infancy *gradient of anxiety* can show up in adulthood.

Sonia starts thinking about dating but says, "I can go so far, and no more. I have to be in love before I do this. I'm too religious." But gradually she sneaks in a little more (for example, after a few drinks at a party she allows something sexual to go on) and then, perhaps through therapy, can relate her reaction of regret and shame back to specific experiences of parental prohibition. It is somewhat easier for her to work on changing her assumptions in therapy than in the cases described above. Maybe she eventually starts allowing some tenderness, maybe a bit more sexual activity, and breaks out in eczema.

Mood plays a large part in learning a function, even if it is about something entirely different that coincidentally and continuously happens during the same learning period, such as constant tension between spouses or an ever-present critical grandparent while learning how to walk.

Finally, here is an example of the multiple ways a primary caretaker's mood and behavior around a common late infancy routine might, when repeated, influence future development:

Many years ago, this writer observed a mother feeding her 15-month-old in her highchair. As the ritual began, the baby screamed, "No, no, Mommy!" already putting up a big, squirming fuss. Her mother was so phobic of mess that she had covered herself in a trench coat and latex gloves. The baby wore an oversized bib. Her mother couldn't tolerate anything on her baby's face, carefully aiming the spoon into the frantic baby's mouth. If the food managed to get in at all, her mother would forcefully rub a wet washcloth around the baby's mouth if anything leaked, which it usually did. The baby's mouth and chin were chapped and irritated. Her mother's behavior certainly didn't evoke cooperation; it evoked a fight.

Not only was eating a horrendous experience, so was exploration and experimentation. The infant was not allowed to play with her food at all: couldn't explore the texture of a crumb or roll a pea around on the highchair table and pick it up with her hands. If there was *any* inclination to experiment with any morsel in sight, her mother cleaned it up and reprimanded the baby. She couldn't try out anything. She couldn't experiment. She couldn't be spontaneous. One could only wonder what would happen during fingerpainting in nursery school: oh, no!

I have not had the opportunity to know this child as an adult. Chances are she is severely self-revulsed and probably has a terrible time enjoying meals. She might be super careful about keeping things clean or might have taken the opposite tack, keeping things messy and dirty, all the while proving to herself that she is indeed a repulsive, unlovable person. She then would be fulfilling the early parental expectation that she is and will always be a mess. Having been forbidden to explore objects around her, at least in the observed situation, she is probably hesitant, if not severely anxious, about learning something new, particularly about the physical world.

Maybe she has enjoyed more positive experiences with people and alternate validators along the way. Hopefully, then, she is now more comfortable with herself and the world, but this was certainly a rough beginning to witness.

THE ORGANIZATION OF THE SELF-SYSTEM

The organization of the self-system is gradual, starting from birth and accelerating with increased perceptual-motor acuity in late infancy. However, it is still in rudimentary form.

Without question, a major influential phenomenon in being educated to become a person by those who matter the most to the infant is the avoidance of anxiety whenever possible (Sullivan, 1953, p. 152). The major function of the self-system is to avoid challenging the restrictions of one's primary caretaker(s), whose moods of affirmation and derogation have laid down marching orders of how to be a functioning human being.

The self-system is composed of experiences that are available to consciousness, or awareness. Many experiences easily come into awareness. The person attends to them without experiencing disorientation, without requiring a drastic reorganization of the person's ability to function. The person's self-system is the total of all those experiences (Pearce & Newton, 1963, p. 14).

There are two major functions of the self-system. One has to do with needs, the other with security. The self-system creates the ability to focus attention so that the self can function at all. Simultaneously, the self-system limits needed functions if the experience of them creates anxiety, which amounts to the loss of a feeling of security. So one needs the self-system to maintain the organization of thoughts, but that organization can restrict needed functioning if it makes the parenting one(s) anxious. In this way, the capacity to focus attention is affected by the anxiety gradient. If a parenting one is anxious about a particular behavior, so is the infant, it is posited, to the same degree.

The self-system includes all functioning that allows a person to participate in life at all, including assumptions that restrict a person from participating as fully as the person might. The self-system strives to avoid anxiety-provoking experiences that include functioning previously forbidden by the primary caretaker(s), but it also engages in productive, already validated functioning. "[T]he self-system can be described functionally as the structuring of consciousness for the avoidance of anxiety" (Pearce & Newton, 1963, p. 15). It is resistant to change, but it also includes productive functioning, so change is still possible.

There are things in focal awareness, and there are things in marginal awareness. Then there are things not available to consciousness at all. *All* of which are part of one's *personality*, all of which motivate. Although the individual is unconsciously motivated by dissociated experiences, the self-system does not include what is out of awareness. Some experiences are more accessible to consciousness than others. When a therapist takes a history and goes into great detail, a person begins to remember things not remembered before. They were *not* part of the self-system until the therapist began asking into, for example, the historical motivation for a particular adult behavior. So the process of inquiry can expand the self-system. The ability to remember more is motivationally determined. The therapist's curiosity is one motivation that may stimulate an increased range of memory during history taking. Curiosity is also validation. When the therapist is curious about something in a person's life that has not seemed important, they begin to pay attention to it; this new attending may stimulate memories previously relegated as "unimportant" to surface.

> Jeff characterized his early years as very isolated, with sadistic but disorganized parents. In response to his therapist's continued interest in alternate validators, he began to remember how he had walked out of his house at three to visit other homes in the neighborhood. The neighbors welcomed him, fed him candy, and made much of him before returning him to his parents, who had barely noticed he was gone. He did not mention these memories of exploring and reaching out to more friendly adults for the first two years of therapy because "they just didn't seem important before."

As a person's life changes and they expand the range of functioning, new memories may also begin to appear, usually related to the new range.

"Memories" of late infancy show up in dreams, moods, and marginal thoughts.[8] Compared with later memories, they are vaguer, not very verbal (though more verbal than in early infancy), and not as coherent.

Learning goes on in focal awareness or in marginal awareness, *out* of awareness (not in the self-system), possibly reemerging into awareness later with greater or lesser anxiety.

> Mindy was very active, exuberant, and unafraid as a toddler, jumping on laps, tumbling, and play wrestling with kids and adults. Soon her parents, because of their own preoccupations and phobias, became concerned that the play was sexual or would be interpreted as sexual. They exhibited a great deal of anxiety

about it, limiting her interaction with other kids and refusing to take her to the playground. Limitations were gradual, starting in late infancy.

Over time, Mindy became sedentary and depressed, shunning opportunities to interact more than casually with people. In her late twenties, she decided to lose weight by joining a gym and reconnected with that toddler experience with a certain amount of pleasure. After a few sessions of wary enthusiasm with her trainer, she got lost walking the few blocks to the gym and had to rely on her GPS. She experienced the anxiety that comes with challenging earlier parental prohibitions, manifested by a breakdown in the function of getting from one place to another.

It can take years for dissociated functions to reemerge, usually with a mixture of pleasure and anxiety. Depending upon the degree of parental anxiety around any of the toddler's behaviors, effects can be dampening. Reemerging late infancy functions, such as curiosity and more mobility or exploration of the self and others, can be experienced as very anxiety provoking, bad, dirty, or evil. Then the thought to be more active in life often emerges only in dreams or lower states of awareness, such as under the influence of liquor, and often in a paranoid mode.[9] A person considers such actions as "badly" motivated, echoing in adult language parental moods from early on: "I am a sex fiend" or "I am basically hostile."

The pressing need for late infancy functions to reemerge may arise later with some soul-searching with those who might appreciate the value of the person's spontaneity and curiosity. In focal awareness, such behavior can be reevaluated in a safe space, such as in therapy, and properly reintegrated into one's life. For example, Mindy initially refuted her friend's recommendation to join a gym: "I won't get there because I'm just lazy." She delayed engaging a physical trainer: "I don't need someone to babysit me!" Through therapeutic inquiry, she began to wonder why such thoughts prevent her from getting things going—and, once she finally started her regimen, she began to understand why she got disoriented walking to the gym after a few workouts.

The Development of the Personifications of the Self

All personifications, experiences of oneself, are contained in what is experienced as *my Self*, distinguished by the fact that one can feel it; it is self-sentience. The sense that "I can feel myself" starts to develop as the baby's perceptual-cognitive system develops, establishing a border between what is "me" and what is "outside of me."

The early infant experiences "good-me" and "bad-me,"[10] having to do with what the infant experiences as the "good mother" and the "bad mother." Think in terms of something mommy really values, "I'm a good eater" or

"I'm a healthy person" or whatever it happens to be, and rewards the infant. That becomes "good-me." Then there are things that feel bad when they are done around mommy, but one can do them indirectly. That's the beginning of the development of "bad-me." In adulthood, some people feel that much of what they do is "bad" or wrong in some way, so they do a great many things with guilt, self-loathing, and/or discomfort of some kind. As part of the late infant's self-system, these conscious experiences can linger even into adulthood. For example, as Mindy started to enjoy her active, more limber self, she noticed she was self-conscious and felt that people thought she was seductively showing off her body.

Those things which are just not part of *me*, the "not-me," coincide with severe anxiety. "Not-me" is avoided at all costs, but the command to avoid it has been dissociated. All one knows is don't go near it.

> Roger, whose needs for comfortable cuddling and exploration of his own genitalia had been met with severe prohibition as an infant, talks repeatedly about his high school experience when the boys talked about girls and girlfriends. He would think, "I'm glad I'm not going through that. It just doesn't concern me. I can't see why they get so excited about it." Complete obliteration: "Not-me." As he becomes more hopeful in therapy, it begins to bother him that he keeps himself away from an activity shared by many in the human race. He becomes wistful: "Gee, perhaps I can do this." Or, "It would be nice if I could do this, but I can't." He begins to find ways to let that happen, but it goes slowly, with much discomfort and dread.

The personification of "good-me" goes a long way in educating the older infant. It could be in all sorts of realms: cooperating with the caretaker while being dressed, or while learning how to feed oneself. This kind of education also goes on in other significant areas. For example, if the baby, as part of developmentally natural and normal imitation of sounds, starts singing with music playing in the home, and happens to be in a musical family, then musical "talent" gets validated very early. Everyone may believe that the young person was born with this talent as if there were "musical genes," when actually it's because the toddler is surrounded with music and rewarded with their own pleasure and parental pleasure in their pleasure.[11] It's true of a multitude of functions; many people assume their "talent" or skill is inborn, not recognizing that it was a pleasure that was repeatedly validated by parental delight with their enjoyment.

> Stephanie brought into her session her 21-month-old infant, who was doing quite well for a child not yet two. He was already saying some short sentences, for example. He also liked to draw with a Magic Marker in exuberant abandon, because he was that age. Stephanie and the therapist were cooing about it, and

> the therapist realized with delight that her own first impulse was to say, "Oh my God, how fabulous!" That's the kind of ability that does develop exponentially when a parenting one or significant other takes pleasure around a particular activity.

> Lauren, an artist with an adolescent son, described in therapy how she started to support his painting, scribbling, and drawing when he was a toddler. She described her steady support and the stories she told him about her own artistic experiences and the artists she knew. He is now a very fine artist. It's hard for her to grasp that she had something to do with that.

> Wolfgang Amadeus Mozart started composing at five. His father was a very prominent violinist and composer, so Wolfgang was surrounded by music from early infancy and most likely before, in utero. His imitative beginnings at three were, of course, recognized and considered precocious. Leopold started tutoring him, making music fun and imbuing him with a rigorous work ethic. The child's "talents" were first validated by his immediate family, and then by the world at large when, at six, his father took him on tour. Although his life was short and tumultuous, he composed over 600 works and was a major influence on subsequent composers, particularly Beethoven. Although his sister had a similar musical upbringing, as a woman she had to marry instead of pursuing a career.

People are born with a staggering capacity to learn and accomplish. Whatever important parenting figures validate with pleasure is allowed to grow; other endeavors get tossed, over time, into the nether land of "not-me" or partially grow but stay underdeveloped or undeveloped in "bad-me." Through experience and later interactions with others that matter, one can expand "good-me." And through brave perseverance, perhaps with the help of therapy and/or extended family members, significant teachers, groups, friends, and/or partners (or even a character in a book or a media personality), one can struggle to uncover early behaviors that went into "bad-me," that is, only partially validated ones, and struggle to expand them. The person, in effect, has developed a new meaningful audience for a function originally shunned as "bad-me." That's the therapeutic work: to clear away the underbrush, the forbidden "bad-me" adult rationalizations, many rudimentarily formulated in late infancy.

Continued Development of the Self-system

The late infant, being a consummate imitator, integrates the body language and intonation of those around them. Often attributed to heredity, their gestures and vocal intonations sound the same as their parenting one(s).

A common type of miseducation is when the primary caretaker(s) and others in the "inner circle" assume that the baby takes after somebody. "Oh, we knew it all along; he takes right after Grandpa Harry, who hanged himself, so he must be just as crazy and suicidal. It's in the genes." Anything that the child does that vaguely fits is proof. Over time, this assumption gets projected onto the toddler, who is still really just being a curious and developing baby with age-appropriate mishaps and successes (Sullivan, 1953, p. 175).

It is also a time when the sense of self as the reflected appraisal by others becomes more clearly formed: "I am a good person" or "I am fearful" or "pretty" or "aggressive" or "angry," etc. This view of self is open to expansion, largely depending on what validation is acceptable from a gradually wider world for the growing person.

For example, the primary caretaker(s) might assume that the toddler has a will and then treat them as if they were willfully naughty. Then they are broken in, like a pony, to not be so self-willed (Sullivan, 1953, p. 173).

> Leslie was attracted to Skittles in a mini mart, picked the package up, and started to unwrap it. Mom, embarrassed because others were watching, snatched it out of the baby's hand and scolded, "We don't steal!" Years later, her mother explained to her that she had to drive the devil out of her child because she was willfully stealing; she had to train her baby. She literally used the word "devil" and claimed that the child had been born a thief. When toddlers pick things up from candy counters and neighbor's yards, they are simply wanting something and going after it with cleverness and determination.

These unfortunate cases exemplify the *personification* of the infant; Sullivan asks what the parent expects of their infant. It's the misperception of who the infant is and should be. The infant develops a self-image that reflects the parental perception of who they are (1953, p. 175).

Of course, most adults whose assumptions matter to the baby have positive expectations, too. It's a range. When there is an assumption that the toddler is smart, for example, toys include colorful cloth books and easy computer games. The adults relish the toddler's enjoyment of these toys, appreciating their curiosity and explorations in a babyproof environment. Leslie's excitement over finding colorful candy in the mini mart, reaching for it and trying to unwrap it are indicative of intelligent exploration and discovery. The child is a curiosity engine, not a thief.

LATE INFANCY FUNCTIONS AND RESIDUALS IN LATER LIFE

Many excellent books and articles discuss functions achieved within each developmental era. One outstanding source is *Conditions of Human Growth* (Pearce & Newton, 1963). The authors list the "residuals" in later life when things don't go well during a particular developmental era, some of which have been discussed in this and other chapters.[12] Of importance in late infancy is the relationship to objects and various aspects of mobility, visual-motor skills, and crawling/walking, all closely related to the late infant's relationship to the object world. For example, among the functions learned in late infancy are the mastery of space and objects and learning how to cherish things. If this is done poorly through interference of some kind (perhaps the house is not babyproofed and the caretaker(s) is constantly saying, "No! Don't touch that!"), the adult residual might be a poor notion about personal property or a compulsion to go on shopping sprees and keep stuff the person doesn't really need or use (Pearce & Newton, 1963, p. 90). If the toddler's self-image is persistently undermined, the adult residual might be self-revulsion and/or a preoccupation with "body beautiful" (Pearce & Newton, 1963, p. 89).

SUMMARY

The toddler's interpersonal experiences with their primary caretaker(s) are crucial in their personality development. The early self-system, particularly as it develops in late infancy, is to varying degrees quite strenuously put together. This obvious phenomenon is unfortunately too often ignored or underplayed in much contemporary therapeutic work. People are indeed brought up by people; there is no blame to be cast on any caretaker when a therapist probes a person's history. Caretakers were brought up by people too, and everyone grows up within culture(s), traditions, and socio-economic conditions. There are also natural and human-made disasters—pandemics, wars, civil upheavals, forced migrations, economic and political emigrations, imperialism, colonialism and occupation, racism, classism, enslavement, and genocides—devastating generations upon generations of lives.

A multitude of positive experiences can and do challenge and change unfortunate consequences of late infancy experiences. Starting in late infancy and continuing as the child grows into adulthood, the self-system can be very positively challenged and changed by, for example, babysitters, other later caretakers, teachers, coaches, neighbors, friends, friends' parenting one(s), and groups. In adulthood their self-system can be further influenced by, for example, professors, colleagues, lovers, and political organizations that raise class consciousness. For some who are more isolated from direct contact with people beyond the immediate, most cherished caretaker(s), positive experiences can come from movies, television, books and magazines, popular songs, and social media, to name just a few.[13]

Interpersonal experiences teach. As in any developmental era, growth is always possible. No one is hardwired, permanently trapped by whatever occurred during the early years. As they mature, people can and do make up for "unfinished business."

NOTES

1. Discussion of late infancy primarily relies on inference and observation because we do not have direct access to what the baby is thinking and feeling.
2. The toddler's words have meaning but are still highly "parataxic," private between the parenting one(s) and the child. See Mullahy (1980) for a comprehensive explanation of speech behavior from late infancy into childhood.
3. Sullivan uses the terms "good mother" and "bad mother" to denote the infant's *felt* experience of a mothering one who is or is not relating to its needs, rather than a moral designation (1953).
4. For a fuller discussion of attachment from a neo-Freudian orientation and related early research, see Bowlby (1982).
5. In discussing how one function is a prerequisite for the next, such as crawling before walking, it is necessary to keep in mind how and to what extent the child's needs are met. A caretaker of a deaf child or one born with cerebral palsy benefits from an understanding of what all children need. Figuring out how to provide for the needs of a differently abled child or one born under unfortunate conditions, in most instances, depends mainly on who the caretaker(s) is and what opportunities are available in a particular community or society. See the introduction to Developmental Eras.
6. Rudimentary musical skills are observed in early infancy as well (Malloch & Trevarthen, 2018).
7. The term "self-system" was coined by Sullivan (1953).
8. The barrier between fully conscious and marginal thoughts is very permeable. Restrictive thoughts, perceptions, and feelings lying in marginal awareness can be called up in moments of potential expansion of the self-system to limit that expansion or can help identify and clarify for the person some obstacles to greater need satisfaction—to potentially clarify one's despair. These marginal thoughts are part of how one sees oneself and the world, representing assumptions about oneself.
9. "Paranoid" in this context is not entirely what is commonly accepted as a diagnosis in the *Diagnostic and Statistical Manual* (2013). It defines a despairing conviction that departs from what is true in reality. It is on a continuum from a false assumption that regulates one's life (like, "I'm a loser") to the florid paranoid psychotic belief that aliens are in control of one's mind (as described in the *DSM*).

10. "Good-me" and "bad-me" and "not-me" are terms used by Sullivan to denote a *feeling about self*, not a moral designation. The same is true of the terms "good mother" and "bad mother," *felt* experiences of a mothering one who is or is not relating to a baby's needs, as explained above.

11. Also, in utero, the person must have been surrounded by music.

12. Residuals are functions not adequately consolidated in a particular developmental era that affect how one functions in later life. The term as defined here was coined by Pearce and Newton (1963, pp. 83, 89, 94, 102, 107, 113).

13. In many wonderful instances, parenting ones do change, grow their own self-systems, or have a more positive reaction to their child when they reach a later developmental era. However, this more positive influence may be difficult to integrate because earlier, more influential interpersonal interactions can easily fall back into place like well-oiled cogs on a wheel. People in therapy sometimes say, "But my parents aren't like that anymore." However, no matter how much a primary caretaker(s) has changed in later years, the *formative* years have the most influence on the self-system. For the self-system to expand, they must understand the *effects of early upbringing*.

Chapter Four

Childhood

The Widening World

Childhood is the developmental era from approximately two-and-a-half to four years, starting with the emergence of communicative speech and the need for playmates (Pearce & Newton, 1963, pp. 91–93).

Like infancy, childhood is a period of rapid growth, physically and in personality development.[1] All previously learned functions, to the extent that they are not significantly hindered, continue to expand through validation from the primary parenting one(s) and other significant caretakers. Chief among these are rapid refinement of mobility; manipulation and cherishing of objects; continuing maturation of communication through dramatization, gesturally and verbally; development of articulate speech; interest in peers; and never-ending curiosity about the world. Western culture refers disparagingly to the period of early childhood development, along with very late infancy, as the "terrible twos." It may be "terrible" for adults whose personalities may be too restrictive to take pleasure in the challenge of a fast-moving, increasingly chatty, experimenting, demanding, and questioning little person. For most parental figures, the child's liveliness may be experienced with pleasure and as an opportunity to grow beyond their own current limitations. The child's *joie de vivre* demonstrates the inborn human need to manifest every capacity. The child matures while simultaneously adapting to expectations and demands of the parenting one(s), who are training their child in what is socially acceptable.

DEVELOPMENT OF ARTICULATE SPEECH

The development of articulate speech[2] is a major step in the child's growth. Its importance in movement toward full human potential cannot be overstated.

As verbal language development surges, the child's major mode of communication shifts from empathy in infancy to the dramatization of feelings. Any interaction between a child and another person may include all three modes of communication—empathy, dramatization, and articulated speech—with one or more modes predominating in any given experience. Although speech may be clear and articulate, in childhood it is used for dramatization more than precise, factual communication, which only develops during the next era, the juvenile, where it is consensually validated and understandable to a much wider audience of people. Often, especially in early childhood, speech may remain understandable only to the primary caretaker(s) and gradually changes as the child encounters more people.

Emotional communication remains essentially non-verbal. The child dramatizes emotions through other behavior or uses speech dramatically.

> Four-year-old Jenny's parents recently separated. In fantasy play during a psychotherapy session, Jenny suddenly picked up the "Daddy" doll and loudly scolded: "Bad! Go to jail!" She shoved the doll under a pillow.

During childhood, children communicate by crying, drawing, lying down and screaming, or saying "more" after licking the applesauce bowl clean, fully expecting more applesauce to appear by "magic." The child learns that particular sounds affect what happens next. Mainly through repetition, trial and error, and testing out new words and sounds, the child learns the language of others. Vocabulary increases, sentences and short paragraphs are formed, and under fortunate circumstances, connectedness to others is enhanced.

The goal of all learning across the life span is the promotion of growth. The capacity for verbal communication is a powerful tool in progressing toward that goal. The maturation process of this capacity begins at birth, when the newborn first hears their own voice. That process accelerates significantly in childhood when the child must learn to adapt to their new environment in order to thrive.

Understandable speech becomes increasingly central to that adaptation and leads to the experience of consensual validation in the juvenile era. Speech enables people to acknowledge each other and to relate to each other with varying degrees of intensity and intimacy. When not satisfactorily integrated as part of one's personality and without sufficient corrective experience (alternate validation), a lack of emotional connectedness to others develops, adversely affecting the person's growth.

Human growth is bumpy because the immature human's growth opportunities are primarily controlled by adults, who are usually concerned with avoiding disruption of their own self-systems. Children benefit when they are encouraged to say what they like and dislike, satisfy their curiosity by asking questions, and tell someone where they hurt or what they are thinking or feeling.

An adult's earliest memory usually refers to the childhood era when the child is very focused on learning to talk (Pearce & Newton, 1963, p. 92). The earliest memory is a rudimentary, symbolic formulation of the child's perception of the world, their place in it, and the nature of their relationships with significant people. It unwittingly serves as a template for later experience. Recalling and examining one's earliest memory as an adult is useful in clarifying significant aspects of current problems in living. For example, the earliest memory of an isolated, lonely 25-year-old woman is of an empty swing in an empty playground. In therapy, discussions of this memory and related historical experiences of isolation enabled her to notice how and why she organized her life to emotionally mimic the desolation of that earliest memory.

With the acquisition of articulated speech, the child can tell another person about experiences, dreams, and nightmares. If shared with the parenting one(s), the dream content can provide a window into what is going on with the child not readily apparent during waking life. For example, a five-year-old reports a dream two months before starting school. During waking life, the child does not appear to be anxious, and when school is mentioned, he proclaims, "I'm a big boy! I'm going to school!" However, in the dream he is trapped in his mother's belly and can't get out and has to live there for a whole year. A possible interpretation is that the child is anxious about going to school and separating from his mother, but at the same time, he would feel trapped at home if he didn't. His anxiety resonates with his mother's anxiety about his starting to leave the nest. They are outwardly exuberant about his sprouting wings, but inwardly would be more exuberant if it could be postponed another year. Although they would probably not admit such feelings (they may not even be aware of them), they actually might be ashamed of their own possessiveness.

LEARNING AND ANXIETY

The development of the child's personality, specifically their self-system, originates in their relationships with their parenting one(s) and/or other primary caretakers. The child is constantly learning about the world and their place in it. This can be observed directly, as with the ability to distinguish shapes, recognize objects and people, or run and climb. Other learning can only be inferred, such as what the child learns from glancing at the parenting one(s) to determine if a particular behavior is acceptable or will be met with their forbidding gestures[3] and/or forbidding words, moods, or actions. If the behavior is unacceptable, the child feels anxious, and the satisfaction of the need is incomplete. The need is distorted, and its satisfaction is relegated to the restrictive arm of the child's self-system.[4]

Sullivan calls this experience learning by anxiety or by the "anxiety gradient" (1953, pp. 151–153). According to him, learning by the anxiety gradient is a major way humans learn to be acceptable to the primary caretakers(s), by gauging how much satisfaction they can achieve before too much anxiety is aroused in their caretaker(s). In the childhood era, the caretaker(s) also attempts to deliberately instruct the child in how to "behave" in ways generally acceptable to the culture in which they live. This instruction, of course, is filtered through the perceptions of the caretaker(s). Repeated disapproval over time and lack of alternate validation establishes a behavior pattern that makes satisfaction of a particular need difficult way past childhood.

In the following example, Agnes's mother considered her daughter's exuberant pleasure as socially inappropriate.

> Agnes was admonished by her mother for being loud (acting "crazy"), i.e., displaying enthusiasm. Other forbidding responses to Agnes's expressions of pleasure were frowns, explosions of anger at something extraneous, and visual and auditory expressions of irritation and contempt, until Agnes "settled down." In response, as a child, Agnes learned to temper her demonstration of pleasure by making it undetectable. She found that it was tolerable to her mother if she simply said she liked something flatly, in an even tone of voice, or if she sought out enjoyment of something out of sight and earshot. As an adult, Agnes was very measured in her expression of pleasure, and perceived as deadpan. She found it difficult to express positive emotions to peers, who found her very serious and difficult to please.

With learning in the presence of less severe anxiety, the child learns to discriminate between allowable and unacceptable behaviors in the presence of the parenting one(s). If a particular behavior is not allowed, the infant or child may nevertheless experience some satisfaction through sublimation: using the "anxiety gradient" to satisfy an otherwise unacceptable need in a manner the parenting one(s) can tolerate. Sullivan (1953) defines sublimation as a substitution out of awareness of a behavior pattern that provokes anxiety in the self-system for one that is more acceptable but still partially satisfies what caused the trouble in the first place. "In more fortunate circumstances, symbol processes occurring in sleep take care of the rest of the unsatisfied need" (p. 193).

At a few months old, and continuing into childhood, the infant manifests sublimation. Avoiding anxiety impedes the simplest, completely satisfactory activity (Sullivan, 1953, p. 114). The individual learns to chart a course by the anxiety gradient. Simple performances that would relax the tension of some needs have been made more complicated to avoid becoming more anxious.

> There was a concerted effort to make Bill stop touching his private parts when he was two. He responded to the constant verbal and non-verbal directives obediently, but soon developed an itch at night and found that he could scratch himself and satisfy that itch. It somehow calmed him. The prohibition and the behavior to circumvent the prohibition allowed Bill to satisfy his need with less anxiety. The need to masturbate returned in adolescence, but Bill was secretive about it. He was more comfortable with somebody else touching him than touching himself.

If the infant or child experiences severe anxiety from the primary caregiver(s), learning does not occur. Instead, there is amnesia, as if one sustained a blow to the head. The behavior of the child is thwarted, and the experience is dissociated and relegated to the unconscious. Consciously, it is as if the experience never happened.

SELF-IMAGE

As a child develops a sense of self in the world, they, most significantly in relationship to the parenting one(s), are also developing a self-image. The child experiences this sense of self as "This is who I really am." Developing from their unconscious, dissociated needs, it artistically reflects the limitations to growth beyond the acceptable. One's self-image is not usually in focal awareness but may be revealed in dreams, nightmares, fantasies, and other behaviors.

> An otherwise happy-go-lucky three-year-old dreams he is drowning. His favorite cuddle toy jumps in the lake to save him but cannot. As confident as he appears to be when awake, his nightmare illustrates that in his less focused and despairing state he sees himself as helpless, alone, and frightened.

As a description of "who I *really* am," the self-image is a compressed, symbolic expression of one's despair that they could never be different. If a caring adult knows this important information, helpful action may be taken. In the above example the newly divorced parent, upon being told the nightmare by the child, became more keenly aware that the child was more troubled than they knew. Their child was "drowning" and desperately needed help beyond their ability to provide it. They found the child a therapist. Interpersonal theory further infers that the very act of having a dream that highlights a serious obstacle to growth can release some tension in the dreamer if it is shared and suggests that the dreamer has perspective on their own despair. One can also use their nightmare restrictively, especially if they assume it is a statement of immutable truth.

The concept of self-image is also useful because it helps explain how a negative and despairing self-appraisal forged in childhood may erupt into awareness throughout life whenever the status of previously dissociated, unsatisfied needs is seriously challenged. One's self-image is used as a shield to protect the integrity of the self-system, thus avoiding anxiety and the potential for growth.

RELATING TO AUTHORITY

Attitudes toward authority begin in childhood (Pearce & Newton, 1963, p. 92) when adults comprise the child's significant interpersonal world; this world expands to include babysitters, relatives, friends of the parenting one(s), neighbors, preschool teachers, and others. Important patterns develop, such as compliance, defiance, and the degree of dependence versus independence from the primary caretaker(s), that determine the nature of the child's relationship to authority figures. "No," "later," and "why" are powerful additions to the child's vocabulary. The parental response is central to the child's perception of authority.

During this period when relationships to authority figures are developing, the primary caretaker(s) is focused on "socializing" the child. One aspect of this socialization process in Western culture and many others is punishment, which may be accompanied by pain or humiliation. With or without the administration of pain, the unfortunate lesson the child learns, if not corrected through subsequent experience, is that they must perceive and relate to authorities as fearsome powerful beings. The lesson becomes firmly embedded in the restrictive aspect of one's self-system.

RELATEDNESS TO OBJECTS

Fueled by their curiosity and supported by parental validation, children move toward mastery of their coordination of the physical world through manipulating and exploring objects. Intense relationships develop between them and toys, blankets, books, dolls, stuffed animals, and, potentially, anything they can reach, walk to, grab, or pick up. Children will touch, feel, smell, and taste these objects; they may even take them apart. These experiences help set the stage for the enjoyment of lifelong learning, beginning with curiosity and continuing to mastery.

Certain objects may become cherished favorites, such as a particular blanket or stuffed animal the child insists on sleeping with and wants with them at all times. Children are comforted by these old "friends." Some parenting ones feel threatened by the intensity of the child's feelings for Mr. Bunny. They ridicule the child or outright prohibit the relationship between child and bunny, managing to "lose" him and then criticizing the child for "making such a big thing out of it" or disparagingly referring it as "Dirty Mr. Bunny." This can devastate the child, who misses the toy animal they are so emotionally connected to. The child also feels anxious by the parental disapproval of Mr. Bunny and, through close association, disapproval of the child.

Relationships with pets have the potential to be an additional source of delight and comfort for the child when there is mutual playfulness. A relationship with a pet may help lay the groundwork for future friendships. Additionally, the child has the opportunity to observe, from a distance and with a new perspective, how important people in their lives relate to living creatures.

NEED FOR PLAYMATES AND PARALLEL PLAY

Although the primary caretakers remain the child's most significant interpersonal experience, by three or four years old the child's interpersonal world undergoes a major expansion to include relationships with peers. The child continues to see itself as a child in the world of adults, but there is a new, conscious interest in being with other children. Presented with the choice of playing in one of two sandboxes—one with no children and one containing other children—the new arrival to the playground is likely to choose the sandbox with other children, although they are all strangers.

The children in the sandbox may or may not directly interact with each other, but the mere presence of others enhances their play experience. When children interact, their newly developing ability for the use of words is very helpful in encouraging and sustaining these newfound relationships. The child begins to learn to share toys, and practices rudimentary forms of compromise with the help of friendly adults. The interest of the child is not only the activity but also the presence of other children, making the activity more enjoyable and interesting. Pearce and Newton (1963) call this interpersonal experience "parallel play" (p. 93).

Parallel play represents an important and necessary step in the child's ongoing growth toward increased independence from the parenting one(s) and toward future development of relatedness to others with different levels of intensity and intimacy. It is an important early experience with humans who are the same size as the child, along with a sense of being in the world of peers.

As parental validation is required for the child to cherish objects, it is crucial that parenting one(s) encourage and take pleasure in their child's small but highly significant interest in and movement toward peers. The child of a self-centered parenting one who rationalizes their disapproval of their child's newfound interest by saying, "Don't hug her. She's dirty," experiences more difficulty moving toward peers.

In adulthood, if all goes well, everyone is perceived as a peer. If parallel play is not integrated, the adult again feels like a child in a world of adults, reinstating a parental/child pattern from childhood that limits options to what the primary caretaker(s) allowed.

SUMMARY

The childhood era (from approximately two-and-a-half to four years) begins with the need for articulate speech and extends to the conscious need for playmates. The primary caretaker(s) remains the most significant relationship(s) in the child's life as they learn according to what is expected by the caretaker(s). Other major areas of development during childhood include relationships to objects, pets, and authority. Mobility and physical coordination continue to develop rapidly. The child's experience is focused on learning to adapt within the family environment while simultaneously being introduced to aspects of the culture into which they were born. In this era, new people in the world outside the family, both adults and other children, become important as alternate validators. The child becomes involved with playmates.

NOTES

1. Personality is "the relatively enduring pattern of recurrent interpersonal situations which characterize a human life" (Sullivan, 1953, pp. 110–111).
2. Including sign language and other alternate modes, such as communication boards.
3. See chapter one.
4. See chapter nine.

Chapter Five

The Juvenile Era

Group Experience and the Political Arts of Relating

The wider world of people outside the family starts in childhood—preschool, babysitters, neighbors, family friends, store clerks—but then expands substantially in the juvenile era along with one's view of self and one's place vis-à-vis other people. The child begins relating to peer groups and learns the political arts of managing relationships within those groups. This era starts at approximately four and culminates in the consolidation of a *chumship*, when one values and identifies with a close friend. However, the learning of political arts and expanding skills in navigating human relationships continues throughout life.

The function of parallel play learned during childhood continues, with varying degrees of success, to be part of everyday experience throughout life (watching movies, going to concerts, working side by side with others). The juvenile perceives, communicates, and relates with others based on commonly recognized social principles more generally understood, consensually validated,[1] and based on cause and effect, rather than the childhood mode of relating to authority.

Each juvenile's household has its own limitations and peculiarities as the socializing influence, along with cultural idiosyncrasies and standards of value that might restrict or benefit the juvenile as they grow up. What has been learned there begins to be open to question and, when necessary and possible, to remedy or expansion (Sullivan, 1953, p. 227).

In the United States, the juvenile generally starts some sort of schooling around four or five.[2] The new, vastly expanded interpersonal opportunities can be staggering, depending upon how prepared the juvenile is for the outside world. They are suddenly exposed to adult strangers they must listen and answer to, along with a wide variety of other juveniles, each bringing to the burgeoning juvenile society their own particular family orientations to living. The juvenile's response to this new environment may vary markedly from enthusiasm to wary watchfulness, shyness, and apathy. The process of adjustment to juvenile interaction is gradually learned, each juvenile eventually fitting into a role which is adopted based on prior experience in the household setting as well as the realities of the new group interactions.

Increased exposure to adult authority figures such as teachers, aides, librarians, coaches, school bus drivers, religious instructors, choir masters, family friends, and counselors (if the juvenile is fortunate enough to also attend afterschool, day camp and/or sleep-away camp) allows them to compare the styles of these authorities to those of their parenting one(s). The childhood sense of powerlessness in face of the absolute power of the parenting one(s) can be gradually tempered by awareness of the different ways people react to authorities. Now it becomes possible to view authority figures as human beings with their own strengths and weaknesses rather than implacable, god-like beings. Not only are there many authorities, each with different characteristics, but there are one's peers, who have their own varying opinions of these people and provide the juvenile much more perspective.

In the juvenile era, the ability to navigate one's place in this new interpersonal mixture forces them to learn new rules to please adult authorities and fit in with peers. One begins to widen one's conception of who and what is important. The environment exposes them to new ways of interacting; rules may be based on generally accepted principles, not dictated without reason. If asked why it's important to cross the street only when the light turns green, the younger child might answer, "Because mommy said to wait" or "Because that's what you're supposed to do." The juvenile who has learned a more consensually validated response based on cause and effect might say, "Because if you don't, you might get hit by a car." Concepts of fairness also become important. Much of juvenile team sports, whether or not managed by adults, involves hammering out the rules of engagement generally accepted as just or correct by the group.

This era is essentially characterized by the struggle between the dictates of the parenting one(s) and the new experiences available to the juvenile. A lot depends on the tools the emerging juvenile has garnered so far to make use of these new experiences, as well as the limitations they bring from their own upbringing that prevent the inclusion of new experiences.

Depending upon the degree of restrictiveness around rules in the household grouping, the new schoolchild has the opportunity to be exposed to and learn from rules that are perhaps more understandable than those at home, along with a different set of consequences for violations. In some homes, for example, there might be double standards and arbitrariness for how to discipline different siblings, stepchildren, and/or genders. The rules may arbitrarily change depending upon parental moods (for example, exhaustion after a difficult workday). The rules outside the home, more generally acceptable to more people and communities, are potentially less confusing because of a more rational system of rewards and sanctions.

Depending upon how a child is treated in the home, the new environment can be startling. If one has been brought up to feel privileged and lacking rules, it is shocking to be required to be an ordinary member of the peer group in the classroom or schoolyard and follow the rules of, say, taking turns or having to raise one's hand to talk or go to the bathroom.

If there were interpersonal deficits that burdened the child before the juvenile era, they may be discarded or at least lightened in this new milieu. Assumptions about other people, as well as the roles and actions specific to the juvenile's home, can be challenged in this much-expanded world. Differences among children and among adult authority figures are noticed more by the juvenile. If they have grown up with feelings of being alone and powerless in a world of hostile authorities, those feelings can be challenged by juvenile interactions. For example, in a discussion about their home experiences, a juvenile from a restrictive home may hear criticisms from a peer or peer group concerning bedtimes or using social media.

If the juvenile has the opportunity to visit a friend's house or have a sleepover, they can garner alternate experiences. They might notice that there are adults who don't require children to finish everything on their plates. There is some room for questioning family rules.

The experience during the juvenile era also depends upon the wider culture the family lives in and at the school the juvenile attends. If the values of the parenting one(s) and the teachers happen to be quite similar, or if the community in which the juvenile lives is almost identical to the atmosphere at home, there is less chance for the juvenile to be exposed to and think about a wider world. The rules may or may not actually be more rational. In a home atmosphere where there is fighting and arbitrary punishment, say, of a scapegoated sibling, a schoolyard with fighting, retribution, and scapegoating will hardly bring anything new to that juvenile's self-system. Sometimes they unconsciously re-create the home situation at school, inviting the same treatment. A juvenile who is picked on at home might behave in a way that invites scapegoating by the other juveniles. If the teacher is harsh, picks favorites, or is demeaning, the world of authorities is potentially hardly different from what the juvenile already knows. If a teacher demeans a juvenile who has been scapegoated at home, they could reinforce the juvenile's low opinion of themself.

But if the juveniles in the schoolyard talk about that teacher and compare notes about the teacher's mood and the friendlier mood of the coach or of teachers in other classrooms, the juvenile has a chance to reevaluate the teacher's view of their status. The juvenile also has the chance to think about the notion that authority figures can be different and can be criticized. This is perhaps the first time their parenting one(s) might be brought down a few notches: maybe they are not as all-powerful as they once seemed. Regardless, blows to self-esteem in the classroom may be less devastating when compared to the juvenile's experience at home, where the parenting one(s) historically responsible in infancy for their very survival and existence matter significantly more than anyone else.

Alternately the role of the parenting one(s) in the juvenile world can be crucial in helping orient and support the youngster, particularly in situations in which the wider world is discriminatory and hostile because of race, religious, cultural, and class differences; physical and emotional challenges; and sexual orientation. The historic struggle for community control of public schools, spearheaded by parents, is an example of parental involvement in demanding a school environment that enhances juveniles' skills and self-esteem.

If the juvenile happens to be the offspring of a town luminary or someone the teacher feels is prestigious, they may get special treatment and not learn to be a regular member of the classroom group of peers, not to mention that the teacher's prestige orientation can alienate them from peers. Similarly, the juvenile whose parenting one becomes the coach for the school or community sports team is often set up to view oneself as set apart and possibly as the victim of the other juveniles' envy.

STORING "UNACCEPTABLE" EXPERIENCES FOR LATER

When positive new school or afterschool experiences that would be met with strenuous parental disapproval at home occur, often the juvenile notices them, but may deem them stupid, dangerous, or immoral. They may not remain in consciousness, or the juvenile may not consciously notice them at all. These experiences are stored[3] in the integral personality and may be remembered in a very different light later when one's life has significantly changed and made them more tolerable to be integrated into their self-system.

They can draw on such experiences later and, having now remembered them, try them out in a different context. That is, they can experience them later, however obscurely, if there is important validation for them. Often an experience is remembered during therapy. An adult can rediscover a positive juvenile experience and now allow it to be integrated into their self-system.

Something other than what the parenting one(s) has approved of can occur, particularly in groups the parenting one(s) already approved of, such as a sports team or the cast of a church play. Although there might not be a well-integrated conscious adjustment of perception, if it's relevant to the juvenile's need, it still can be remembered later.

If the juvenile does not have the opportunity for such corrective experiences at school or in the neighborhood, and if they don't occur at home, later functioning in the world becomes much harder. Therefore, whatever happens in the outside world, what community they're in, whether it's accepting of them, is crucial. A juvenile of color in a racist white community, a differently abled juvenile in a derisive neighborhood, a Jewish juvenile in an anti-Semitic area, or a juvenile having trouble figuring out their gender identity has an exceedingly difficult time collecting alternate experiences to store for later if there is no support from family, school authorities, or other community groups. The oppression continues the experience at home: If one is put down at home, in the extended family, and in the neighborhood, then goes to school and is put down there, there is less hope for a truly positive juvenile experience.

However, the cultural and familial environments are rarely identical. While similar experiences may happen at school, the adults and kids there do not have the same strenuous emotional investment as the parenting one(s). The juvenile can feel that. Once they are out of parental sight for seven hours five days a week, when they have never been away for so long before, it's a whole different world, not controlled totally by the parenting one(s). It's never total; it's a continuum. The degree of control and the degree of opportunity varies, depending upon the environment and upon what the juvenile learns though reading (assigned in the classroom or secretly passed from juvenile to juvenile), television (for example, seeing a revered sports figure "taking a knee"), movies such as *The King's Speech* (about a stammering royal), video-sharing platforms, and social media.

Moreover, there's usually something that will be a little different in school because nobody comes from the exact same family with the exact same values and prohibitions. The juvenile is usually going to find peers who potentially share something in common.

COOPERATION, COMPETITION, AND COMPROMISE

Increased exposure and continuity with peers comes simultaneously with an increase in the need for specific interactions with peers, as opposed to the more generalized parallel play of the childhood era. There is a difference between the enlivening but diffuse experience of building a castle in a sandbox next to other children who are similarly engaged in their own projects (parallel play) and the more complicated processes involved in jump rope with two turners and a line of jumpers taking turns while singing in unison to the rhythm of jumping. Parallel play for an adult might be watching a game of basketball on TV with others in a sports bar, versus the juvenile experience of playing basketball on a team, involving shared, mutually agreed on strategy, a recognized set of rules, and specific roles for each player.

The new juvenile gradually learns from peers and authorities to follow rules of group participation, the give-and-take of fairness, and rules of winning and losing, along with competition, compromise, and cooperation. They also learn that it is fun to care about the successes of the group: the team's score in game, building a sturdy snow fort, a group science project in school, or the jubilation of the cast after a well-performed school play.

Cooperation, competition, and compromise without the loss of self-esteem for the sake of group spirit become important in the juvenile era. In juvenile society, all is organized to accomplish a goal in a cooperative situation. In that spirit, the juvenile becomes attuned to the needs of the others of the group.

Competition involves pitting one's skills against another or others using agreed-upon rules of engagement. In the childhood era, the individual plays side by side with another child or engages in winning in a game by all costs, even insisting that their opponent (usually an older child or adult) let them win, or by cheating. It is self-centered playing without following the rules. The juvenile learns that winning is more fun if the rules are followed.

Juvenile competition can be a test of one's skills compared with another's. It can involve emulation of the other's skills and joy in participation with the other, even when the other's skills are perceived as greater. The greater skills of the other can become a source of inspiration to do better, or even simple admiration. The goal of personally winning is less important than matching oneself against one's rival. In competitive activities, a rout on the field is less fun for the winners than an evenly matched game. Honing one's skills is a fun learning experience. In contrast, the competition of the childhood era focuses on winning, no matter what. In adulthood, that kind of "cutthroat competition," with its focus on going after the competitor, is a product of the failure to learn how to enjoy matching one's skills against a competitor in the juvenile era.

Compromise involves giving something up for the sake of achieving a common goal that is experienced as important and worth the sacrifice. The clearest example is the process of taking turns. If there is one bicycle and three children, the best way to happily play together is to share it. It is difficult for a younger child to learn to compromise. Childhood is a "me" era, and often no amount of adult persuasion will stop feuds over, say, who gets to go first in line at Chuck E. Cheese, short of threatening discipline or promising an after-lunch treat. To give in and let the other go first can feel like a loss of self-esteem, suggesting that the other somehow deserves more. The juvenile learns that the team will have a better chance of winning if they aren't first at bat, or that one doesn't lose self-esteem because they must pass the basketball to another who has a better shot. Compromising does not mean losing. They learn that they get something more from compromising than not: compromise with honor, without loss of self-esteem.

Juvenile cooperation involves awareness of the needs of others to accomplish a task or reach a goal, including capacity to empathize with others, grasping cause and effect, having foresight, and compromising. The juvenile forms alliances and empathizes with others in a spirit of "fairness, justice and equality" (Pearce & Newton, 1963, p. 101).

The juvenile wants to feel like a member of the group and demonstrates conscience and commitment to the group's welfare: enlightened self-interest (Pearce & Newton, 1963, p. 101). Group functioning takes precedence over individual preference. The group's interest becomes each member's personal interest.

The concept of cause and effect is learned in the juvenile era. It is the basis for enlightened self-interest and cooperation. What are the consequences of my actions? If I insist on riding the only bike all the time, I won't have anyone to ride with. The "enlightened" juvenile might suggest that others bring their bikes outside so all can ride. If that is not possible, they know that the choice is between taking turns or riding their bike alone.

IDENTIFICATION WITH THE JUVENILE GROUP

A primary goal for the juvenile is experiencing group membership. Identification of belonging expands beyond the family constellation to the new juvenile group. If there is parental support for juvenile functioning, the juvenile is comfortable with group participation and can try out roles different from the one(s) assigned at home. If not, there is a tendency to assume a role within the group similar to one at home.

A juvenile who is in a group or on a team but feels they must be the head of the team, or is overly concerned with their personal role, is not working toward being a fully integrated member caring about the team for its own sake. An example is the bully who, rather than valuing team spirit, has a winner-take-all attitude. Another example is to immediately strive for being the team star. A good player is an asset to the group cause if they act with team spirit. However, if prestige in and of itself is the goal, the group experience is subsumed under the assumption that they must be the best or the boss to fit in. Juveniles who have been taught to never try for anything unless they can be the best may avoid participating in a team sport, class play, or the school band. The framework of the parenting one(s) remains dominant.

The definition, then, of one who is integrating juvenile functions is a person who identifies with the group. Juveniles cooperate to make the group function well. A juvenile who must be the head of it or control everything is not working toward being a member of the group and loving it for its own sake. Preoccupation with prestige and status is a serious difficulty for those who do not feel like comfortable members of a group. The desire to be the top or the best is not the same as being a leader in the sense of helping the group achieve its goals. Prestige, for its own sake, is a residual[4] from the childhood orientation to all others as authorities (Pearce &Newton, 1963, p.94). It is intolerable for a child to lose a game, even to an adult. To a successful juvenile, losing is a chance to learn from the winner how to get better. A successful leader recognizes superior skills and acknowledges them for the good of the group. The preoccupation with prestige and status is the hallmark of a person who is still working on achieving juvenile group membership in adulthood. It is a very common affliction. The successful juvenile is one who has integrated competition, cooperation, and compromise, and a solid feeling of group membership, a lifelong task for many.

MOVING INTO THE JUVENILE AS A NATURAL INTERPERSONAL NEED

If a juvenile is extremely isolated, does not attend school, or is homeschooled without much opportunity to interact with the outside world, their interactions with imaginary friends often become more cooperative. Perhaps inspired by movies or online games, the juvenile is ready for more interaction with groups of juveniles, even if they are only fantasized juveniles, animals, or super-heroes.

> Jen, isolated from others, fantasized about being with other children. They start building a log cabin, more kids get interested, and they build more cabins. Then they decide to build a fence around the cabins, like the forts in Westerns. The fort is self-sufficient; no grownups are allowed. It becomes a cooperative community of kids. In Jen's fantasy she is organizing a life consisting of a community of friendly people all working together to make something that excluded people who didn't love them. The elaborate fantasy went on for several years.

The memory of even minimal group interaction may be dissociated for years, but it moves into awareness when a new opportunity for juvenile experience arises.

When Brandan was five, their mother didn't enroll them in kindergarten. Their parents were derogatory about other people. Their mother insisted that other children in the school were inferior and uncultured. Their father was a professor who considered his colleagues "petty" and "just interested in using people to get tenure." The family put a sign on the door at Christmas to ward off carolers disturbing their "superior" way of celebrating the holiday. Brandan had some group experience as a student and stored these experiences away like acorns for the future.

Brandan avoided group participation in later years. Eventually, and with some trepidation, they accepted a job in a laboratory as a biologist to earn a living. They eventually sought out therapy. Through therapy, precious memories of group experience as a student resurfaced. After considerable anxious experimentation, they can cooperate and compromise comfortably with their project team at work.

The individual who remains isolated throughout the school years has little opportunity to learn alternative ways of interacting with the real outside world from peers (and other adults). Even if the child is kept isolated, some nuclear families are part of an extended family and join gatherings with cousins, aunts, and uncles. These gatherings are the only occasions in which the young person learns to play with others close in age. Siblings in an insular family might be very far apart in age, so they don't learn group play as well as they could potentially learn from extended family gatherings with cousins. With rare exceptions, none of these experiences are as valuable as games in the neighborhood playground, play dates, and, of course, school, but hanging out with siblings close in age and/or with the extended family gives the person opportunities to learn how to play games with rational rules, for example. Even if the extended family is insular and reinforces what goes on in the nuclear family setting, playing games with cousins is better than nothing.

Then there are nuclear families with twins and/or other multiples or several children very close in age because of adoption, foster placement, etc. In such homes, it is possible that the parenting one(s) teaches the children the juvenile skills of competition, cooperation, and compromise. In addition, older ones might be called upon to assist in caretaking the younger ones, including helping with homework and bedtime. Games and toys are often organized to be shared; taking turns is crucial. These children might come into the juvenile era with more juvenile skills. However, it is still the nuclear family. With exceptions—such as when the family exposes children to external experiences and ideas—whatever is learned under the rubric of juvenile behavior in the home prior to outside group experience still lies under the influence of the parental values, with few opportunities to check out the wider world of differences.

CONSENSUAL VALIDATION

Emotional content during the juvenile era revolves around group relatedness, with the individual striving to achieve comfort within the group. Communication with peers is crucial. Toward this end, the juvenile increasingly tries to express thoughts and feelings to peers with language. They seek appropriate words and phrases to achieve group goals, with the focus on consensually validated speech. Idiosyncratic words and phrases within the confines of the immediate family give way to expressions accepted by the group. Whereas the child's mother learned to understand the child's personal word for an object, that won't fly with peers (or the teacher, for that matter). The new juvenile learns rather quickly to toss out "baby talk" for agreed-upon language, consensually validated speech.

ROLE-PLAYING

Ideally, school teaches juveniles that there should be respect for all and everybody is treated equally. Some children come from families in which there is a hierarchy of who are the "good" and "bad" people. If the school pushes this child to be in a group espousing the notion of freedom for all, the child might role-play believing it while striving to be the leader of the group, bringing prestige to the child and to the child's family. Actual membership is avoided. On the other hand, role-playing can have beneficial effects because it places them in a position of needing to act "as if" they are a group member; then they can learn a bit about what that experience is like. Role-playing is pretending to be a member while feeling like an outsider or acting as if all the others equally matter—because the teacher insists—when in fact the conviction is that some are more acceptable than others. In contrast, taking on different roles from the one experienced at home might include talking up in class, when at home the child had to be "seen but not heard," or joining the school glee club, when at home it was assumed that the child was tone-deaf. The role one assumes can feel unreal, but as one tries it on, some experience and some conceptual expansion of what is possible are gained.

> As a shy adolescent, Jenny encountered a camp counselor who asked her how she made friends. She told her that she watched what people did and if they were friendly and asked to be her friend, she would let them. Her counselor told her that the only way to make friends was to plunge into it without abandon. Jenny was shocked but tried it in a new school. She said "hello" to almost everyone. She was soon surrounded by all kinds of people, found she could make choices from the people she had gotten to know, and developed a core group of friends.

OSTRACISM

One of the most strenuous motivational aspects of the juvenile experience is the fear of ostracism. If they master the feeling of being a truly participant group member, they can risk trying to challenge or oppose the group, even if it means being excluded from that particular group, because there are other groups to join (Pearce & Newton, 1963, p. 100). The availability of different kinds of groups in a school or neighborhood setting is important in developing juvenile skills. The child who is academically successful but awkward physically might have a hard time joining an athletic team but might find a haven with other "nerds" playing computer games and developing blogs. That adjustment can be successful if there is no emphasis placed on loss of prestige connected with being a "nerd" versus a "jock," or vice versa. In communities where there is emphasis on prestige via social class, income, nationality, or race, the issue of ostracism can be very troublesome. Much then depends on the importance the school and the community place on the need for belonging in each child. The support the family gives the juvenile in their search for group membership is also very important. This can be in the form of finding appropriate opportunities for group experience and encouraging participation, as well as being sensitive to the juvenile's needs and preferences.

Physical differences such as being differently abled can also create ostracism from groups at school and in the neighborhood. The burden is on the family, community, and school to create a genuinely inclusive social milieu. If needed, adults must find alternative sources for their juvenile's group participation.

The severity of the devastation wrought by ostracism to the juvenile's self-esteem is largely dependent on the relative fragility of their self-esteem coming into the era. If the parental figure(s) validated the child's needs up to this point, self-esteem will be less fragile in the face of ostracism and bullying.

A good deal of stereotyping gets "stamped-in" during the juvenile era (Sullivan, 1953, p. 238). This stereotyping, which might be learned from the parenting one(s) and/or the wider society, is usually related to the disparagement of other people. It is a major obstacle to growth during the juvenile era. The youngster struggles between the dictates of the parenting one(s) and the newly available experiences. A lot depends on what tools the emerging juvenile possesses to use in the new experiences, and what deficits the juvenile has that prevent their inclusion.

In Sullivan's (1953) words: "If you have to protect your feeling of personal worth by noting how unworthy everybody around you is, you are not provided with any data that are convincing evidence of your having personal worth" (p. 242).

It is even more strenuous when the larger community perpetuates the stereotyping. "[A] great many juveniles arrive at preadolescence with quite rigid stereotypes about all sorts of classes and conditions of mankind. . . . [I]t's hard indeed to avoid organizing—accessible to awareness—crude classifications of people, performance, and so on, which really are irrational and which later become troublesome stereotypes" (Sullivan, 1953, p. 238).

Racism, which embodies numerous stereotypes, is a destructive force as it occurs in the juvenile experience, creating hierarchies and divisions between groups of children.

MASTERY OF INFORMATION

Reading widens the juvenile's understanding of the world. Juveniles can experience intense identification with fictional characters and be influenced by biographies and autobiographies. They also can become enthralled with movie characters or actors, as well as those in electronic media. After being exposed to whatever the household has offered in the realm of entertainment, juveniles have exposure to not only new types of stories and topics in school but also the often-diversified tastes of the households of other juveniles. In addition to visits to schoolmates' homes, this exposure may be from simply exchanging ideas, books, and electronic media the juveniles bring to school.

For many, movies and books are perceived as having catapulted them into a better future. As one woman noted, "*Nancy Drew* (Keene, 1959) helped propel me beyond my shyer juvenile experience, because Nancy Drew drove a car. No female in my family ever drove a car. And I thought, 'Wow!'"

Juveniles become intensely involved in mastery of abilities and devote a considerable amount of time to the task. Athletic skills blossom and propel many juveniles into team games and competitions. They master computer skills, do science projects, tinker with electronics, and learn music. Such mastery can lead to finding like-minded juveniles and eventually forming their own group, such as a band or an astronomy club. Validation for particular interests often starts at home prior to the juvenile era through the nuclear and/or extended family, a godparent, or a babysitter. The mastery develops further as the juvenile learns skills at school; joins a team; gets validation from coaches, schoolmates, and teachers; and visits the homes of other juveniles who are into the same endeavors. In addition, the internet provides opportunities to receive validation for projects.

Sometimes the juvenile does not get a chance to stay at a location long enough to learn from the new interpersonal environment; for example, the family frequently moves because of job or military relocations. If the previous environment was particularly hostile, this could be an opportunity for the child to start fresh. Or, having begun to learn one set of rules to negotiate, the child is thrust into a new set (or even into a foreign country with a new language and customs). The need for continuity of relationships that allows for greater understanding and possible intimacy with one's peers is important, but so is the knowledge that there is a wide variety of possibilities to choose from.

The relationships formed in the juvenile era build the basis for an important network in which to develop more skills and greater intimacy with peers and authority figures. If the continuity of these relationships is disrupted, the functions learned within this context may also be disrupted. In addition, constant relocation can cause despair about making and keeping friends with the consequence of "why bother?" The following is an example of such disruption and its effect on later functioning, as well as family obliviousness to the pressing social needs of the children:

> When Julia was in the third grade her father took the family to London on his sabbatical, where she and her siblings were enrolled in a neighborhood school. In the United States she had just begun to gain mastery in jump rope. She was also beginning long division in class. These were important skills that gained her acceptance with others at school. While in London, she and her siblings were negatively singled out by the teachers and other juveniles because they looked and sounded different and didn't play the same games. They were also behind in schoolwork. Julia and her siblings banded together in self-defense, learning to rely on each other for support. This became the basis for a lifelong pattern of unquestioning loyalty to each other with a concomitant distrust of "outsiders."
>
> When they returned to the United States the next year, Julia discovered that the juveniles in the playground had already progressed from jump rope to double Dutch, jumping over two ropes turning in opposition to each other, and she was far behind them in skill. She never mastered long division and many of the other academic subjects covered in the previous year. Upon her return, she withdrew even more from other peers. Years later, in therapy, she complained of feeling inadequate and having a lifelong regret that she had never learned how to do double Dutch or long division. They were proof of her inadequacy. She distrusted co-workers and sought human interaction only from her siblings and spouse. The memory of her year abroad returned to her awareness after some time in therapy, and she began to understand the effects of frequent relocations on developing group membership and friendships. Inadequacy, isolation, and sadness were learned over the years.

OBSTACLES TO SUCCESSFUL INTEGRATION OF THE JUVENILE ERA

There are myriad ways the primary caretaker(s) might interfere with the juvenile comfortably having school and afterschool opportunities for alternate ways of functioning in the world. Parenting ones who participate in the juvenile's school activities may take a positive interest in the child's life by coaching, helping out on school trips, or taking a job in the child's school. However, such involvement can be problematic depending on the degree of comfort the parenting one has with other workers at the school, the juvenile's experimenting with roles different from what was learned at home, the juvenile's choice of friends, and the juvenile's expansion of functioning beyond the parent's own abilities.

For example, coaches who are the parenting ones of team members must avoid favoritism toward their child, who must not appear "special" or "privileged." Adults whose mothers worked as the school nurse, teacher, or school aide in their schools have described feeling that they couldn't make a move without the information being reported back to their mothers, putting a damper on exploration of new roles.

In U.S. society, there are at least two other hindrances to successes in the juvenile era. Child abuse occurs much more in the home than elsewhere. In 2012, according to the U.S. Department of Health and Human Services' Administration for Children and Families (2103), four-fifths (80.3 percent) of perpetrators were parenting ones, 6.1 percent were relatives other than the parenting one(s), and 4.2 percent were the unmarried partners of parenting one(s) (p. 76). However, the home as a haven in a dangerous world is still a widespread belief. Accordingly, children are often restricted to their residences, which often offer much fewer opportunities than the park, playground, or street. School-aged children are sometimes barred from public playgrounds or parks by parenting one(s) who are afraid for them. They may have children to play with in the same building or on prearranged play dates (usually with one other child). But the group experience is lacking. Nevertheless, if there are resources available and financial considerations are not obstacles, juveniles can enroll in afterschool programs or participate in organized group activities such as athletic teams or performing arts groups, providing extremely valuable experiences.

A major hindrance to integration of juvenile functioning involves unfortunate school policies. Partly the result of the Bill Gates approach to education, programs such as No Child Left Behind and Race to the Top have led to an earlier focus on academic achievement at the expense of socialized play, physical education, and creativity. Standardized tests, teaching to those tests, and sanctions for not doing so have become increasingly pervasive. The elimination of music, art, and physical education cuts off access to valuable areas of mastery for many children moving into the juvenile era.

When famed jazz bassist Ron Carter was growing up, there were music classes in his Ferndale, Michigan, school. He was presented with an array of instruments and chose the cello, his entry into a long music career.[5] Since then, funds for such programs have been cut, making it very difficult for poor students to even attempt such a career.

THE BURGEONING SHIFT OF PRIMARY AUDIENCE

In the juvenile era, the sense of childhood powerlessness in the face of the absolute power of the parenting one(s) is gradually tempered by the awareness of other ways of doing things and the importance of the perceptions of other adults and juveniles. But the parenting one(s) remains the primary audience, with their powerful messages of what is acceptable and unacceptable still very much the juvenile's motivating forces. There is a whole new world of people now, primarily other juveniles at school and at play, and other adult authority figures, but the do's and don'ts of the parenting one(s) still prevail. After all, not only has the child been under the influence of the primary caretaker(s) since birth, but the child goes back home to that caretaker(s) at the end of the school day. The limitations of the parenting one(s) are still paramount.

The juvenile questions parental assumptions, but even if those assumptions turn out not to be useful anymore, they are not discarded. Challenges to earlier assumptions may temper perceptions and be incorporated, but parental dictates still rule. Sometimes there is shame about the parenting one(s), a need to distance oneself from them in public to feel acceptable to the peer group. The juvenile who begins to challenge the limits of the family may do it defiantly or secretly, but with a sense of guilt. The audience is still the parenting one(s). Functioning beyond the limitations of the family might feel like role-playing until the primary audience in a person's thinking changes.

The chumship experience of emotional identification with an admired peer in preadolescence is a prerequisite for a *major* move beyond parental ways of being in the world. If there is no empathic identification with another human being beyond the parenting one(s), newly learned behaviors are implemented to get along in the wider world, but the new insights do not have the emotional resonance to replace or alter previously cherished childhood assumptions.

WHAT HAPPENS NEXT

Many people remain juveniles for much of the rest of their lives. Some do not quite consolidate juvenile functions (although managing to role-play juvenile functions while not quite feeling like a true member of society) and remain in some sort of amalgam of the childhood and juvenile eras.

Some of the new juvenile learning may be unconsciously stored in the integral personality until the individual is ready (if ever) to bring them into consciousness and use them.

No matter how long a person lingers in the juvenile era in order to master identification with the group, one is not capable of loving another human being as much as one loves oneself unless a feeling of true membership in the group, and in the human race, is achieved first. For example, if a person marries and has a family but still feels like an outsider in relationships with other people (in the community, at the workplace, in the bowling team, at the PTA meeting), then the relationship feels more like an alliance in a potentially dangerous world. If the individual does not view themself as an equal member of the human race, they do not progress from unconsolidated juvenile membership to preadolescent mutual cherishing, which, in turn, is necessary for more integrated loving relationships during late adolescence and beyond.

Moreover, if the person has not learned from juvenile and preadolescent experiences, they perceive others according to the original parental opinions of people (Pearce & Newton, 1963). This is fine if the parenting one(s)' feelings about people are useful and inclusive, but in that case the person has been able to connect with the juvenile community and one or more best friends in preadolescence and has learned even more from those experiences. Without juvenile and preadolescent experiences, relationships tend to be organized as they were in the childhood home, with the spouse and/or people in the workplace and community perceived as people from the person's childhood family. For example, the boss is the irrational authoritarian, the colleague is a competitive or envious sibling, or one's spouse is the perennial nag. Of course, in many instances, the individual has unconsciously organized the marriage or the workplace to mimic the family constellation, provoking fights with colleagues and neighbors, or choosing a spouse who in fact turns out over time to actually be like that person's mother, a "nag."

The adult may be exploitative, manipulating others as objects for their own ends. Many adult juveniles remain devoted to norms of the juvenile era but have not learned to feel like a group member. They mistake power, prestige, and achievement for membership.

If one remains enmeshed in the juvenile and does not also comfortably integrate the functions of later eras, the adult can become a perpetual juvenile:

always competing with others in trying to get ahead at all costs or compromising one's own needs, rarely standing up for oneself, to avoid an argument. These are well-integrated juvenile functions they inappropriately use in later interpersonal interactions. Such behaviors make it difficult to grow beyond the juvenile. They make competition and group participation a chore instead of fun and cut off empathy with others. Relentless competitiveness and/or fear of ostracism stop a person from progressing to the next stage of development: identification with and admiration for a peer. They promote instead the seeds of deterioration to childhood functioning.

SUMMARY

The juvenile is the era in which the political arts of cooperation, competition, and compromise without loss of self-esteem are learned under the rubric of understanding cause and effect and enlightened self-interest. It is a vast expansion into the wider world beyond the parental home, into learning how to relate in that world.

The juvenile era is essentially a struggle between the assumptions and training of the parenting one(s)—that is, the self-system(s) of the parenting one(s), from restrictive to expansive—and the new experiences available to the youngster. The deficits the emerging juvenile still retains from prior years impede the inclusion of new experiences. The parenting one(s) who has developed past the juvenile era recognizes and accepts their children's discoveries and is enthusiastically willing to grow in new directions with their children.

Navigating the juvenile era and learning from this extended interpersonal environment, with all its opportunities for broadening one's experiences in life, are profoundly crucial in one's development, even if specific juvenile functions are not successfully integrated during this period. Useful experiences forbidden by a child's self-system are stored in the integral personality and available for emergence into conscious implementation whenever the individual is ready to make use of them.

NOTES

1. This is called the shift from *parataxic* to *syntaxic* thinking (Sullivan, 1953). Also see Mullahy (1980) and Pearce and Newton (1963), particularly the chapters on modes of communication and the juvenile era.

2. U.S. children can enter a setting such as daycare or preschool before four. Learning juvenile skills in these settings is much the same as in kindergarten but tied to the

development of language and motor skills. At two, the child is more firmly rooted in the childhood era with idiosyncratic, personalized language that is only understood at home, and self-centered ways of relating to peers and adults. The teacher organizes activities such as games, crafts, etc., in a preschool or daycare setting. In this process, parallel play is paramount. This experience of shared fun in the presence of other children is the bedrock for all future learning of juvenile relatedness. It is what makes the learning of juvenile skills, such as taking turns and other forms of compromise (with honor), worthwhile. Until there is integration of parallel play, the child is not ready to take on the more arduous tasks of the juvenile era, including cooperation, compromise, and competition. The child who stays relating to peers in parallel-play mode has no thought about team spirit or group identification.

3. Storing experiences in the integral personality for later use—because they will make an individual too anxious to integrate them into the self-system at the moment—is different from dissociation of heinous experiences such as physical and/or sexual abuse. The latter are often relegated to that unremembered place in order for the child to continue in life without conscious interference—although they generally interfere with a person's life in ways that are not yet available to conscious understanding. The integral personality might make those events available to the older individual, often when the individual is emotionally stronger because of positive experiences (Pearce & Newton, 1963).

4. Residuals are functions not adequately consolidated in a particular developmental era that affect how one functions in later life. The term as defined here was coined by Pearce and Newton (1963, pp. 83, 89, 94, 102, 107, 113).

5. From a talk Ron Carter gave at "Only at Merkin with Terrance McKnight," September 28, 2019. Also see Ouellette (2017).

Chapter Six

Preadolescence

Falling in Love with a Peer

MOVING FROM THE JUVENILE ERA INTO PREADOLESCENCE

The major preadolescent interpersonal project is to develop a loving[1] relationship with a peer they admire and identify with. This friendship prepares the preadolescent to eventually embrace, even more than before, a world of people wider than the world of the primary caretaker(s).

The development of the capacity for intimacy, along with the capacity for empathy, is a complex process that begins in infantile experience with the primary caretaking one(s) and builds from there from developmental era to developmental era. In each era limits are established based upon the limitations of the primary caretaker(s),[2] poorly consolidated earlier functions, and lack of opportunity. Accumulating residuals[3] affect how one experiences later eras, how they can continue growing in preadolescence, adolescence, and adulthood. Despite these complications, how does one develop the capacity for true peer intimacy with people other than the primary parenting one(s)? How does one learn to love an ever-widening world of people?

During the earlier juvenile era, a person develops and consolidates the experience of group membership. Unless they can make up for poorly consolidated juvenile functions later in life, they are, to varying degrees, self-centered and childish in their interactions with other people.

To the degree that juvenile functions are consolidated, a person moves beyond "me" as the center of the universe to identification and membership with one or more specific groups. Caring for and identifying with a group paves the way for the preadolescent era, usually between eight and puberty. Now a person begins moving toward at least one emotionally intimate best friend[4] without relinquishing the need for and continuance of team identification and involvement. The friendship is their first loving relationship outside the immediate framework of their family (Sullivan, 1953, p. 245). This interpersonal intimacy is closeness without a sexual component; it allows for all aspects of self-worth to be validated (Sullivan, 1953, p. 246).

When the young person connects with a special peer, it's the first time they feel someone else's deepest needs are as important as their own. Characterized by a great deal of trust and confidence, the friendship differs from those in earlier eras. It also does not involve manipulation or competitiveness. Developing outside parental assumptions, it usually involves secrecy and privacy. With that freedom and inner drive to harness that freedom to expand their self-systems, the friends explore the wider world and reevaluate heretofore cherished assumptions about it. They are growing each other up, inseparable in that project (Pearce & Newton, 1963, p. 105). The preadolescent starts being intimately attuned to another person's wants, not figuring out how to do something to get what they want for themself, but instead how to make their best friend happy and support their prestige and self-esteem (Sullivan, 1953).

This collaboration between two mutually cherished preadolescents who identify with each other goes a long way in raising one's self-esteem. It really matters that someone who is loved is reciprocating that love.

In connecting with another peer who is so much alike, boundaries kind of fade. The two young people learn to talk freely with each other about anything and everything, knowing each is feeling and struggling with the same issues: interest in and confusion about their almost pubescent bodies; hopes and dreams about the future; mutual interests and validation in the mastery of skills; perceptions about family, teachers, schoolmates, and mutual friends. They engage in long discussions, often completing the other's sentences because they think so much alike. If one is happy, the other is happy; if one is hurting, the other is too. They can giggle and weep, share excitement, and bring new experiences to each other without evoking envy or competition. They are inseparable, and if their parenting one(s) allow, they sleep over at each other's houses as much as they can. They might exchange tokens of mutual esteem, a bracelet or locket, symbolizing they are absolute and forever pals. They're in love.

For some, it's the first opportunity to talk about the (often) taboo topic of gender identity, why they are gendered male or female, and what that means if they feel different from their gendering. This topic is easier if both are similarly confused, but in the best of worlds, they talk freely about these feelings no matter what. Sexual urges have not yet become paramount; both are simply thinking deeply about things. (The taboo about preadolescent same-gender friendships is discussed below.)

More recently, forthrightness about LGBTQIA+[5] issues, including gendering and gender-affirming change, might make it easier for them to freely discuss those issues with each other, particularly because of social media and mainstream coverage.[6] It also depends on how difficult it is to stray from parental and community values, even in best-friend discussions. This friendship is so valuable that a young person may desperately not want to risk losing it.

SAME-GENDER CHUM

Sullivan emphasized "same-sex" chums. His criterion reflects the attitude that was prevalent in the early 20th century, that boys are more like boys and girls more like girls. Today there is no need to make that distinction. The preadolescent chum is learning they are no different from this other human being; one human being can love the other, no matter what; and the feeling goes both ways, without complications of sexual urgings. This major point is consistent with Sullivan's (1953) one-genus postulate: "everyone is much more simply human than otherwise"[7] (p. 32).

Nevertheless, in the current culture, there still tends to be a divide between male and female, so preadolescent experience often does divide along gender lines. But not always. It cannot be overemphasized that the issue is less about gender than about mutual identification, admiration, and tenderness. It's possible for preadolescents of all genders to be best friends. They all reap the benefits.

Heightening Self-Esteem and Expanding Awareness of Others

Identifying with a best friend and realizing that their friend is valuable allows a person to recognize their own value as a member of the human race, paving the way for an ever-expanding capacity for close friendships. Consciousness of membership in the human race starts during the childhood era, at the integration of parallel play, but in preadolescence it is more profound, having to do with heightening self-esteem and considerable expansion of awareness of others.

Preadolescent chumship enriches already-growing awareness of the surrounding world; now personal concern evolves into concern about the greater world, making use of increased skill sets that enable greater social and political involvement, greater identification with all peoples. Preadolescence is the era of considerable expansion of knowledge about and interaction in that larger sphere.

Major Changes in the Self-system

The best friend is becoming almost as important as the original source(s) of affirmation. Consequently, the self-system significantly changes in its expansion beyond the original frame of reference. In this mutually cherishing relationship, they are preparing for an ever-expanding self-system, one that can continue embracing a myriad of mutually validating tender relationships. They, as equals, experience mutual peer *inter*dependence. They learn about freedom of choice, association, and commitment, all crucial for developing into a mature adult (Pearce & Newton, 1963, p. 107).

Preadolescence is a short phase when compared to other eras. Nevertheless, it is "probably rather fantastically valuable in salvaging one from the effects of unfortunate accidents up to then" (Sullivan, 1953, p. 227). The self-system has a grand opportunity to significantly change and is "of incredible importance in saving a good many rather seriously handicapped people from otherwise inevitable serious mental disorder" (Sullivan, 1953, p. 248).

Timing of Preadolescent Chumship

This preadolescent experience can occur at any point later in life. However, until it happens, the individual has difficulty moving past juvenile values to realizing that individuals matter in the way that mutually cherishing, loving individuals matter. A crucial therapeutic task is determining where the person is developmentally. Many people first need more experience with juvenile group identification; when that happens a person, no matter how old, can look toward developing the kind of best friend that characterizes the preadolescent era, with all its advantages.

Then comes adolescence. The one-to-one relatedness, if consolidated in the chumship, now expands the capacity to love, to form deeper, integrated partnerships. Adult loving relationships have to do with how successfully preadolescent and adolescent interpersonal experiences are integrated. The gender and sexuality of a partner is a non-issue. The ability to develop the capacity for peer intimacy with at least one person other than the original parenting one(s) is *sine qua non*. Blechner (2009) summarizes Sullivan's general observation: "[M]ental health is not so dependent on the specifics of one's sexual desires per se; instead, whatever one's sexual desires, mental health depends on whether one can integrate them successfully with another human being" (120).[8]

While functions develop in an orderly sequence based on emerging needs and earlier learning, they also develop in and around the limitations established by the self-system, within the restrictions of the parental world view, along with whatever alternate validation is present and deemed "acceptable."

Acquisition of new functions is based on opportunity, but it does not always seem to be orderly. One's functioning occurs within one's self-system's restrictions according to what is possible. There will be detours and accommodations and, therefore, residuals of unlearned areas of functioning that skew later learning. People are always playing "catch-up" with themselves to expand their capacity to grow in all areas of living. Human growth is like a river, flowing around obstacles and seeking expression via the area of least resistance. No two people are exactly alike in terms of the accommodations they must make to form intimate relationships. In human functioning, there is no reason to think any one path of flow is better.

Intimacy Panic

Consequently, culture and adults significant in the individual's upbringing play a significant role in how well earlier developmental eras become consolidated. A preadolescent who makes a same-gender best friend can, and often does, bump into clichés and taboos about same-gender closeness. Intimacy panic[9] often interferes with the need to develop a chum, and one or both individuals might bid a hasty retreat, fearing that there is something terribly wrong with what they have been doing. The panic is very unfortunate; it can cause an individual to be uncomfortable moving toward any loving relationship. Convinced that they are "weird" or "disgusting," they avoid friendships with anyone. If the push for chumship arrives later, in adolescence or in adulthood, because it was never or poorly consolidated in preadolescence, the panic can also be a very unfortunate inhibiting force. Inculcated and promoted by contemporary society, it is a disastrous stumbling block for anyone's growth and development—and a convenient cover-up for fear of intimacy.

The parenting one(s) might be uncomfortable with the preadolescent moving toward emotional intimacy with another. The preadolescent friendship is more intense than any the parenting one(s) has observed before, causing a burgeoning of interests far wider than previously, which might be threatening the limits of the parental self-system. To the extent they do not validate a burgeoning chumship, it is developed with varying degrees of guilt and hesitation, perhaps with repudiation. It may not happen at all.

If, for whatever reasons, moving toward chumship arrives in adolescence when pubescent sexual needs may be loudly pushing for satisfaction, the situation can become more complicated. If the friends are the same gender, depending upon the degree of homophobia within the family and community, the relationship can be fraught with guilt, which can interfere with the friendship. Nevertheless, the experience goes a long way in developing the capacity to be in love with other people (Pearce & Newton, 1963, p. 109).

Integrations of preadolescent chumship and of adolescent relations are often burdened with a great many residual deficits interfering with consolidation. There are probably very few people who manage a fully satisfying chumship or beyond. With exceptions, adult intimacy is generally fraught with some struggle, no matter the gender and sexuality or asexuality of the people involved. People are all playing catch-up at the same time. Nevertheless, how or when they play catch-up, or with whom, is beside the point.

No matter what, the development of the capacity for intimacy, not the gender, sexuality, or asexuality, of the partner, is crucial. The bottom line: developing a true preadolescent best friend, whether in preadolescence or afterward, is a prerequisite for loving adult relationships. It helps if chumship is consolidated during preadolescence, but better late than never. In addition, preadolescents can have somewhat intimate relationships that are repudiated later, short-lived or deteriorate, but they can have loving relationships later with some limitations based on that early experience. Adult relationships can also improve based upon additional elements of chumship experienced later in life that a person can piece together.

SUMMARY

The preadolescent chumship, no matter when it happens and no matter how well consolidated, is a prerequisite—as vital as crawling before walking—for achieving loving adult relationships, as imperfect as they may be. The chumship experience can be acquired later, even after marrying, so partners can learn to love each other, rather than marrying the concept of marriage, playing house, and worst of all, organizing a household and family that mirrors whatever the dysfunctional aspects were in their childhood homes. After all, the preadolescent chumship is the first loving relationship that is *separate* from whatever might have been restrictive in the original household. To not experience it at all, no matter how old a person is, puts them in danger of repeating history, not growing to experience an ever-widening quality of living. People do not need to shed useful aspects of their original upbringing; they need to reevaluate and discard troublesome ones.

In whatever way the adult sexual or asexual relationship emerges, getting on with the project of loving—growing each other up—is worth the strenuous project of understanding the need for the kind of love that exists in the preadolescent chumship and working toward it, even if the adult is chronologically way past that developmental era. For many it means visiting even earlier eras of development (with adult projects and experiences) to find ways to be comfortable with peers. For some, it means learning how to enjoy parallel play (such as taking an art class), a prerequisite to enjoying the juvenile functions of team spirit (such as joining a baseball team or a political group project), a prerequisite to having a closest best friend or friends with whom private thoughts are finally unabashedly shared. All these projects can be taken on as chronological adults, with the knowledge that people grow unevenly and quicker than the time it took to become chronological adults. The projects can be lots of fun. When adults develop and experience close friendships that satisfy preadolescenct needs, they have the chance, going forward, to make informed decisions about whom they choose as loving partners.

NOTES

1. The use of the word "love" has to do cherishing, validation, and tender relatedness to the other's needs, not the traditional meaning of romantic love.
2. There is always room to grow beyond the original primary caretaker(s)' self-systems. The word "limitations" does not denote criticism, but a rather fluid conceptualization of the parental self-systems based on the primary caretaker(s)' upbringing and opportunities for changing their own self-systems.
3. Residuals are functions not adequately consolidated in a particular developmental era that affect how one functions in later life. The term as defined here was coined by Pearce and Newton (1963, pp. 83, 89, 94, 102, 107, 113).
4. Sullivan emphasized "same-sex" friendship, consistent with when he wrote and lectured.
5. Lesbian, gay, bi, trans, questioning/queer, intersex, asexual/agender/asexual/ally, and others. The acronyms and language are constantly in development.
6. Although, as of 2022, "don't say gay" legislation has complicated the issue.
7. With this principle, radical for his time, Sullivan was emphasizing that "homosexuals" and people diagnosed schizophrenic must be not be placed in a category of "other" and treated as such. In the current social climate, not only must his one-genus postulate be reasserted, it must particularly call attention to "recently acknowledged complexities in gender identity, development, and both the vulnerability and resilience of transgender communities; in other words, a greater understanding of the diversity in the human condition" (Taffel, 2020, p. 17). This applies to all peoples who are oppressed and whose common humanity must be emphasized.
8. As discussed in chapter sixteen, for asexual people, sexual attraction is on a continuum from no sexual urgings to sexual attraction once the person forms a strong emotional connection with someone else. It cannot be assumed that asexuality is a problem requiring treatment. Likewise, it cannot be assumed that not feeling romantically attracted to anyone (a-rom) is a problem requiring treatment.
9. Sullivan used the term "homosexual panic," reflecting the era in which he theorized. The terminology is constantly changing. At the point of this writing (2022), we are using the phrase "intimacy panic."

Chapter Seven

Adolescence

Precursor to Independence, Emergence of Sexuality, Need for Partnership, Intimacy—A Work in Progress

PRELIMINARY COMMENTS

A major change in interpersonal relationships occurs from preadolescence to adolescence. Until then, the primary caretaker(s) has been the audience for all interpersonal relatedness. They have been powerful authorities, and perceptions are formulated within their framework. To the extent that previous additional relationships have been validated, valuable social skills have been learned. The preadolescent chumship, if successful, is the first time another human being becomes almost as important to the growing person as their parenting one(s), but the chum doesn't take the parenting one(s') place as the primary audience.

If all goes well, with the emergence of adolescence around the time of puberty, the adolescent's view of their parenting one(s) and their relationship begins to shift. For the adolescent, parental limitations in relatedness to others becomes clearer. If the parenting one(s) is also growing and changing, there is less struggle, but it still exists as the adolescent begins to discern differences between the parental self-system and the wider world of opportunities and attitudes. Depending on the history of the parent-child relationship, the clearer perception can result in contempt or compassion for the parenting one(s), or a mixture of the two. From the parental point of view, the adolescent's attempts to grow beyond their current ability to relate might be perceived as threatening or inspirational. The parenting one(s) may have continued to learn how to relate to others more successfully than in the first, say, 10 years of the adolescent's upbringing. In that case, the parenting one(s) can continue to be a valuable source of validation. However, gradually, the parental voice is no longer alone. They must learn to be one of the many potential validators in the adolescent's life and no longer demand center stage.

With the possible exception of early infancy, adolescence in many cultures is the stormiest developmental era. Early infancy encompasses the transition from the womb to the outside world and the beginning of life. Adolescence marks the transition from the family to the world at large. If there is to be continuous expansion of personality, the adolescent's additional primary validators necessarily become people who can provide experience and support for what has not been learned from their caretaker(s). Parenting one(s) are often crucial, helping to organize practical aspects of the adolescent's life, but they are unable to remain primary validator(s).

Some parenting one(s) are invested in how the adolescent appears to the world. Their shortcomings and awkwardness, because of lack of validation for previously unvalidated needs, can expose the shortcomings of parental child-rearing efforts and become a source of embarrassment or chagrin.

In earlier times, depending upon the culture, children by the age of 12 were often thrust into a world much wider than the nuclear family. Rich or poor, by mid- or late adolescence they went into the factory, boarding school, early marriage, military, monastery, or convent. They may also have lived in a much larger group: aunts, uncles, grandparents, and cousins, as well as other members of an extended group. In most cultures, adolescent rites of passage in their early to mid-teens symbolized transition into adulthood. This social structure remained relatively stable from one generation to another until the 20th century.[1] What makes the current time different, at least in the United States, is the extremely rapid nature of change in the society at large. The world the adolescent experiences can be very different from their parenting one(s)' experience of it. In addition, with major cultural and religious exceptions, family structure has changed from a multi-generational family or clan to the nuclear family, and very often, a single-parent home.[2]

Simultaneously, in current society the adolescent is still dependent economically, practically, legally, and emotionally on their parenting one(s). In the current, rapidly changing culture, no longer organized by clan or extended family, it's still necessary to begin growing beyond the parental view of the world, which has been formed and delimited by the parenting one(s)' own self-systems. Sometimes the older adolescent is designated to assume adult responsibilities at the expense of school and afterschool socializing (to take care of younger siblings or an ailing parenting one or to replace a deceased or absent parenting one and take over financial support, for example). However, despite these real issues, if the adolescent is to become an independent, self-sufficient young adult, they must continue expanding their interpersonal skills. They must learn to find validation in the world beyond family.

This shift is extremely anxiety provoking to the adolescent and the parenting figure(s) because of a major contradiction in adolescence. At least temporarily, the adolescent usually remains financially, legally, and emotionally dependent on the parenting one(s). With some exceptions, they continue to live at home. They are still in school and will probably need to continue education or training for almost another decade beyond puberty if self-sufficiency is to be attained. The same exists for many legal rights; depending upon where they live, their legal rights are not recognized until the age of 18 or 21. This inevitable conflictual situation creates an almost perfect storm in relations between parenting one(s) and adolescents that may be very difficult to negotiate.

Parenting an adolescent is usually an extremely tough job. To be helpful to the adolescent, a parenting one(s) has a monumental task. They must find ways to reduce conflict and leave room for the adolescent to continue growing, while providing material and emotional support and guidance based on their greater experience and perspective. All must go on while the adolescent is exploring interpersonal relatedness beyond what their parenting one(s) has already taught them.

Adolescents have many ways of relating that were not available to their parenting one(s) when they were growing up. One is the digital world. Using various forms of messaging, social media, and interactive games, the adolescent has, unlike the previous generation, expanded opportunities to form relationships with an ever-widening range of people. They are also more rapidly exposed to new ideas. In mandating that the adolescent limit their "online time," their parenting one(s) may be curtailing important online connections. There are also real reasons to be concerned if the adolescent retreats into the digital world to avoid people or to interact with internet predators posing as friendly new contacts. Parenting one(s) must help them make informed decisions about whom to interact with online and how much time they spend on their devices without interfering with academics and meaningful social interactions, even though digital. That is, when the parenting one(s) feels competent to do so.

Another major change is the attitude about gender expression, gender identity and sexuality.[3] While the Gay Liberation Movement in the United States started to have impact in the 1960s, and acceptance of LGBTQIA+[4] people continued to increase over the next 50 years, it has only been over the last 20 years that the concept of choice about one's gender expression, gender identity, and sexuality has become, with major exceptions, more routinely acceptable and has entered popular thinking in the United States. In this atmosphere, the adolescent may feel more inclined than their parenting one(s) to explore their own gender expression, gender identity, and sexuality, perhaps with varying degrees of inner conflict, including unspoken guilt and shame, and/or overt, sometimes charged, arguments within the family circle.

In short, current social expectations and peer pressure that may conflict with parental value systems are powerful influential forces.

However, the adolescent growing up in the modern world is not a tabula rasa. Adolescents seek satisfaction of heretofore invalidated and forbidden needs that could not be met by the parenting one(s). At the same time, they are limited by the strength of the security operations that have been established very early to restrict the satisfaction of those needs. The adolescent takes the risk of moving beyond their parenting one(s) but is governed by the limits of their own learned judgement and anxiety.

The parenting one(s) also must learn how to tell the difference between their own awareness of the wider world and their fears about it, and develop respect for the ability of the adolescent to exercise judgement. The goal is to foster independence, not fearfulness.

The same is true of the adolescent's life choices of affiliation and identification. Any group affiliation outside the family circle has the potential to provide new opportunities for expansion. Their choices may appear bizarre to the parenting one(s) and even dangerous, but the young person is focussed on exploration of new and different ways to relate. They are trying to find methods to achieve autonomy and satisfaction in the world. In this instance, as in many others to be discussed, parenting one(s) must find ways to share their knowledge of the world, and of potential pitfalls, to avoid obvious disastrous consequences, simultanously respecting the adolescent's choice of affiliation. In some ways, the adolescent may have greater knowledge of the world, knowledge their parenting one(s) may not be aware of.

Some examples of how this might play out:

> A young man, Bill, grew up in a physically and sexually abusive foster home. He joined a local neighborhood gang that engaged in various risky and antisocial activities. Bill found a sense of structure and mutual support he had never experienced before. While the gang fought enemies and preyed on non-members, his experience was an important transition from an extremely destructive home environment to one where he could learn tools for living. He eventually developed more constructive and socially acceptable non-gang relationships.

> Ted, raised in an extremely restrictive home environment, was allowed to try out for a local theater company, largely because his mother fantasized he would become famous and support the family. Once accepted into the company, he could spend long periods without his parenting one(s)' scrutiny and oversight. He met many new people and traveled abroad with the troupe, learning many interpersonal skills and garnering hope he could successfully leave home.

> Lisa's mother refused to let her attend college away from home. However, she won a scholarship to an Ivy League college, wresting permission to attend on condition that she return home after college. At school, she guiltily formed relationships and tried out skills she could not have attempted at home. After college it was difficult for her to return home; she quickly accepted a job in another city.

Parenting one(s) must respect their adolescents' choice of affiliations, simultaneously monitoring their judgment to prevent innocent miscalculation. In situations that require intervention, a parenting one(s) needs to intervene non-judgmentally. Also, adolescents may move into new areas of relatedness beyond parental experience, so perspective and intervention from an outside, relatively neutral source may be helpful.[5]

PARTNERSHIPS, SEXUALITY, AND INTIMACY

Inevitably, the adolescent will explore sexuality. In addition to sex education at school, they can benefit from whatever the parenting one(s) is comfortable sharing. It's also helpful if the adolescent can seek out information elsewhere, including the internet.

Adolescence begins with the emergence of sexual functioning evidenced by structural physical changes as well as, for many, the felt experience of sexual urgings. For asexual people, sexual attraction is on a continuum from no sexual urgings to sexual attraction once the person forms a strong emotional connection with someone else (The Trevor Project, 2021). At the same time, the need for peer intimacy emerges, depending on the individual's experience in prior developmental eras and with intimacy in the preadolescent chumship. They must learn how to manage these strands and how they relate to one another. There is no ideal combination of the two. It is often expressed in the search for partners, defined here as collaboration between peers for mutual satisfaction, not necessarily a committed two-some.

The choice of partner, the quality of relatedness, and the mode of sexuality or asexuality engaged in with the partner can begin to interact and even collide with the larger social world beyond their family. They are negotiating with larger social issues, including economics, kinship structure, ownership, status, gender and sexuality, convention, and morality, all of which impact their choices regarding sexual or asexual expression and intimacy.

The Emergence of Sexual Urgings

While there may be interest or experimentation prior to full-blown adolescent sexuality, biological development of adolescent sexual urgings, when they exist, is dramatic and inexorable. In addition to the emergence of secondary sex characteristics, there is increased hormonal and autonomic responsiveness and heightened sensitivity of genital and other erogenous zones. This makes preoccupation with sexual urgings much more central. As with the need for food and air, sexual need (if it manifests) is experienced with some urgency. It is one of the most powerful forces, next to loneliness, that propel adolescents out into the world.

The need to sexually touch and to be touched in some fashion often collides with highly developed social norms prohibiting such touching. Consequently, adolescents must find a path around the myriad existing social norms preventing the satisfaction of their sexual needs. Usually, the process is only partly conscious.

As with any other function, sexual relatedness must be learned and requires practice. Within the ongoing restrictions of family and society, the adolescent who experiences sexual urgings must learn techniques of achieving sexual satisfaction. Masturbation is a helpful preliminary, allowing a person to get in touch with their own body, its timing, and manner of response unencumbered by success or failure with another person. Masturbation, a necessary precursor to successful sexual relatedness, also develops confidence in the ability to reliably give and receive sexual gratification. Once achieved, it allows the person to be more accurate about how to relate to a partner (Pearce & Newton, 1963, p. 112). Often frowned upon socially, the adolescent usually seeks and needs privacy, free from social observation and disapproval.

However, masturbation as the exclusive means of satisfying sexual need may be used to avoid satisfying the need for sexual intimacy with another person (Sullivan, 1953, pp. 170–171).

Experimentation with various partners is an important vehicle for increasing experience with sex. But it is often considered promiscuous or sinful, so the adolescent may secretly experiment. Nevertheless, it is needed to develop skill.

Sexuality occurs in an interpersonal context. To satisfy it, another person, real or imaginary, is required, even with masturbation. The choice of partner, the way the partners interact, and the social setting in which the interaction goes on are all aspects of the function of sexuality. However, with few exceptions, the broader society has established standards about what kind of sexuality may be acceptable. Adolescents strive to discover their own sexuality within that set of standards, or they eschew the standards altogether. The adjustment required to express one's sexuality despite or within social restrictions is one of the adolescent tasks. For most, finding privacy for such exploration is often herculean.

Anxiety about Sex

The primary caretaker(s) are indispensable early validator(s) of taking pleasure in one's body and physical contact with others. Cuddling is a major component of the function of sexuality. Much of adult sexuality is experienced in an intense, non-verbal, "parataxic," i.e., non-logical way. Intense pleasure or intense loathing and feelings of rage, joy, or grief, for example, are all part of the experience and are reflections of a very early time when one was a naked infant and touched tenderly or not.

Frequently, as the person grows from infancy through the developmental eras, there is likely to be some dissociation of the sense of touch because of various social prohibitions. With the emergence of puberty, however, there can be a re-emergence of sensitivity, which is anxiety provoking, dependent upon earlier restrictions and prohibitions as well as current responses.

Examples of social obstacles to healthy sexual expression:

- *Primary genital phobia* (Sullivan, 1953, p. 61): a phobic response to one's own (or another's) genitals, as if they were not part of oneself, accompanied by intense anxiety, loathing, and terror.
- *Ridicule:* coming from anxiety about adolescent fledgling attempts at experimentation.
- *Segregation of the sexes:* limiting knowledge of the "opposite sex."
- *Pejoratives:* words that disgrace sexually curious adolescents and warn them away from curiosity and exploration, creating divisions between "good" and "bad" people.
- *Misogyny:* role differentiation and polarization between genders setting different standards for consent and choice.
- *Homophobia or transphobia and derogation of gender variation:* derogation of same-gender or other partnerships as legitimate; a restriction on the need to explore and experience pleasure in a partner.
- *Possessiveness:* ownership of rights to association with the partner is a pervasive dampener of enthusiasm and pleasure.

Some Restrictions Based on Interpersonal Deficits in Development

If a person has not yet begun to see themself as an equal member of the human race, i.e., has not yet integrated childhood parallel play or juvenile feelings of membership, the advent of sexual experience may be experienced in infantile terms, evoking powerful mood-memories[6] so that new sexual experience takes on powerful significance beyond the current. The partner may be experienced as much more powerful, as the "good mother," romanticized into someone capable of giving infinite pleasure and tenderness. This often quickly turns into the "bad mother," entrapping and smothering, or punitive and capable of all kinds of evil, depending on the nightmarish moods evoked from a person's history (Pearce & Newton, 1963, p. 113). To cope with these moods, the functionally unprepared adolescent can withdraw sexually, recoil from the experience, fight back, or take revenge.

Or the unprepared adolescent "falls in love frequently" only to discover an experienced deficit in the new love each time, which feels like a betrayal.

Intimacy and Partnerships

Prior to preadolescence, interaction with peers occurs in the form of parallel play, becoming a sense of belonging to the human race as a whole and the negotiation of the political arts in the juvenile era, with enlightened self-interest plus the feeling of membership in specific groups. In all these experiences, the major reference point is always the parenting figure(s) providing the framework within which the growing person experiences all other relationships.

A major shift begins in preadolescence with the discovery of a chum who is experienced as admirable and, simultaneously, as very much like oneself. The chum's needs become as important as one's own. That is a sea change, becoming paramount in adolescence with the advent of gender identification, sexuality, and integration of partnerships outside the family circle.

This developmental transformation takes place with inevitable deficits (residuals[7]) depending on the quality of or lack of previous validation. Previous interpersonal residuals affect later functions, providing limits that restrict each person in the process of forming new relationships.

Development from adolescence onward continues in the context of primary relationships, providing validation, cherishing, and tenderness. The parenting one(s) continues as the backdrop for the adolescent's perceptual framework, but the ideal parental role has changed from validating new functions to being a coach and facilitator for the emerging young person attempting to make up for functions not previously validated by them. This new parental role includes sharing experience and expertise, and providing financial support, advocacy, and enthusiasm for the adolescent's expansion into areas the parenting one(s) has not yet ventured. It's an opportunity for them to allow the adolescent to point the way to broader, previously inconceivable interpersonal experience. The parenting one(s) might also be inspired to expand their self-systems. Everyone can benefit.

The adolescent's choices of intimate relationships are attempts to expand their ability to relate to and function in the world delimited by the parental perceptual framework. The newly developed frame of reference is usually not far from the parental. It's often observed that people choose marital partners who resemble their parenting one(s). Expansion is gradual, despite the major shift of primary validator from parenting one(s) to peer. However, once that shift occurs, potential is open-ended.

Partnerships and Other Intimate Relationships

The adolescent begins a search for relationships that provide support for functions not previously validated. This can take many different forms. Sexual urge is often part of the motivation for the initiation of relationships. It is certainly one of the most powerful motivations to seek out relationships beyond the family. The adolescent also needs to find peers who can validate functions beyond the ones their parenting one(s) can fathom. The validation of functioning is no longer the sole responsibility of the parenting one(s).

Intimacy

Validation, cherishing, and tenderness can be summed up in a single word: intimacy. Sexuality and intimacy are often intertwined and confused with each other. Relationships based primarily on the satisfaction of sexual urgings (in reality or in rumination, conscious or unconscious) occur with great frequency, especially during adolescent exploration of the new world of sex. People also engage in sexual integrations or at least fantasize about them (consciously or unconsciously) throughout life.

It is possible for the adolescent to form sexually satisfying relationships providing validation, tenderness, and cherishing in other areas as well. The process of growth generally happens in the context of relationships with others, each working on making up their own deficits in functioning. These relationships can occur simultaneously to others; they can be short term, integrated around specific projects, or long-term partnerships. They remain productive as long as each person expands their capacity to relate. If a relationship no longer serves the needs of both, there are many possible outcomes. The relationship can simply end, with each partner moving on to other projects or more unfortunate outcomes. Here are examples of both:

> Two people meet at summer camp, both connecting with strangers, exploring new experiences. They can share adventures, sexual and otherwise, learning new skills together. At the end of summer, the relationship may lose its allure with the advent of returning to school and/or home. Optimally, both partners may separate as friends with fond memories of each other or remain friends but more distant than before. Each has learned something they can apply to their ongoing experience.

> Less fortunately, one or the other partner feels abandoned by the other at the end of the summer and is focused on feelings of rejection, disillusioned about forming intimate relationships: "They always end." The other partner might feel guilty for getting on with life or, even worse, dutifully maintain the fiction that the summer relationship still has the same function. This might result in many exchanges, each paying more and more attention to how many times one texts the other or "likes" their social media posts. In the world of electronics, communication becomes an easy weapon in the war of reproach and recrimination. The relationship morphs into each keeping track of how many days, hours, and minutes there are between texts as proof of love. Or each one's Instagram presence becomes a battleground, with each partner monitoring just who appears in the other's posts. The original excitement of learning how to kayak together, skinny dipping, or sleeping under the stars morphs into each policing each other's actions and making sure that expansion to new friends and experiences stays limited by the outworn commitment. Each begins to "discover" or invent proof that the loving relationship they experienced was a fluke or deception. A loving relationship turns into what can be called a "hostile integration" (Pearce & Newton, 1963, pp. 193, 197–216), locking together each other's security systems.

In addition to asexual intimacy, there are myriad new possibilities not involving sex at all in which an adolescent can begin to recognize and satisfy previously unmet needs and experience emotional intimacy. Examples are experiences with a co-worker, team member, study partner, teacher, mentor, advisor, counselor, choral or drama director, or coach, all productive platonic collaborations involving commitment to projects that provide satisfaction and new learning.

All relationships, sexual or not, are productive as long as their life project or projects continue to provide satisfaction for both parties, directly or indirectly. These relationships should expand the personalities of both partners. If not, they begin to restrict each other's satisfactions and, as described above, to become an integration of each other's security operations, i.e., hostile integrations (Pearce & Newton, 1963).

INDEPENDENCE

In adolescence, establishing and maintaining self-sufficiency becomes paramount. Competence depends on the consolidation of earlier learning, starting with the organization of perceptions, comfort with the learning process, visual-motor coordination, and communication and social skills. One's position in society and self-image are often pivotal in adolescent choices. Social class, race, gender, and sexuality are all significant. The parental orientation and that of the larger society may or may not be in unity on the question of adolescent choice. In fact, that choice may be determined by partnerships they develop, with or without the blessings of the parenting one(s) or the larger society. The story of Billy Elliot, a coal miner's son who becomes a leading ballet dancer, is a case in point.[8]

Vocational choice is, however, often limited by the need to earn a living despite personal preference, how one sees oneself and one's prospects and socio-economic pressure. In Western society, the gap between rich and poor is exponentially widening. Educational opportunities are increasingly limited to those who can afford them. In the United States, the school-to-prison pipeline is a reality (Taras et al., 2003, p. 1207; Wald & Losen, 2003, p. 11). The capacity to form relationships with others who validate a way out of poverty and helplessness is essential for establishing self-sufficiency. The stakes are very high and there is passion behind the strength of such relationships. Adolescents often form crucial relationships within the context of a larger group of associates.

The formation of intimate relationships with peers continues as the adolescent begins to work toward independence but is still in some way dependent on the parenting one(s), financially and (usually) emotionally. Financial dependence forms a major dilemma, especially if they continue to perceive the parenting one(s) as an authority with more than financial and practical power.

Adolescence must also be understood in terms of the current declining economic situation. Young people who drop out of high school to work at a low-paying retail chain may achieve a modicum of financial independence but have severely delimited their futures. The adolescent who takes up drug dealing risks imprisonment or death despite substantial short-term financial gains. Even with an advanced college degree, unemployment looms in today's economy. There are many stumbling blocks to deal with in the current socio-economic climate, particularly for oppressed peoples: people of color, women, im/migrants, LGBTQIA+ people, and people with disabilities.

The parenting one(s)' role is to be available for advice if needed or requested and to provide financial support, if they can, and encouragement. They can only be available to the degree they can accept the adolescent's right to independent choice. The primary role is to be friendly, non-intrusive, and encouraging, as well as willing to share one's greater knowledge of possible pitfalls such as sexually transmitted diseases and infections, early pregnancy, or encounters with the law. The parenting one(s) has life experience and sometimes can help financially. Friendliness consists of being accurate about what is needed and supplying it or finding resources to help. Insistence on a particular career regardless of the adolescent's preference is a common pattern of inaccuracy and unrelatedness to their needs with major consequences for later life. On the other hand, withholding important practical information about career choice is equally inaccurate and unfriendly.

Sometimes parenting one(s) who live out their fantasies through the young person may advocate career goals without seeking guidance from more knowledgeable sources.

> Wanda's parents advocated specialized conservatory training in music for their daughter but failed to consider how she might earn a living before becoming a coloratura soprano at the Metropolitan Opera. Wanda chose a more practical undergraduate degree and was able to earn a living while still pursuing her vocal career.

Financial help is a tricky proposition. Parenting one(s) may be asked to sign financial loan forms for college or provide a stipend while the adolescent completes essential education. It may mean providing money for a vital medical procedure, a security deposit, or bail. If they can, they might finance the first few months' rent until the young person finds a way to start paying on their own. It does not mean an indefinite availability for loans or financial support with the possible attendant reproach and control of the person's behavior. Sometimes, because the adolescent is not learning independence under their roof, the parenting one(s) asks the adolescent or young adult to move regardless of whether they're able to be independent. Sometimes that means finding a good drug rehabilitation program. Or it might mean sending them to more available relatives or friends.

The parenting one(s) needs to see the adolescent in a new way: as independent. They need to let go of guilt or fear of their own parenting one(s) and make their own decisions about how to help the adolescent become independent of them. If the parenting one(s) begins to grow past their own previous limitations, they can more easily accept the adolescent's.

Leaving Home

Geographical proximity to the parental home in late adolescence and early adulthood can reinforce whatever restrictions had already developed while the child was growing up, especially if family members see each other every day. Then the notion of growth in ways that would precipitate independence from the parenting one(s) seems less conceivable. The original audience is too close. Interaction between the adolescent and parenting one(s) who is unable to validate independence creates severe limitation on the person's concept of self as independent.

The project of "leaving home" begins in early adolescence (in many cases, probably before). It may become inevitable because of impoverishment or parental death. It often starts in fantasy, really a form of planning, part of adolescent assumption of responsibility for their own growth. The more the adolescent can assume that responsibility, the less they feel a victim of parental dictates. Much, of course, also depends on societal restrictions governing adolescent freedom to make choices about how their lives will go.

The age of legal independence varies from state to state in the United States and differs vastly in cultures. Often the adolescent's independence begins long before it's legal. Or they may continue dependency on the parenting one(s) late into life, determined by the degree to which the adolescent can organize perceptions and learn practical and social skills. That, in turn, depends on whether the functions of social relatedness have been validated. These include the ability to relate to strangers; exercise the political arts of compromise, competition, and cooperation; and form collegial and intimate peer relationships.

There are many ways for older adolescents and young adults to leave home, for example, college; international student programs, apprenticeships, or au pair programs; choirs, junior theater groups, and touring sports teams; as well as residential treatment centers that offer boarding and preparation for financial independence. Some use marriage as a way out, even if emotionally ill-equipped to make that commitment. Others share a living space or, if financially able, rent on their own. Some people leave home via incarceration, drug rehab programs or hospitalization; or, because of harsh socio-economic conditions, some enroll in the armed forces because they offer opportunities to travel, training, and financial compensation.

Supporting the Parenting One(s)

If one or both parenting ones become dependent, it becomes problematic if the adolescent preserves the notion of a parenting one as authority. If there is realistic appraisal, there can be opportunity for growth.

> At 19, Gail assumed responsibility for her terminally ill father and learned to perceive him as a person in need rather than a frightening authority. She supervised his care in a nursing home but did not limit her own activities, including continuing her education. She had always perceived her father as a powerful but distant person. In the process of relating to his needs, they developed a relationship closer than she had ever enjoyed. Had she given up on her own life in the process, she most likely would have lost that opportunity for intimacy because of the resentment that she might have developed.

POSTSCRIPT ON SULLIVAN

The world the adolescent lives in is changing more and more rapidly, especially since the beginning of the 20th century. Interpersonal theory of the adolescent developmental era has also evolved.

Harry Stack Sullivan practiced, wrote, and lectured between the 1920s and 1950s. His most famous clinical work was with people perceived by the larger society as a breed apart. He practiced at Shepherd and Enoch Pratt in Washington, DC, and then at Chestnut Lodge, a psychiatric facility in Maryland. Those on his caseload were often fairly young and diagnosed with schizophrenia after the emergence of puberty. They were incommunicative, enigmatic in speech, and difficult to manage, behaving in irrational and often dangerous ways that required separation and restraint. Sullivan's approach to them was from a sociocultural perspective unusual for his time (currently as well). He achieved markedly successful results primarily using verbal psychotherapy and social manipulation of the treatment environment (Sullivan, 1962; Blechner, 2009, p. 110).

The One-Genus Postulate

Sullivan's (1953) basic postulate in his theoretical approach is: "Everyone is much more simply human than otherwise" (p. 32).[9] This postulate frees the therapist to observe even the most seemingly bizarre behavior and to extrapolate from that behavior what may have caused it; it allows the therapist to identify with the other person.

In his work on the ward Sullivan (1962) chose nurses and attendants who could identify with the young schizophrenic people and relate to them with acceptance (pp. xiv–xv). This work formed the core of what was to become a fully encompassing theory of personality.

Intimacy Panic

In exploring their histories, Sullivan found that many of these young people had suffered a crisis while establishing an intimate relationship with a same-gender partner.[10] This intimacy was not necessarily sexual, but the experience of closeness, admiration, and identification with the best friend was explosive in its effect on the person, who immediately labeled it with what was then seen as the most negative and repulsive word thinkable: they must be "homosexual." This "revelation" sent the person into a tailspin of horror, self-revulsion, and panic, culminating in a psychotic episode.

Therapy involved helping the person understand that closeness to another human being other than their parenting one(s) was forbidden regardless of gender identity or sexuality. Once this was recognized, it was possible to explore earlier severe restrictions in the ability to reach out to and relate empathically with others. The person's first cherishing relationship outside the family severely ruptured their self-system, precipitating the psychotic episode.

Sullivan wrote long before "Gay Liberation" was even on the horizon. The prevailing attitude toward sexual and gender variance was negative and derogatory. It was just emerging from being considered sacrilege or a crime punishable by death. Liberals who defended gay people strove to define it as some kind of illness, mental or otherwise. However, that view created the deplorable perception that sexual variance from the "norm" was a mental aberration. It would take a broad social movement to change the social view of LGBTQIA+ people so that they were no longer a psychiatric category in the *Diagnostic and Statistical Manual of Mental Disorders* (American Psychiatric Association, 1987; Faderman, 2015, pp. 279–297). Now, acceptance of people who embrace their sexuality and/or question the gender assigned to them at birth is requiring yet another social movement. Leslie Feinberg (1992, 1997, and 1999) was one of the pioneers of that movement.

Sullivan (1953) discusses "homosexuality" and "heterosexuality" at length, and occasionally he seems to suggest that "homosexuality" is a less successful resolution for sexual integrations (pp. 263–269). However, he humorously sums up all the possible integrations of sexual interaction by choice of partner, genitalia or other body part, and use of those parts, coming up with "72 theoretical patterns of sexual behavior in situations involving two real partners" (p. 294), adding that probably only 45 are reasonably probable. He finishes by saying,

> I would like you to realize, if you realize nothing else, how fatuous it is to toss out the adjectives "heterosexual," "homosexual," or "narcissistic" to classify a person as to his [*sic*] sexual and friendly integrations with others. Such classifications are not anywhere near refined enough for intelligent thought; they are much too gross to do anything except mislead both the observer and the victim. (p. 294)[11]

He also makes the point that the emergence of sexual desire or "lust," as he calls it, heterosexual or not, is a dynamism that must be integrated into the already established dynamisms of personality, and, further, that in adolescence there needs to be an integration of the total personality into the larger cultural matrix. In other words, sexual urge is a complicated socio-biological function that has many potential patterns of development depending on the essence of who a person is, the vagaries of interpersonal experience, and societal expectations. There is no "correct" or "incorrect" integration. This integration is very complex (pp. 263–296).

Established integrations of sexual functioning may or may not be acceptable to society. There are varying degrees of congruence and antagonism. Some push each partner to expand. Some result in disaster. All have validity.

The labels for LGBTQIA+ people are currently less evocative (with major exceptions) of the horror that existed prior to the Stonewall rebellion in 1969. However, anxiety and psychosis continue to exist, but with different repugnant representations of the "unimaginable" and "loathsome." Symbols of anxious reaction to potential intimacy may change, but if there are restrictions on intimacy, new repugnant symbols can always be found.

SUMMARY

The major dilemma of adolescence is the dependence on the parenting figures(s) for financial and practical support coupled with the adolescent's urgent need for validation and tenderness from peers beyond those who were their primary validator(s) from birth. Relatedness begins to be primarily to peers, but they are still strongly attached to their parenting figure(s). They need to begin perceiving them more realistically as equals, with their own strengths and weaknesses.

Financial and emotional independence are major components of adolescent development that are also dependent on functions the young people have integrated in previous eras. Their deficits now need to be made up by receiving validation from peers and important adults (teachers, counselors, coaches, etc.) in areas their parenting ones(s), because of their own problems in living, couldn't validate. Often, in contemporary Western society, at least, one necessary parental role is to provide financial assistance and support, depending upon their own financial situation.

Sexuality emerges, requiring exploration, practice, validation, and integration. For asexual people, there may be no sexual urgings.

Adolescence is the beginning of the rest of one's life. The goal is to continue expanding relatedness to peers, in widening circles, with greater accuracy and intensity as their life evolves.

NOTES

1. These rites of passage are part of many major cultures and religions.

2. “Single parents are raising one in every three kids across the nation—and single-parent households are 4.5 times more likely than married households to live in poverty” (Annie E. Casey Foundation, 2019).

3. “Gender identity is each person’s internal and individual experience of gender. It is a person’s sense of being a woman, a man, both, neither, or anywhere along the gender spectrum. A person’s gender identity may be the same as or different from their birth-assigned sex. Gender expression is how a person publicly expresses or presents their gender. This can include behaviour and outward appearance such as dress, hair, make-up, body language and voice. A person’s chosen name and pronoun are also common ways of expressing gender. Others perceive a person’s gender through these attributes” (Ontario Human Rights Commission, n.d.). Sexual orientation is “an inherent or immutable enduring emotional, romantic or sexual attraction to other people” (Human Rights Campaign, n.d.).

4. Lesbian, gay, bi, trans, questioning/queer, intersex, asexual/agender/asexual/ally, and others. The acronyms and language are constantly in development.

5. For example, a teacher, guidance counselor, coach, or family friend.

6. The memory of infantile experiences such as pleasure, satisfaction, euphoria, terror, and anxiety are intensely felt and can reappear later in life as if from nowhere and in powerful form as *mood-memory*. Mood-memory can be negative or positive, reflecting actual infantile experience. They can also be dredged up from slightly later experiences (past the age of four or five months) parataxically, when there is still very limited capacity to verbalize and limited ability to orient oneself enough to have perspective.

7. Residuals are functions not adequately consolidated in a particular developmental era that affect how one functions in later life.

8. In this beautiful film, *Billy Elliot*, a talented boy is helped by a sympathetic dance teacher who takes him on as a student, unbeknownst to his father. When his father finds out, he forbids dance lessons but eventually reluctantly agrees to allow him to audition for a London ballet company. A highlight of the film is his father’s enchantment 12 years later as he sees his son leap onto the stage as the black swan in *Swan Lake*.

9. With this principle, radical for his time, Sullivan was emphasizing that “homosexuals” and people diagnosed schizophrenic must not be placed in a category of “other” and treated as such. In the current social climate, not only must his one-genus postulate be reasserted, it must particularly call attention to “recently acknowledged complexities in gender identity, development, and both the vulnerability and resilience of transgender communities; in other words, a greater understanding of the diversity in the human condition” (Taffel, 2020, p. 17). This applies to all peoples who are oppressed and whose common humanity must be emphasized.

10. Sullivan used the term “homosexual panic,” reflecting the era in which he theorized. The terminology is constantly changing. At the point of this writing (2022), we are using the phrase “intimacy panic.”

11. As discussed above, at the time he was writing and lecturing, “homosexual” was a derogatory term.

Chapter Eight

Adulthood

A New Interpersonal Challenge

The crucial difference between adolescence and adulthood is that the adult is now entirely responsible for organizing their own growth. Until puberty, validation comes from primary parenting one(s) and alternate validators acceptable to them. After puberty, despite inexperience and financial and legal dependence, an adolescent needs interpersonal validation of functions beyond parental limits. These functions might include comfortable basic physiological functions, motor skills, the world of objects, and social skills. The parenting one(s) has imparted their full repertoire of relatedness and limitations. Now in adulthood the person has even more freedom to obtain validation for expanded functioning.

This shift does not mean that the young adult must reject what has been learned. It doesn't mean the parenting one(s) has no more to give. Parenting one(s) can be a source of resources, such as accumulated experience, technical skills, or financial assistance. However, if the young adult wishes to expand beyond what was already learned, they must look elsewhere, evaluating, possibly rejecting, limitations set up in the parental context. Human development is always in motion (growing or deteriorating), so the relationship between the young adult and the parenting one(s) may continue to provide validation if the parenting one(s) is also growing. However, the nature of that relationship becomes even more peer-like. If all goes well, the parenting one(s) can be viewed as having strengths and failings, but no as longer the central figure(s) in one's life.

There's a difference between the parenting one(s) as a person or people in the adult's life and the "eidetic" or symbolic parenting one(s). An eidetic parenting one is the image of who was central in a person's life during the formation of their self-system, often bearing little resemblance to the current one. To move past old restrictions, the young adult must identify how they use eidetic parenting one(s) to set up barriers to new experience beyond the limitations of parental and their own self-systems. Then they can challenge and reject the restrictions, seeking out appropriate validators for new experience.

Every human being enters adulthood with unmet needs limited by anxiety. Motivating the adult to expand functioning is the pressure of unmet needs, conscious and unconscious. The project of adulthood is to find methods to satisfy unmet needs in order of urgency, depending on their practical life situations. This pressure exists despite resistance in the form of security operations established to prevent such satisfaction.

There are myriad examples: A person, realizing that they have no knowledge of the world outside their particular town, decides to live in a different city, far from parental scrutiny and other associations perceived as restrictive; another realizes that making friends requires joining a new social group or accepting invitations from colleagues to hang out after work, and that they have remained isolated because they have been too critical of other people; or they decide to go back to school to obtain training and credentials in a more interesting skill. It might mean ending a restrictive early marriage and looking for someone more able to meet their needs. It might mean improving on one's previously neglected physiology by finally getting a tonsillectomy to clear up a chronic strep infection, organizing orthodontic adjustment, or improving their diet and lifestyle to address obesity.

To the degree people notice the limitations of their own lives and what it would take to move beyond them, they can continue the process of making up for deficits from the earlier years before they were responsible for their own growth. As young adults become acutely aware of their areas of unpreparedness for independence, they often become resentful of parental inability to provide validation. At the same time, they can feel intense loyalty to their parenting one(s) and hold on to their actual or eidetic restrictions.

The resolution for this impasse can go in a destructive or productive direction. Destructively, the parenting one(s) might exercise existing legal and financial control over the person's life to prevent independent movement beyond parental limitations. Some examples may be parental restriction of career, school choice, or choice of mate. The parenting one(s) might set overly restrictive, inappropriate limits; relentless, intrusive monitoring; early curfew inconsistent with the person's age; assign unnecessary, time-consuming "chores"; or regulate the person's choice of friends. They might withhold access to funds necessary to purchase equipment, clothing, or education. They may even threaten expulsion from the family, including exile from home without providing assistance for the young adult to establish somewhere else to live. Or they may exercise no restriction on their offspring's current behavior but have much earlier limited the young adult's capacity to seek outside validation to begin with. In such cases, the pattern has been established: even greater dependency exists, and the young adult continues to assume their parenting one(s) is the only source of survival and tenderness.

Other ways the parenting one(s) might restrict the independent action of the young adult, given their lack of experience in the world and their position in it, include derogating the young adult's ability to become important to others, inserting themselves inappropriately into peer interactions between the person and a new friend, complaining they're burdened with the responsibility of organizing the person's life, and derogating their judgement. Or the parenting one(s) might bemoan their own misfortunes, forcing the emerging adult to feel responsible at the expense of carving out time to garner new experiences.

A more positive, constructive resolution by no means out of reach is for the parenting one(s) to acknowledge the person's growth beyond them—acknowledge their own deficits and emulate their offspring. They can make available their financial and legal resources, if possible, as well as their practical life experience. While the parenting one(s) can share information about perceived pitfalls and dangers of certain choices, they should refrain from exercising control over them. They need to get on with their own growth projects so that the issue of envy[1] is non-existent or less central in their interactions with the young adult.

THE PROCESS OF GROWTH IN ADULTHOOD

A shift in the nature of validation occurs in the move through adolescence to young adulthood. Before puberty, the direction of validation of perceptions is from the validator to the child. The parenting one(s) validates the direct perceptions of the child, providing a framework, an orientation to life. As discussed in the chapters on the juvenile and preadolescence, some perceptions have been altered by experience outside the parental framework but are still more or less governed by those of their parenting one(s). By puberty, their orientation has been weakly or not so weakly consolidated, including their attitudes toward others and themself and their beliefs about what is possible. After puberty and into young adulthood, the person grows and adds to that framework by absorbing new experience and validation through "identification, participation and sharing of the reference points" (Pearce & Newton, 1963, p. 121) of peers. The young adult grows by intensely engaging in and identifying with the activities of others they see as peers. To truly be part of the activity, they must be able to empathize with the others as part of sharing the experience.

Young adults are usually very aware of the degree of preparation they have already garnered for adult human interaction. Sometimes, as a solution, they continue looking for parental validation and guidance. However, those attempts can be frustrating and become a form of reproach to the parent(s). In any case, the time has usually passed for such validation from the parenting one(s) to be effective since it was needed at a much earlier age when they were not available to provide it. Such validation is in fact available via adult interactions with others. Even if the parenting one(s) has grown enough to validate new experience, the young adult still might confuse them with the earlier, limited, eidetic parenting one(s).

Obtaining validation for previously forbidden functioning is the major project of adulthood throughout life. Such validation comes via the sharing of projects with others who are similarly engaged. Essentially, adult life is a process of engagement in such projects centered around goals shared by others. Motivation for such projects comes from the need to expand one's ability to function beyond the restrictions established through puberty.

For example, the young adult might be deficient in the juvenile functions of participating in a group using the political arts of competition, compromise, and cooperation. This may play out in the young adult in several ways: an inability to participate without getting into squabbles over finding mutually satisfactory solutions in a relationship or in the workplace, or by being a bully or being scapegoated in groups and never feeling like a member. Rather than looking for support from their parenting one(s) to advise or defend, the young adult needs to find those groups that share their excitement about something. In the process of sharing, they begin to find validation for participation in the group and to learn the political arts of being in a group, all striving for the same goal. The type of group can vary widely: a band, a sports team, a political group, a hobby group, residents in a rehab center, or even a gang.

As the young adult becomes more independent and begins to grow more reliably among others, resentment and embarrassment about parental limitations may diminish. If the parenting one(s) has shifted their focus to their own growth projects and no longer seeks to limit the growth of the person, resentment on either side may no longer exist. At that point, the relationship is more peer-like and proceeds based on shared history and whatever mutual projects the parenting one(s) and the young adult may share. For example, a parent finally decides to join Alcoholics Anonymous or enters a drug rehab facility, kicking a longstanding dependency. The young adult and the parent might then feel freer to work on their separate growth projects.

Projects of Young Adulthood

Contemporary Western culture has paved a specific route for how a person assumes an adult role in the world. However, the series of tasks or milestones in the years subsequent to adolescence vary widely. Some include leaving home, achieving financial independence, preparing for and engaging in satisfying work, building a social network of peers and establishing an intimate partnership, raising children, and/or providing validation for others' growth. Within the organization of the current Western social environment, achieving these goals is assumed to be a prerequisite for a satisfying life. Most young adults feel pressure, even urgency, to complete them. Nevertheless, the list is not exhaustive of all possibilities for adult projects.

Leaving Home

As discussed above, the young adult is now responsible for their own growth and must seek validation from people beyond what is conceivable to their actual or eidetic parenting one(s). Now the task involves organizing the means for obtaining that validation, which can be awkward, if not impossible, under the parental roof. Learning new functions requires privacy from parental purview. In addition, the power of earlier eidetic parental deficits in living remain in one's head, possibly eclipsing everything, no matter how much the parenting one(s) may have changed. Therefore, the distracting omni-presence of the current parental audience exacerbates the difficulty, derailing the young adult's attempt to immerse themself into a new set of perceptions, associations, and audiences.

Much has to do with the mood of home as it is experienced by the young adult.

> Susan reminisced: I remember when I was at CCNY, a wonderful college with no dorm. It was a year before I moved away from home into my own apartment. I would get up early, about 6:00 a.m., and arrive at school in time to have breakfast with my friends when the cafeteria opened at 7:00. By the time I finished breakfast, the library was open, and I would head there if I didn't have a class. When class was over, I would be back at the library to study or at the cafeteria to hang out with friends until it closed at about 10:00 p.m., after which I went upstairs to the Math Club meeting. I wasn't much of a mathematician, but the Math Club met very late. I would hang out there until the meeting ended around 11:00 p.m. I was usually in a pretty cheery mood until it was time to go home. I remember the long, cold, nighttime walks down the hill to the subway. I thought about how cold and tired I was, how much work I had to do, and how long it would take before I could live on my own, without a constant sense of drudgery and oppression. By the time I reached the Bronx, my step had slowed, my back had hunched, my head was bowed. I was in a mood ready to be viewed by my family.

Every home has its rhythms, its routines, and its moods. For the young adult to continue exploring possibilities of further personality expansion, they must break free of the mood of home, no matter what that is. To do so while still living at home is very difficult. Fortunately, in addition to marriage, opportunities for leaving home include forging one or more intimate partnerships either sequentially or simultaneously (see below), getting a job and moving in with roommates, going away to college, or joining Job Corps or a touring performing group. All possibly provide opportunities to further explore one's potential far from the parental purview, real or imagined, of the earlier upbringing. The project is particularly tough for oppressed groups and people with severe financial hardships. Economic problems in the family may cause the young adult to stay home in order to support the parenting one(s) and other siblings, foregoing their own further education and career plans. Young adults desperate to leave home might feel forced to make choices that are far from optimal, such as joining the military or the police force, camping out on the streets, or finding a homeless shelter. Or they may choose to live with a partner's family.

Obviously, one can physically leave home but never expand beyond the limitations set in earlier years. There is a difference between physically and emotionally leaving home. However, physically being away from the dominant mood of home and the daily reminder of one's limitations can significantly set the stage for potential growth.

Some people feel they should work out their problems before leaving home. Even after moving geographically away from home, people rationalize maintaining their connection with parenting one(s) as if in formative years, as if their restrictions remain.

> Joan, a successful executive who called her mother four or five times a day, insisted that if she didn't call, her mother would call her; she was just heading her off. The notion that she might limit her daily obligation to her mother filled her with nameless dread.

A similar misperception, that a parenting one won't survive without the person, equally maintains the restrictions. There are many rationales: for example, "they might die tomorrow, and I will regret not visiting."

However, visits home do provide time or space to form perspective on restrictive patterns or to forge a more productive relationship if the parenting one(s) is also growing.

It is more difficult if one marries to leave home, delaying life plans because of the financial and time-consuming responsibilities of child-rearing (see below).

Financial Independence

Being financially independent, with all that implies, is closely related to leaving home. Despite having a good job, one might still choose to live at home, impacted by the mood there and hampered in their ability to relate differently outside. Or one can live separately and still be wholly or partially supported by the parenting one(s).

In a friendly relationship between the parenting one(s) and the young adult, the parenting one(s), if able, may use their greater financial ability to subsidize initial living arrangements until the young adult is able to be financially independent. Or their parenting one(s) might be in a better position to finance tuition or training. But the accompanying mood is key. Optimally they provide financial subsidy with no strings attached.

Having the ability to support one's own projects in living provides a heightened sense of liberation. One can make choices without looking over their shoulder. At the same time, with financial independence comes the need to exercise foresight, budget, and set priorities for one's life.

If an adult is still being subsidized by the family and can't support themself, there is the concern that their choices will not be supported by their family and that they still need permission from the parenting one(s) to make important life choices: school, career, living arrangements, location, romantic partner(s), a car. This can be very hampering indeed. Also, if one is marginally self-sufficient, continually asking for or borrowing money from a family that attaches strings to their support can limit project choices and the intensity to pursue them. In both instances, the family may overtly or covertly ridicule them for not yet being financially independent.

Sometimes the parenting one(s) requires the young adult's financial support. While that arrangement can promote a sense of accomplishment, "proof" of one's adulthood and competence, it can also severely limit independent plans for expansion of their own education or training.

With exceptions, it is increasingly difficult for most people to earn a living wage. In today's economy in the United States and elsewhere, the issue of financial independence looms as an ever-greater problem for many people, limiting feelings of independence and autonomy.

Productive Work

In the current organization of class society, with its vast differences in accessibility to resources such as education, training, mobility, etc., many people have little or no possibility of finding a way to obtain paid, productive work they find fulfilling. Many settle for an income no matter the job, feeling they have no other option. This may even occur in well-heeled families when the parenting one(s) expects the person is to follow in their footsteps by obtaining the same kind of job or pursuing the same kind of career regardless of preference. It's important to be able to tell the difference between prestige and fulfillment.

However, there are many ways to organize productive activities, even when access to what is seen as the "charmed circle" is blocked. Because of the necessity to maintain economic independence, a person may be forced to devote a large amount of time to unsatisfying work. However, if they organize more meaningful activity after work, the sacrifice is more bearable. It might even be possible to slowly change careers by continuing their education part time and/or using a portion of their income to finance it. One has something to look forward to. Hobbies, activity groups, and shared projects of all kinds are essential; they make life meaningful and with purpose. It is also important that such activity is shared with others.

In the United States, more and more people cannot find work that would support them independently and remain partly or fully financially dependent on the parenting one(s), creating hardship for all. The push for independence, however, does not go away and people pursue other solutions. The young adult may find another source of financial help, such as a godparent, or may seek out grants, loans, welfare, or disability assistance from the state or other institutions. Some may use social media, such as GoFundMe, or pool resources with other likewise financially constrained peers to establish an independent living situation.

Intimate Partnerships

A major preoccupation of almost all young adults, and many older people as well, is finding a "soulmate" to establish a household, raise children, and share life.

However, lack of social skills inhibits finding a partner. In Western culture, at least initially one needs to feel comfortable meeting strangers (that is, unless one accepts the choice of a religious matchmaker or weds the "best" spouse, vetted by the family). A person needs to take pleasure in activities with others to establish relatedness and the kind of sharing and camaraderie required to establish partnership(s) that promote growth. In summary, they must enjoy experience with people in parallel play/work, juvenile group membership, and close preadolescent friendship.

The search for the "perfect" partnership may turn into a search for the "good mother," which is illusory and quickly turns into finding the "bad mother" when the partner doesn't live up to one's fantasy (Pearce & Newton, 1963, p. 123). The person romanticizes the perfect intimate relationship, which repeatedly falters because they have not yet learned the prerequisite functions. One cannot skip a developmental era on the way to intimate adult relationship(s). They repeat dysfunctional patterns, unconsciously interfering with mastering the earlier functions, such as simply feeling like an equal or feeling like a member. If a relationship begins to feel more than their self-system can handle, more potentially mutually satisfying than they have ever experienced, they may find ways to scuttle it or manipulate the partner to break it off. The self-system remains unchanged.

Sometimes a young adult feels the obligation to fulfill what is perceived as the family obligation to "make a good marriage" and produce the expected grandchildren and lifestyle. Then the choice in partner and lifestyle can have less to do with meeting one's needs for further growth and relatedness and more to do with maintaining the status quo and satisfying perceived parental and societal demands.

> Ellen's father never tired of explaining to her that he married her mother because he had had sex with her and so was obligated to marry her. He made no secret of his contempt for his wife, openly had affairs, and thought she was stupid and conventional. Her mother, on the other hand, stolidly bore his contempt and did her duty by keeping the house clean and the children clothed and fed, even finding a job to support the children as Ellen's father slid further into alcoholism. It took her mother 10 years before she finally kicked her husband out. Even then, she continued to behave mechanically with Ellen and her siblings, seeing her relationship with them as an obligation, but never a pleasure.

In the above example, with variations, the goal is to maintain the status quo rather than meet one's needs for people in one's life. In such relationships, one's defenses are strengthened against new experience and the conviction that nothing will ever change for the better. The result is usually deterioration rather than expansion.

In other cases, partners are chosen out of a desperate desire to get away from home with the concomitant fear that there is no real place to go. This is more like a jailbreak or acceptance of a lighter sentence and a new, hopefully less onerous prison.

There is also the very strong attitude in the culture that if one is "single" or childless, one is inferior, not grown up, and even to be pitied or matched up with someone. The push to find a "soulmate" is very strong. A person in a friend group who remains single is often not seen as being as mature as the married ones. The coupled friends might already have at least one child, are preoccupied with child-rearing, and are much less available to their friends, particularly the single ones without children.

Another pattern might be partnership in which each member increasingly communicates only with the other; no new meaningful outside contacts are allowed. They assume the relationship fulfills all basic needs without the necessity for new experiences which might "threaten" the relationship. They are primarily focused on keeping the relationship going, no matter what, emphasizing faithfulness and permanence over mutual relatedness to needs and shared exploration of new possibilities.

More hopeful and productive relationships grow out of the recognition that people need a broadening range of people. Growing up implies organizing an audience that validates the possibility of having more satisfaction in life, not just onerous duty. That is, the young adult needs to realize that to gain true independence and productivity, one needs an increasingly larger circle of other people, not just a soulmate. One finds closeness to other people by sharing projects oriented to growth. This might mean that before one finds the "love of one's life," one needs to be comfortable with people in general and feel needed, as a member in projects with goals all members share. With this shared membership and mutual cooperation strong bonds of intimacy develop since each needs the other to accomplish the goals for all. Depending on the situation and the importance of the goals, strong relationships can flourish and last for years, even a lifetime, if the sharing of mutual projects continues to be productive. The experience paves the way for one or more productive life partnerships, if that is ultimately what one decides to pursue.

Some examples might be the relatedness that develops in a group of students studying for exams, a labor union local on strike, a writing group, a sports team, the cast of a repertory company, a band, or a political action group. Sometimes the intimacy of working together lasts a short time, say, a limited run of a summer stock production or the duration of a crisis, such as a strike. Sometimes, however, as people collaborate, more projects emerge as important and long term and discoveries are made about people that lead to even more reasons to continue to work together productively. The major determinant is whether one feels more alive and more of a sense of satisfaction in the presence of the other(s), despite issues that may crop up.

However, it would be a flat contradiction of reality to say that intimate relationships only develop in the context of a group project. In the contemporary world, there are numerous ways to meet people and test out the possibilities for intimacy. Online dating, for example, is a useful way of meeting people and forming relationships. Nevertheless, a young adult who has gained experience in the process of developing cooperative, collaborative relationships is likely to be more hopeful and self-confident in the process of finding a partner, no matter how they go about it.

One of the prerequisites for any successful relationship is mutual respect for each partner's participation in projects that may not include the other. For example, a union leader may form a relationship with a lawyer, who is not part of the union, but they share a close, cooperative relationship raising their children. For that project to be successful, each would have to respect without resentment the other's schedule and the need to hang out with fellow union members and fellow lawyers. At the same time, the two would have to relate wholeheartedly to their children's needs, finding ways to make it all work, with nobody left out. In that situation, each partner would not only learn to work smoothly with the other, but each would, by necessity, expand their world to include the other's friends with whom they can relate in their own way, expanding their world to include more and more people.

The same interpersonal needs apply when there are concurrent intimate partners. In the not-so-distant past, polyamory and open relationships in many countries were vilified. As with LGBTQIA+[2] people, these relationships were formed in secret. If they went public, they often endured varying degrees of oppression, including contempt, ostracism, and job loss. Depending upon where they live, people in polyamory or other open relationships are becoming more accepted in the world as of this writing in 2022.

Parenting Children

Parenting children is a significant, life-changing project. But it's still a project, and as with any project it involves sharing with other people with the same goals. It involves the process of finding validation for heretofore poorly validated or forbidden needs as well as the exercise of already integrated functioning in the service of further expanding relatedness.

Parenting children can be used productively and restrictively. On the productive side, it can affirm one's own adulthood in the ability to take responsibility for relating to the needs of children. It validates the feeling that one is a legitimate contributor to the continuity of human history and future. An aspect of this continuity is the development of a sense that one belongs, is a member of the human race, and, by parenting a child, contributes to the continuation of the human race (Pearce & Newton, 1963, pp. 128–129). How people organize to become parents has also broadened as the definition of family has expanded to include LGBTQIA+ people.[3]

Raising children is a great opportunity to revisit empathically one's own early experiences, including areas in which one needs further validation for unmet needs. One becomes closer to one's own inner experience, more in touch with what has been missed, what one has avoided and repudiated and, nevertheless, needs.

Parenting a baby immediately raises the urgent need to broaden one's interpersonal base to have more people in one's life. Conventional wisdom, now less prevalent, is the paradigm of the husband-and-wife couple sufficient unto itself. This paradigm has probably never been viable as a completely independent entity and is becoming more and more obsolete as the culture changes.

In areas of caretaking in which the new parent(s) is inexperienced or anxious, the need for friendly suggestions without judgment becomes crucial. This may be via a friendly, non-judgmental parenting one: a grandparent, midwife, baby nurse, babysitter, doula, or knowledgeable friend, for example. Access to medical personnel is, of course, crucial. Many young parents form friendships with other parents of newborns and share parenting without a sense that they have failed to do it on their own. The frequent presence of other friendly adults provides validation for the infant and growing child when the parent cannot. It lightens the burden of responsibility and provides an indirect mode of validation for the parent as well. Using the grandparent(s) as babysitter and alternate validator can be helpful, particularly if the grandparent(s) has had positive parental experience themselves, and if they have expanded in their lives in ways that allow them to enjoy the process of relating to their grandchildren. On the other hand, if the grandparent(s) has deteriorated in their ability to function, they can have a deleterious effect on the ability of the new parent(s) to relate to the child's needs if those needs make the grandparent(s) anxious. The new parent can also learn about one's own upbringing from noticing when their parenting one(s) is uncomfortable with their grandchildren, particularly if there is an obvious contrast between their behavior and how other people relate to the new baby.

Restrictively, new parent(s) can become self-centered and preoccupied with their performance as caretaker(s)—concerned with looking good instead of relating wholeheartedly to the baby's needs, instead of admitting when they don't know what to do or finding someone who does, or learning to relate, no matter how awkwardly.

One can dissociate one's ability to empathize with the baby and instead play a role of "responsible parent" as they may imagine might be expected by their own parent(s), thus missing their child's cues and using the failed methods one grew up with instead.

> Paul was having trouble with his five-year-old daughter, Joanne. He found himself engaged in power struggles with "her over simple" activities of daily living. He brought the problem into therapy after a particularly bitter struggle over getting Joanne to school. In a session, he revisited his own childhood history with discipline.
>
> He had become anorexic, refusing to eat to the point of hospitalization. He casually mentioned that anorexia was his way to satisfy his need for control. Then he remembered that his battles with his daughter were often about who was controlling the situation: very often Joanne would have a tantrum if Paul refused to let her engage in some harmless ritual before she complied to his morning routine. It had to be his way, which is exactly what his parents did to him. He remembered that things got easier for him at boarding school when he was allowed some time to organize his life himself, even if it bent the rules

a little. Maybe that was the problem with Joanne. She needed to have some control over how she ate breakfast or dressed in the morning. Paul remembered how he would sit in front of a plate of uneaten oatmeal by himself. He was not allowed to leave the table until he finished all his food, and he began to sympathize with Joanne. Then he thought, maybe it was OK to let Joanne wear her princess crown before putting on her shoes and socks in the morning or to allow her to rip crust off the toast before eating it for breakfast. Maybe he didn't have to win that struggle.

SUMMARY

Adulthood opens opportunities to make up for what was lacking in the years leading up to and including adolescence. No one emerges into adulthood having integrated all potential functioning. People all have residuals[4] in functioning, probably at every level of development. The difference is that the adult must organize their own opportunities for growth.

Simultaneously, moving beyond the self-system's boundaries created in the earlier years of life creates anxiety, disorientation, and usually terror in its various forms. The process is a dialectic of opposing forces in which one's needs are pushing for greater satisfaction while one's security system is pushing for increased restriction. One can grow or deteriorate, depending on the strength of validation and experience one garners to overcome the strength of the security system. The opportunities, should one choose to take them, are limitless. In fact, young adulthood is the beginning of the potential for greater choices if a person has the courage to challenge their self-system's status quo.

NOTES

1. See chapter thirteen on unconscious parental envy.
2. Lesbian, gay, bi, trans, questioning/queer, intersex, asexual/agender/asexual/ally, and others. The acronyms and language are constantly in development.
3. With the anti-abortion ruling of the United States Supreme Court in 2022 (*Dobbs v. Jackson Women's Health Organization*) and "don't say gay" legislation in some states, same-sex marriage came under threat in the United States. In the same year, Cuba passed a new "Family Code," which, in addition to affirming the right to free abortion, honors the wide variety of family structures. Among its provisions are the legalization of same-sex marriage, the right for same-sex couples to adopt children, and assistance with surrogate pregnancies.
4. Residuals are functions not adequately consolidated in a particular developmental era that affect how one functions in later life. The term as defined here was coined by Pearce and Newton (1963, pp. 83, 89, 94, 102, 107, 113).

PART II

Personality and How It Works

Chapter Nine

The Self-system

The self-system[1] includes all conscious experience functioning productively and restrictively. One major facet of the self-system is the organization of perceptual-cognitive functioning, focusing attention in order to do anything at all. The self-system's restrictive apparatus uses selective inattention to avoid awareness of anything threatening to disrupt the historical connection between the primary caretaker(s) and the infant. If a primary caretaker is uncomfortable with a need, so is the infant, to the same degree. So dependent upon adult(s) for its survival and functioning, the infant makes necessary cognitive and behavioral adjustments to restore that vital connection.[2]

Developing within the newborn's interpersonal milieu, the self-system accelerates with increased perceptual-motor capacity in late infancy, although still in rudimentary form. Through adolescence and beyond, the self-system gradually forms relatively stable patterns. Strenuously pulled to stay connected to those originally responsible for survival and ability to function, the self-system resists change. New validated experiences challenge it to expand, to organize subsequent learning in the process of integrating new functions.

Productive functions are experienced as "good-me," the restrictive as "bad-me."[3] "Good-me" later in life might be "I'm healthy and I like to work out." "Bad-me" might be "I'm not very bright and I shouldn't aspire to a job requiring intelligence."

"Not-me," not part of the self-system, are needs dissociated according to the infant's and growing person's experience with parenting by significant others. One's self-system is limited depending on how much is dissociated. Its limitations are maintained by a wide variety of security operations such as selective inattention, and diversionary and substitutive preoccupations. Security operations, a major part of the *security apparatus*, shield a person from awareness or acceptance of forbidden, dissociated needs.

A dynamic struggle exists between the push to grow, to expand one's functioning, and the self-system's restrictive aspects.

ROOTS OF RESISTANCE TO CHANGE

The self-system provides the organization for functioning, allowing one to live in the world from minute to minute with minimal distraction. If a person experiences a challenge to the self-system, say, by suddenly recognizing how they set up distancing maneuvers with others, they cannot function as usual. They can become disorganized, fall apart to some degree.

> Barbara notices that she consistently ignores her colleague's invitations to happy hour. Having had the thought that this colleague might be simply friendly, without "ulterior motives," she finally accepts the invitation. Suddenly she becomes awkward around other people, unable to interact.
>
> In therapy she remembers, as the small child of her very isolated mother, trying to talk with the child across the street. Her mother became extremely anxious and yanked her into the house. She must not talk to strangers or people who are different: "They only want to take your toys!" Because she was so dependent upon her mother's goodwill, any break in their relationship felt dangerous. She learned to avoid putting her mother in that state by building reasons to avoid friendships. The "reasons" are part of her elaborate security apparatus developed by her self-system. This paradigm continued. In the schoolyard she didn't play with other children because they were "thieves" and from the "wrong kind of family."
>
> In adulthood, she talks to a potential friend at the obligatory company holiday party. On the way home, she becomes disoriented, gets lost, and feels as if someone is following her with a gun. Even though she talked to a "stranger," she is not as vulnerable to her parent's admonitions as she was when a child. But her self-system's restrictive apparatus—that aspect of the personality mustered to maintain the status quo—is also powered by infantile experiences when her mother was, for whatever reason, not attentive or unhappy with her. Because she was totally dependent for her very survival upon her primary caretaker, these mood-memories[4] are powerful deterrents to change.

In therapy she learns that accepting the challenge to make a friend initiated the expansion of her self-system by rejecting her restrictive fears. Through interpretation she recognizes her unfounded fearful reaction: it's "dangerous" to make a friend (she will lose her early connection with her mother). Now she might reject resilient earlier marching orders and expand her self-system. Or her self-system might reassert itself: she might decide the therapist is talking though her hat ("Don't you know? New York *is* a dangerous place!").

> Jenny, a physics professor, never thought of herself as creative ("Art is for right-brain people! Besides, I'm a 'Type A' personality. I have no time for simply fooling around, let alone getting messy."). A colleague inspires her to take pottery classes a few blocks from her apartment. New worlds open as she delves

into the mushiness of the clay; she meticulously adds the classes to her busy schedule. The following week, she wanders around and around looking for the studio. Forgetting she has GPS, she texts her colleague, who gently teases her: "It's on the next block. I guess the creative bug got you loopy!"

The struggle to expand or further restrict the self-system is dialectic, depending upon the balance of forces in a person's life: friendly validators, new opportunities, education, increased availability for alternate interpersonal experience, or the opposite.

When one expands their self-system, requiring reorganization of their perceptions and behavior, they experience anxiety, feelings of disorientation, and uncanny emotions, often including dread and horror, coupled with the temporary loss of functioning involved in struggling to reorganize. The uncanny emotions stem from original experiences of disruption from the parenting figure(s) in the process of coming up against original restrictions.[5]

It's like building a new muscle at the gym. It aches for a while, but if one continues exercising, it becomes stronger and no longer hurts. Now they can move onto more rigorous routines that make use of this stronger muscle. Or the person stops because the pain is discouraging; the muscle weakens over time.

Understanding this phenomenon is essential to the therapeutic process of helping people recognize the need for and acceptance of new "unacceptable" experiences despite anxiety. Anxiety comes with the territory of change, especially in the adult striving to grow beyond strenuously held assumptions limiting their life.[6]

Positive functions can temporarily go haywire during the disorganization that comes with change and reorganization. Cognitive functioning is temporarily disrupted, as well as any recently learned functioning. People forget things, they lose things, they confabulate; they have some trouble until they can manage reorganizing their self-system. To return to the example of not being allowed to make a new friend, if the person starts to make a friend on the job, their self-system can become disorganized and thinking can fall apart; they might forget the person's name or "inadvertently" not recognize who sent a text and delete it, later deciding the potential friend has "ghosted" them.

The degree of disorganization is on a continuum. On the milder side, meeting people at a new job might make a person who has been trained to isolate become more disorganized. They can't find the restroom. They walk into the conference room on their way to the restroom. They leave their coffee cup in the microwave and wander around looking for it. It's a very different scenario for somebody who has had very severe restrictions on their right to have friends with anybody outside the limited parental/familial circle. That person might become strenuously disoriented and disorganized, as many young people do upon moving away for a job or starting their first year of college not in commuting distance from home. This kind of severe disorganization happens most prevalently from adolescence through young adulthood when they are thrust into new situations with strangers and possibly into more intimate relationships. Their world falls apart during periods when opportunities for new experience and learning is greater. Other examples include having a baby, experiencing a mid-life crisis, or coping with retirement.

This chaos or disorganization can be resolved in a restrictive way if a person reformulates their perception of the validating person(s) and validating experience(s) in a paranoid way; systems of logical thought give way to the logic of despair.

If the person has a support system of friends, a validating group, and/or useful therapy, disorganization and paranoid formulations can be more easily tolerated and recognized as temporary, coming along with the territory of change. Their self-system reorganizes and expands to varying degrees. The person grows.

Disorganization can be mild, where one forgets their password; or it can be massive, in which a person is frozen in a state of paralysis, unable to decide how to move or think coherently. The degree of disorganization depends upon how much of a challenge there is to one's self-system.

In therapy, disorganization of thinking processes might manifest after a strenuous session in which, for example, a severely depressed person critically examines a deeply held false assumption. Their self-system rattled, they miss the next session, having temporarily lost the ability to function. When the therapist says, "It's at 5:30," the individual is easily reminded, and says, "Oh yes. I'm sorry. I forgot."

RECALL AND FORESIGHT

In early infancy recall might involve the experience of hunger, hearing oneself cry, and the experience of nipple-in-lips. If all goes well, the emergence of the nipple produces the expectation that hunger will be satisfied. The first experience of recall and foresight, the beginning of parataxic perception, operates on the principle of contiguity of events. The self-system utilizes parataxic perception and symbolism in its formation.

Sullivan (1953) illustrates a restrictive expectation: the infant rubs its anus. Because of a parenting one's repeated horrified reaction, the infant feels something horrible will happen if they do that, so they don't anymore, or they do it in a way that avoids strenuous parental prohibition (p. 153).

Recall and foresight initially organize a primitive form of learning not necessarily conscious but very effective. The child navigates to get needs met around the productive and restrictive capacities and limitations of the caretaker(s). Sometimes prohibitions are obvious. The young child learns useful lessons, for example, don't eat food on the floor and don't kick the dog. However, they avoid many behaviors because of implicit parental responses such as forbidding gestures.[7]

Parental rules can also be more complex: "You can only be friends with your sister and your cousins. Never trust anyone else!" Making a friend outside those rules would disrupt the self-system. The power of such prohibitions goes back to the infantile experience of trying to get satisfaction from the primary caretaker(s) when a function that was extremely threatening to the primary caretaker(s) and disruptive of the infant's relationship with them could be fatal to the infant if it went on long enough. A person's defiance of parental restrictions in a later developmental era, depending upon the severity of the challenge to the self-system, can still evoke anxiety.

SELF-IMAGE

When one examines their self-image, they may be able to understand how they limit experiences as dictated by their self-system's limitations. The self-image is primarily in marginal awareness, but periodically in focal awareness. It is a person's symbolic condensation of how they view themself: a symbolic encapsulation or representation of what one believes is possible or not possible for oneself in life. Many memories are poetic or symbolic statements of one's self-image.

> When Harriet thinks about riding a bicycle, she remembers her grandmother, a primary caretaker, repeatedly warning her, "You'll be killed if you ride a bike, but alright, do it if you dare." Consequently, she mostly avoids riding bikes, but when she does, she pedals with serious misgivings. Her self-image is: "I am a bike rider with misery and terror." Her self-image is a condensation of both the potential for growth and the restrictions. It resides in marginal awareness and can more or less easily be brought into consciousness when the opportunity presents itself.

MARGINAL AND FOCAL AWARENESS

Levels of awareness are on a continuum. Experiences in focal and marginal awareness reside within the self-system. Outside the self-system are experiences not available to consciousness, that are dissociated.

Dissociation is also on a continuum. Some dissociated experiences are more accessible to consciousness than others. For example, when a therapist takes a history, pushing the person to recall specific details, they may remember dissociated experiences. The content was *not* part of the self-system until the therapist began asking into, for example, the historical motivation for a particular behavior. This inquiry can expand the self-system, but not without arousing the security apparatus.

> Paula, a young trial lawyer suffering from bouts of guilt and self-disgust, recalled an image of her mother grimly scrubbing feces off her legs, muttering, "When will you learn to use the potty?" She was able to connect this two-year-old memory with numerous other memories of shame over her inability to quickly master toilet training, as well as other "defects of character." This vivid memory was useful to her in beginning to pinpoint the origin of her often-paralyzing bouts of guilt and self-recrimination as well as her inability to recognize her own competence. However, in the process of remembering and making connections, she simultaneously became remorseful about thinking ill of her mother and extremely preoccupied with competence as a trial lawyer. Temporarily, her guilty ruminations, her *security operations*, increased. During therapy it was possible to bring this juxtaposition of insight with the increase of symptoms to her attention and to integrate the new information into her self-system.

Learning also takes place in focal and marginal awareness. It may even occur *out* of awareness (not in the self-system) and then can reemerge into awareness at more propitious moments with greater or lesser anxiety. The ability to remember more is motivationally determined. The therapist's curiosity may stimulate increased range of memory during history taking. Or, as a person's life changes and the person expands their range of functioning, new memories may emerge, usually related to the new functioning; the self-system is changing, expanding.

> A relatively isolated person begins to remember positive interactions with other children as they now, through therapy, begin to focus on making friends. Or a person, despite much hesitation and trepidation, finally starts driving lessons with the encouragement of a friend, and they remember going to horse camp at 10 and successfully learning how to ride in spite of misgivings.

Understanding the role of the self-system is crucial to the therapeutic process, as discussed below.[8]

Levels of awareness are constantly changing. The barrier between marginal and fully conscious thoughts is very permeable. Restrictive thoughts, perceptions, and feelings lying in marginal awareness can be called up in moments of potential expansion of the self-system to limit that expansion or to help identify and clarify some obstacles to greater need satisfaction to potentially clarify one's despair. These marginal thoughts are part of how one sees oneself and the world. They represent assumptions about oneself. Most dramatically, despair can come up in nightmares or nightmare moods.

> Martin thinks about applying for a better job and has a nightmare about desperately trying to run but being unable to move; his legs are stuck, and when they get unstuck, he keeps crashing into obstacles. His despair: he has limited or no mobility. So what's the use of applying?

> Iris, a fairly isolated woman, has the thought she might search online for a "meet-up" group in her hometown. She then has a nightmare that intruders break into her apartment and stab her. Her despair: strangers are dangerous, so don't go online and look for a group of people with mutual interests.

Such restrictive thoughts come up during therapy; all are expressions of the conviction that life can't possibly get better. In therapy, the heretofore forbidden expansion of the self-system may be more possible. These limitations, despairing thoughts, and nightmares, experiences of the self, can be accessible to awareness and are often made more accessible. They may not be welcomed because they are usually despairing and unpleasant when pulled into focal awareness, but now there is the possibility of critical examination in the light of day.

For example, when the therapist comments on a person's childhood memory, the person might become uncomfortable, but they understand the interpretation.

> Iris's earliest memory, at about four, is looking out her window at children playing across the street in a neighbor's front yard. In her isolation, she feels peaceful and happy. In therapy, as an isolated adult, she hears herself recite this earliest memory, and her therapist wonders about the very early feelings of "peaceful" and "happy" when alone with her nose pressed against the glass. When her therapist gently challenges her well-cherished *tranquil-while-alone* assumption thorough interpretation, she may begin noticing her need for people or her resistance to being with people, which has been dissociated. Now the self-system can be disrupted. The status quo has been challenged, and the security apparatus of the self-system might struggle successfully to debunk the interpretation and prevent change, or it might be unsuccessful in that struggle and allow change to happen.

The recognition of one's symbolic operations or thinking processes or stream of consciousness can start the examination of one's self-limitations at the onset of self-system expansion. Taking away the power of one's dearly held assumptions disrupts the self-system. It then moves successfully or unsuccessfully to maintain its prior organization.

UNDERPINNINGS OF THE RESTRICTIVE ASPECTS OF THE SELF-SYSTEM

Dread associated with challenging the limitations of the parenting one(s) usually goes back to infancy, when things were more precarious, more a life-and-death issue. It comes from the underpinnings of the central paranoia: the infant's early fear of death, disorganization, and a loss of tenderness with disruption from the mothering figure(s). It has devastating power and is usually in marginal awareness, but becomes more focally conscious in moments when the limits of the self-system are challenged.

While a person may be motivated to allow in as much new experience as possible, one also must function in everyday life. When the status quo is challenged and the self-system is disrupted, the person is unable to function to varying degrees depending on the level of prohibition and disorganization required to admit the new experience and functioning. The self-system strives to keep the person together by reasserting old assumptions.

The most challenging is learning how to balance the two: to grow beyond the current self-system and yet function in the world. Mastering this capacity and allowing new learning into one's personality is integral to growing. Human growth beyond the original restrictions is possible; unmet needs can be met through experiences with friends, books, teachers, classes, media, therapy, or any new validation that gives an opening to the person's integral personality.[9]

OPPORTUNITIES FOR EXPANSION OF THE SELF-SYSTEM

Expansion of the self-system starts with any opportunity of new experience beyond the limits of the infantile experience with the parenting figure(s). For example, as the older infant crawls and then walks without the assistance of caretakers, real opportunities appear for the expansion of the infant's world. Adults can help by providing the toddler with "childproofed" areas where they can safely explore. They can provide toys and puzzles the toddler can explore independently. People in the toddler's world who allow for comfortable exploration—including their parenting one(s), siblings, alternate validators, even pets—provide opportunities for expansion. All depends upon the degree to which the primary caretaker(s) allows or restricts what the toddler can do and/or whom else they can feel comfortable being with.

The toddler might have fewer opportunities to expand their self-system because of adult limitations: They are kept from toddling around or exploring things beyond the arms of the parenting figure(s); they are kept from relating to people more available, tender, experienced, or simply different from the original caretaker(s). When the child moves from late infancy to childhood and juvenile eras and beyond, opportunities continue to expand, if permitted. At the dawn of each new developmental era—with new people, new experiences, and new capabilities in each—opportunities for expansion become more obvious. In the transition from early infancy to late infancy, the toddler is introduced to the world of objects and increased validation from the parenting one(s), alternate adults, and other children. From late infancy to childhood there is increased interaction with other children who are seen as peers during the process of "parallel play" in preschool or on the playground, for example. In the transition from childhood to the juvenile, opportunities for experience increase with more complex interactions and a sense of belonging to groups outside of the family, on the playground, in neighborhood streets and parks, at school, in camp, and in team sports and afterschool classes, to name a few.

The parenting one(s) who might have been uncomfortable with an utterly dependent early infant but is more comfortable when the child becomes more mobile, more exploratory, can now be more validating. Maybe the primary mothering one(s), for whatever reason, has expanded their own self-system and is now more available. No matter who is validating, the child is still coping with limitations originally established in infancy. But change can and does happen. It's like building a pyramid of functions; the pyramid can have gaps which may or may not be filled in later, depending on how shaky the base is and the availability of validators. A brick can get inserted in the base, replacing the original instability, because the interpersonal milieu now includes a primary alternate person (such as a sibling, extended family member, godparent, babysitter, teacher) or the primary parenting one(s) has changed and is more available.

> An awkward, shy child is moving from childhood to juvenile functioning. A teacher or paraprofessional helps them make up for an earlier deficit after noticing that they are isolated in the playground. The adult pulls them into a small group of awkward kids and teaches them how to jump rope. Once the child learns how to jump rope as well as the other kids, they rejoin them, becoming, over time, more comfortable with their peers.

In less fortunate instances, the earlier restrictions may create a deficit so serious that eventually it is obvious to adults that something is wrong. There are various outcomes to that scenario. The parenting one(s) may become very guilty but assume the deficit is "incurable." The child may be labeled as shy, a bully, stupid, depressed, or hyperactive. Much depends on whether the increasingly obvious problem is seen as a given, as part of the child's nature, or as a problem amenable to change with remedial experience that slowly expands the self-system.

Depending on their own capacity to function, the parenting figure(s) can be available as a validator throughout the person's adolescence. Once they have taught all the functions they are capable of teaching, given their own self-systems, the emerging adult looks to others to validate new, expanding experiences. No longer the introducer and validator of new functioning (unless they are constantly learning and expanding themselves), the parenting one(s) can be available to provide practical support for more experiences. The relationship is productive if they do not seek to restrict growth. There is still a tendency for the young adult, particularly one still living in their parental home, to consider them an unquestionable authority figure(s), not also with problems in living. Usually, the emerging young adult needs to physically leave home to fully explore and expand their self-system. Leaving home may happen in numerous ways, such as going away to college, getting married, accepting a job in another location, or just moving out.[10]

LOGICAL FALLACIES

To protect itself, the self-system builds a wall or moat of logical fallacies, called the central paranoia (Pearce & Newton, 1963, p. 16),[11] that surrounds and protects the self-system. The logical fallacies are the bases for security operations which vigilantly distort experiences that might challenge the self-system.

For example, the self-system has the capacity to turn a positive experience on its head. If someone starts to have the experience of *not* being demeaned—has a positive experience that challenges the self-system's assumption of, say, low self-esteem—the self-system protects itself by saying, "No, the whole world thinks of you as a loser." These thoughts can get very loud and are quite convincing, and may, to that extent, become more restrictive and rigid. If a person allows the new experience into awareness, the person can expand the ability to function, to relate to people and feel good about themself. Or a person may effectively put a damper on the new experience, reasserting and strengthening old restrictions. There is either growth or deterioration, not stasis. If the person accepts the original restrictive premise, there is no disorganization; the self-system has retained its integrity, and no change leading to a better sense of self occurs. The person even more fervently thinks of themself as a "loser."

If a new experience bursts through that is compelling enough to challenge the logical fallacies, the self-system can become disorganized and despairing moods may erupt. Anxiety rarely lasts very long, but it is almost immediately superseded by attempts to restore the self-system's restrictions. Or the self-system can integrate the new experience and expand to the extent that the self-system's logic can accept the change. A person would be less aware of the experience of reorganization but tend to remember feelings of terror and rage, other uncanny emotions, and a plethora of other unpleasant experiences. It might manifest as a full-blown "anxiety attack" (such as heart palpitations, sweats) or a feeling that one has been hit by an eighteen-wheeler, or a sudden feeling of dread (often at night in the form of night terror or a nightmare). The experience of anxiety is usually very brief. The self-system rapidly employs the unpleasant feelings to stop the reorganization; those feelings remain in awareness, serving to warn a person not to try that change (for example, to avoid accepting a favorable opinion of oneself).

A person can go through all this and still come out of it rejecting the negative thoughts and overcoming the security operations and uncanny feelings. With the help of a positive interpersonal milieu (actual, virtual, or mustered up from earlier positive validating experiences), the self-system accepts the new experience, and growth can take place.

THE INTEGRAL PERSONALITY

So why does any person even risk change, risk debilitating anxiety? Because people also possess an integral personality (Pearce & Newton, 1963, p. 21). Every human being has the capacity to push for satisfaction of needs, no matter how forbidden, no matter how many experiences reside out of awareness.

While the self-system is composed of what one is aware of (experiences either fully or marginally available to consciousness), the integral personality includes, in a more or less organized manner, *all* experience, both unconscious and conscious. Operating since birth, the integral personality pushes to grow, no matter what, continuing throughout life and providing the counterpoint to the security system's restrictive apparatus.

The integral personality is fueled by the energy of pressing needs. In an infant, that can be as simple as cuddling. The need presses (the infant cries) until the need is satisfied. Most needs pressing for satisfaction get met, or the infant would die. Others might only partially get met, so the infant stores the energy of the partially met needs in the integral personality, which searches for other opportunities to satisfy them. The integral personality might have to wait a long time, so the needs may be stored very deep in dissociation. When a need finally gets triggered, say, in adolescence when hormones might be pushing for certain satisfactions, the energy to satisfy that need surfaces from the integral personality and pushes the self-system to accept the opportunity. The self-system may still not allow the need to be met, or it may allow it with disorganization and modification.

The integral personality also makes observations and comments outside of awareness (in dreams or fugue states[12]), often about the security operations that limit pressing needs. These become louder when needs are most pressing for satisfaction, like the unsatisfied needs from infancy and childhood (Pearce & Newton, 1963, p. 21).

If there were no integral personality, the self-system would rule; no positive change would take place. These aspects of human personality are in constant internal struggle; the integral personality pushes to grow, but the central paranoia and security operations ward off its efforts.[13]

All people go through disorganization of the self-system in some fashion each time they grow or change. At a moment when a challenge to the self-system crosses the moat constructed by the central paranoia, one suddenly might become preoccupied and stop thinking about what they are doing. The adult's deep reverie about something else may be a sign of disorganization. Or they forget what they were doing; they went to the kitchen, forgot why they were there, and returned to the living room. Another is traveling somewhere and not knowing where they are. Or a person sits in a chair, thinking about something, several hours pass, and then they realize they've been someplace else in their head, but they don't know where. Or they board a train traveling in the wrong direction. These phenomena are sometimes called "fugue states." The normal organizational functions are not working, and the person suddenly discovers they're not doing what they normally do. They're *making a mistake*, confused. These may not be "senior moments." The phenomenon (even for a senior!) may have been caused by a break in concentration when something new is going on.

What has happened? Instigated by the integral personality, the individual is about to make a change or has just allowed a previously dissociated experience into the self-system (such as comfortable cuddling) and becomes frightened (and might frighten others) by the self-system's disorganization. It may be just this very disconcerting and troublesome disorganization that catapults a person into therapy, where they can gain perspective about growth and concomitant disorganization.

THE SELF-SYSTEM AND THE STRUGGLE TO EXPAND IT

Early physiology can break down when long-held assumptions about oneself are challenged,and the logical fallacies initially fail to work to protect the self-system:

> Dorothy, a graduate student, attended a panel presentation at her first professional conference. As she walked out of the room, she thought, "I can do this," a big-time challenge to her self-system given how she was brought up to think of herself. Suddenly she experienced what seemed like the flu—difficulty breathing, congestion, exhaustion; she collapsed onto a couch, completely unable to move. Not the flu; within a half hour her symptoms subsided.

There was a sudden flash of realization that a major change of her self-perception was possible. She had the thought and then a dramatic physiological breakdown, as if moving in a professional and creative direction would inevitably cause her body to stop functioning normally. At that moment she reestablished deeply held assumptions, her logical fallacies: don't do (or think about doing) anything rash, anything beyond what her parents felt were possible for themselves or for her. She'll get sick and die.

Here are two, among other, similar assumptions she learned and held dear from early on:

> Her mother (whose own self-system made it inconceivable that her offspring could be smart and inquisitive) told her she was reading too much and would go blind, "use up" her eyes. She also warned her not to learn how to ride a bike (i.e., expand her capacity for mobility) because she would fall and have to go to the hospital, or worse, the brakes would fail and she would careen into traffic and die.
>
> As a young adult, she traveled to London to do research for her first book. Flying there (more expansion of mobility, like riding that bike) was a major and traumatic undertaking. In addition, writing a book represented a massive challenge to her self-system given how she was brought up to think of herself and the disastrous consequences of pushing beyond that concept of herself. Recognizing that she was disoriented and distracted, she had to be very careful when stepping off the curb because she kept forgetting that the British drive on the left. Since she had the benefit of understanding that disorganization and positive change are partners (from several years of therapy) she managed to challenge her self-system and continue her research.

If a person knows what is going on, having developed insight into the how the self-system can become disorganized when challenging its assumptions with new experiences, they can have a slightly easier time dealing with the phenomenon, even developing compensatory behaviors to cope with the disorganization.

The disorganization of the self-system may also take on psychotic proportions.

> Matt, a young man in his early 20s, was admitted to the inpatient psychiatric unit because he thought there were earthquakes under his feet. He couldn't move, because if he walked the ground would open up. During the intake and then in subsequent sessions, it became clear that he recently had the thought that he could leave his parents' very restrictive and authoritarian home, i.e., become an independent adult in the adult world. The psychotic sensations probably stemmed from learning how to walk in an atmosphere of intense anxiety. As his history unfolded, it became clear that his mother was only comfortable relating to a little "baby-doll" infant, not to a more independent toddler. Walking away from her would be disastrous.[14]

An acute psychotic break is on the continuum of how disrupted the self-system can become, and how strenuously it tries to keep the original assumptions in place. People walk around with their original audience, their primary caretaker(s), in their heads. Most people's inner thoughts take the form of pronouncements or images of various kinds. When thoughts not recognizable as part of oneself become very prominent, they're sometimes experienced as not coming from oneself. But they *are* one's own thoughts. A hallucination *is* that person's thought because it exists in the person. Nobody else hears it. Some people hear such pronouncements very loudly, such as, "You're no good" or "You're a loser" or more paranoid ones, such as, "Everyone hates you." They are summaries of one's most despairing thoughts, arriving as intrusions of dissociated experiences from early on. They are now experienced as if somebody is actually yelling (or whispering) hateful things to them. These assertions may have been said to them quite frequently in one form or another when they were very little, but in later life they're saying it to themself, very loudly. For example, the person usually doesn't recognize they've been going along feeling disparaged, *not* saying it, not consciously noticing how much they feel hated. The prevalent conviction is a given, like the constant background noise of traffic, not recognized as extraordinary. Now they're noticing they feel that way much of the time (the traffic noise has suddenly gotten very loud and unrelenting). These paranoid pronouncements— forbidding, despairing thoughts residing in marginal awareness—are now fully in consciousness and can become strident and convincing when people challenge their self-systems. They emerge when a person has reached or breached the limits of their self-system and there is the "threat" that they might push beyond them, or they already have pushed beyond them.

Despairing and paranoid thoughts, part and parcel of the central paranoia, are not fully dissociated. In marginal awareness, they can be called up with less effort than buried needs. Emerging into more focal awareness, they are the self-system's responses to intrusion of those dissociated needs now pushing for satisfaction, for admission into the self-system. For example, the positive experience of comfort with cuddling may be in dissociation because comfortable cuddling was mostly forbidden in infancy. The feelings of rage, self-revulsion, or resentment and uncanny emotions are the reactions of the self-system to that dissociated need now trying to find satisfaction.

> When an adolescent whose early formative experiences were essentially devoid of comfortable cuddling[15] first experienced the possibility of comfortable cuddling, she assumed a warm advance by someone was hostile and harmful; she also assumed the person would vomit as soon as they touched her.

In a psychotic reaction, an adolescent whose infancy cuddling experience was very awkward and intermittent might perceive (hallucinate) a potential sexual partner as a vampire or some other kind of monster.

Hallucinations may come with the experience of dissociated needs emerging into consciousness, complete with the terror and rage that accompanied their original dissociation. Or they are the marginal thoughts, which are part of self-system's functions, that become very loud in a person's head if they are beginning to move, albeit unwittingly, against early forbidding parental dictates. Ultimately hallucinatory thoughts contain parental messages, the marching orders from very early on.

A nightmare that awakens a person in a terror state is a brief but powerful psychotic experience.[16] It's a symbolic statement about one's deepest despair. Consequently, it usually occurs when somebody is beginning to expand their self-system. As they do something *positive*, they begin to see the depths of their own despair in a nightmare, which symbolically expresses their deepest-held, central paranoid assumptions in an attempt to convince them that it's *not* possible to change. It's the "Not-So-Fast-Charlie Syndrome."

A nightmare is a function of the integral personality, which formulates the despair out of awareness when one is dreaming. If one were awake and having such an experience for an extended period of time, it would be a psychotic episode. The person who is psychotic may say things that sound like a nightmare. For example, aliens from outer space completely filling their brain with bugs is a nightmare formulation. Experienced in a nightmare, it would be a formation of one's despair that one does not have the right to think, that their thoughts are contaminated by some authority, notably the early dictates of parental authority. Once formulated in a nightmare, that formulation ("I can't think for myself; I am always at the mercy of a higher authority") is accessible to awareness. The dream formulation is the integral personality poetically describing that same experience unbound by one's sense of what is real and what isn't.

To pay attention to one's awake psychotic formulations is to witness the integral personality's formulations. When the therapist says in interpreting a nightmare or an hallucination, "You seem not to believe you have the ability to think for yourself," the person may say, "Yeah, I do feel that way sometimes, like I can't have an independent thought. I know it's ridiculous." Interpretating a hallucination is the same as interpreting the integral personality's formulation in a dream, of recognizing a person's despair. Now, in the process of therapy, the hallucinating person can get to the point of "Here I go again, assuming I'm so dependent on my parent's judgments. I just had another hallucination about that."

When a person wakes from a nightmare and has trouble shaking it, they are in a brief psychotic state. But if a person is simply waking up with a lingering nightmare feeling, they are not psychotic because they're aware that it doesn't make sense to feel that way. It's just the hangover from the dream.

It is a continuum, a gradient. A person wakes up from a nightmare; it takes 10 minutes to realize it isn't real. Or half the night. They're afraid to move because monsters are still climbing through the window. At that moment the individual who is not in a full-blown psychotic episode, but who is in a brief psychotic nightmare state, can understand how it feels to be psychotic for a long period of time.

Children's nightmares start at about three, after the self-system has had a few years to develop into a relatively smooth working machine, and the concept of foresight and recall has really kicked in: *If I do this, then something horrible is going to happen.*

In all these instances, some things can really go haywire in the process of expanding the self-system. Most people desperately want to prevent the accompanying unfavorable stuff from happening. If they do happen, the person, and those around them, can panic. The therapist must not also panic. Varying gradations of chaos come with the territory of change. People can be helped though the crisis and come out stronger because the self-system has integrated positive change. A muscle challenged by exercise aches but is strengthened if the person pushes on. They use that stronger "muscle" to go for more rigorous exercise and grow even more.

It really helps to not fear the chaos accompanying change. Understanding why one is frightened helps make one less frightened. Revolutions pushing for positive change within one's mind, like progressive revolutions within a country, are messy and vigorously defended against, but when they win out, people are in a better place. For the individual, it might mean successfully organizing to get their needs met: becoming less isolated, choosing more positive relationships, developing self-esteem, maximizing one's potential (in sports, creativity, and skills, for example), changing one's lifestyle to improve health and fitness, or organizing for more satisfying employment.

The therapist's job is to mitigate the fallout from the self-system's disorganization, as well as to help the person allow positive change to happen. The therapist engages in positive management of the disorganization, whether it is brief or an acute psychotic break. In the United States (and elsewhere) an acute psychotic break is not likely to be managed well by the mental health system, especially if the person is relatively isolated, too impoverished to afford even the minimum of supportive intervention, and/or faces racism, homophobia, transphobia, sexism, and/or classism in whatever health care is offered. When a person is incarcerated, the situation is even more dire. Without positive management of the disorganization, the self-system is more likely to reorganize back to its original, less useful configuration, and the logical fallacies, the restrictive central paranoia, and the security operations can rule even more vigorously. However, where there are facilities providing safe havens for disorganization and encouragement for developing new social skills, expansion of productive functioning is possible.[17] Such conditions exist in places that provide open-ended social communities or halfway houses for people unable to navigate living in a less protective environment.[18] They organize opportunities to interact socially and work productively in a sheltered environment until the person is ready to navigate the wider world.

When the need for reorganization of the self-system is massive, there can be a longer, more florid period of psychotic experience. The situation is complicated by the overuse of medication, which can cause persistent physiological and neurological changes that can lead to increased dependency on medications and caretakers and to limitations in functioning. In the United States, there are very few resources for people who require a lengthy inpatient therapeutic environment to reorganize their self-system as it accepts and integrates, with positive validation, more positive experiences.

SUMMARY

The self-system, essential to every person's existence, enables and organizes a person's productive functioning but also formulates and maintains negative formulations that prevent participation beyond limits originally set by the primary parenting figure(s).

The self-system, starting to organize at birth and somewhat more systematized in late infancy, has increased opportunity to change as a person moves through childhood, the juvenile era, preadolescence, adolescence, and into young adulthood, when a person ventures more away from home emotionally and/or geographically, providing for additional opportunities for alternate experiences that challenge the self-system to expand.

In order to evolve throughout life to one's full and satisfying potential, it is useful to achieve insight about what resides in a usually stubborn and well-defended self-system, what logical fallacies reside in the central paranoia, how one employs security operations to maintain the security system, and what is possible to tap from the integral personality to make use of experience and opportunities that always present themselves.

The security system, particularly despair, is a kind of electrified perimeter of the self-system. In approaching its limits, one touches those aspects of despair, paranoia, etc., which become activated, like an electric shock, to intimidate them from going further.

People can go further. They can expand their self-systems without having names for the intrapsychic phenomena, even without a clear understanding of what is taking place as they grow. But they must struggle nevertheless, with the help of friends, support groups, and alternate validators, and with or without therapy.[19] Whatever early interpersonal forces pull people downstream are tough to swim against, but people who don't fear anxiety and bring alternate audiences with them as a cheering squad do manage (with struggle) to swim upstream. It simply (well, not necessarily so simply!) does take brave and patient commitment to evolve.

NOTES

1. Coined by Sullivan (1953) and elaborated upon by Pearce and Newton (1963).
2. This example is discussed in more detail in chapter 11.
3. Sullivan (1953) coined these shorthand explanatory terms (pp. 161–165).
4. In adulthood, the memory of early infantile experience can reappear as if from nowhere and in powerful form as *mood-memory*. See chapter 11.
5. See Sullivan (1966, pp. 163–164, 315–316, 320–322, 326–327, 359–362) for discussions of uncanny emotions.
6. Pronouncements such as" just change your ways" or "just think positively" do not actually work in the long run. The self-system's resistance to change is very strenuous, and one can "act as if" for only so long before dissociated needs start pushing for satisfaction and the original forbidden assumptions lying in wait in the self-system interfere. People who are afraid of "looking bad" by becoming disoriented or disorganized have a harder time solidly changing for the better because they always have to be "well put together." Their self-systems hardly expand. In therapy they might say, "Things are getting worse! Look at me now!" or "Therapy has made things even more horrendous!"

7. A forbidding gesture is a non-verbal mode of communication that expresses dissatisfaction or disgust with what another is doing or saying. A person cannot remember the actual gestured message of disgust from infancy, but now, as an adult, they might be able to get in touch with the mood-memory of self-disgust and connect it to stories about their infancy.

8. See a fuller discussion of psychotherapy in chapter 14.

9.The integral personality is the total of all aspects of experience, dissociated and in marginal or full awareness. A fuller discussion of the integral personality can be found later in this chapter, in chapters 1, 10, and 14 and in Pearce and Newton (1963). It is a profoundly complex conceptualization requiring more discussion than is useful in this chapter.

10. Given the current socio-economic conditions in the United States, it has become increasingly difficult for young adults to move out on their own. Joining the armed forces might be appealing; for some, especially the most oppressed, it might feel like the only way out. In many cultures one cannot leave home until they marry, and even then, the requirement might be to live in the same home or nearby.

11. As indicated in chapter 1, the use of the word "paranoid" in this context is not entirely what is commonly accepted as a diagnosis in the *Diagnostic and Statistical Manual* (2013). It is meant to define a despairing conviction that is a departure from what is true in reality. It is on a continuum, from a false assumption that regulates one's life (like, "I'm a loser") to the florid paranoid psychotic belief that aliens are in control of one's mind (as described in the *DSM*).

12. Fugue states (Pearce & Newton, p. 347) are the intrusion of dissociated material into waking life, including both the forbidden functions and the forbidding thoughts that kept them dissociated. See below and chapter 1.

13. For more on the integral personality, see chapter 1 and Pearce and Newton (1963, pp. 186–187).

14. Here are some other possible scenarios of mother-uncomfortable-with-toddler: His mother, only comfortable relating to a "baby doll," might have simply become a helpless bystander as the toddler began to move into areas of danger. Perhaps she didn't childproof the play area or provide comfortable structures in which to explore. Then accidents happen; the toddler crashes into a porcelain vase and gets badly cut or they stick their finger into an electrical socket. Or their mother might have responded to any exploratory action with hysteria and panic, treating every fall as tragic instead of encouraging them to try again. This anxious atmosphere around initial mobility translates into anxiety in later attempts at independent movement, such as leaving home.

15. No infant would survive with the complete absence of comfortable cuddling (Spitz, 1946a), but if they experience some, but not enough, during those early years, the need for comfortable cuddling becomes dissociated. That is, if the infant's demand for more physical contact is, for whatever reason, more often than not repellent to the parenting figure(s), the infant dissociates the need for tenderness in order to keep going without disruption of the self-system. Later, say in childhood, the individual might proclaim that they "hate" hugging. But the dissociation outlives its usefulness

as they become older, and the need can push through, particularly in adolescence, as in this example.

16. See chapter 15.

17. Sullivan's inpatient therapeutic community made use of his interpersonal approach at Sheppard and Enoch Pratt Hospital in Baltimore in the 1920s; it is known for having an 86 percent "cure" rate (Blechner, 2009, p. 110).

18. Long-term residential treatment can function as a safe haven for adolescents from troubled homes. The Richmond Fellowship, a chain that existed throughout England, western Europe, and the United States, provided live-in halfway houses for discharged psychiatric patients (Harris, 1980). However, their scope deteriorated as funds for "Socialized Medicine" (in the United Kingdom it was called "National Health") dried up. Instead, with exceptions, long-term psychotropic medication has become the solution for those who might have benefited from long-term residential treatment, including Sullivan's inpatient ward described in the previous note.

19. If for whatever reasons in one's upbringing, a person finds oneself brave enough to try on new experiences, rock the self-system's boat, they can learn that storms of dread and disorganization can be survived and are worth the positive outcomes of change. One does need a positive audience in or near their rocking boat, either imagined from previous validators and/or from current people in their life. One may think it is better to tough it out on one's own, but without a previous and/or current cheering squad, the struggle to weather the storm can be too daunting. Each survived boat-rocking can prepare a person for the next one.

Chapter Ten

Despair and the Central Paranoia

The newborn is eager to relate to whomever is available. The primary caretaker(s) provides nurturing for survival, growth, and development. The interaction is reciprocal, the caretaker(s) gaining empathic relatedness and satisfaction as infant's needs are satisfied. Despair originates in lapses of relatedness in that relationship.

If a caretaker is for whatever reason unavailable at a particular moment and there is no alternate, the infant experiences a break from the source providing the means for survival, continued functionality, and tenderness, creating intense terror, paralysis, and isolation.

No mothering figure is 100 percent available. Sometimes, alternate caretakers are unavailable. There are always times the caretaker can't relate to the infant tenderly, so everyone has such moments in their history, to varying degrees. Since the infant is totally dependent on continuity of relatedness with the caretaker for survival, the ability to function, and tenderness, the disconnection from that relatedness is experienced as threatening to all three.

A caretaker can be unavailable because of anxiety about the infant's behavior or because of extraneous circumstances unrelated to the infant.

Personally, every caretaker at times bumps into barriers of anxiety, responding with forbidding gestures to an infant's need. The *repetition* of forbidding gestures in response to a need threatens the infant's connection to survival, sanity, and tenderness. They form the basis for creating, as if with barbed wire, a barrier around a forbidden area of functioning the infant and, subsequently, the growing person cannot cross or even approach without severe distress. Despair includes assumptions about trying to satisfy forbidden needs: logical fallacies, the foundations of security operations that protect the self-system from risking change. These fallacies are in marginal awareness unless there is a powerful threat to the organization of the self-system. They can appear in nightmares or psychotic episodes. They are a person's "central paranoia."[1]

The central paranoia is the basis for a person's despair, subsequently elaborated in later developmental eras. It's called central because it forms the lifelong basis for a person's entire defensive structure. It's called paranoia because, like the commonly used term, it is a set of pseudo-logical assumptions that support a false reality.

Repetition of this dynamic is necessary to form the basis for those restrictions. For example, repeated parental disgust with the infant can be the basis for feeling like a disgusting person. As discussed in chapter two, one babysitter, well-meaning friend, or relative who is disgusted by diaper changing and then is no longer welcomed by the parenting one(s) as a helper comprises only a short-time experience among many positive ones and will not form the basis for a person's despairing assumptions about oneself. This formulation applies to the cumulative effects on the developing person in continuous interaction with the primary caretaker(s).

DESPAIR

Despair as expressed in central paranoid assumptions is a compilation of one's worst fears. It includes the fear of death, the fear of disorganization, and the fear of the loss of tenderness. It is often expressed by a symbolic statement about why the anxiety-provoking project can't work, firming up the original limits. They exist in marginal thoughts or dreams, implied in mood, or in realization in focal awareness. It is a formulation that people experience most powerfully when they are on the cusp of growing their self-system beyond what was conceivable; to grow beyond the self-systems of the primary caretaker(s), even long past the original interaction, would threaten very early continuity. Nightmares often occur during periods of change in a person's life when there is greater awareness of previously dissociated needs through new sources of validation, at a turning point toward growth. Nightmares are symbolic statements of despair. They are useful tools in therapy because they reveal or codify the marginal despairing assumptions the person always lives with. In the light of day they can be challenged and connected to break through into something new.

> After leaving home, Sheila had a nightmare that a giant hammer fell from the sky to crush her. She rushed to the other side of the world and the hammer came down and crushed her anyway. Her therapist suggested that her fear was that her parents had such power that, no matter where she went, she couldn't escape them, that is, find a way to grow beyond them.

One or more of the uncanny emotions of horror, loathing, awe, and dread fueling one's despair is connected to one's dissociated self-image, and may be revealed in a dream, a nightmare, or during a flagrant psychotic episode. The timing is specific. A nightmare often occurs after a person seriously threatens the dissociation of a relevant need.

> John passed his PhD oral examination after his second try and was ecstatic. Afterward, he celebrated with friends, feeling on top of the world as he fantasized how this newly earned credential would change his life. That night he had the following nightmare: "I suddenly found myself in a huge maze. I had no idea where I was. I shouted out: 'Is there anybody there?' Dead silence. I frantically tried to find my way out. I was terrified. Totally lost. I cried and screamed. I thought I was lost forever and that no one would ever find me, and I would die in this maze. I woke up, out of breath and covered in sweat."
>
> Seeing himself as lost, alone, and incompetent and feeling helpless to do anything about it was John's self-image. He significantly challenged it when he got his PhD. Through discussion and analysis of the nightmare in therapy, John remembered previously "forgotten" events of his growing up which shed further light on why getting his degree, as well as some other experiences he had, were so fraught with anxiety. His frightening self-concept, as depicted in his nightmare, became a tool that helped him and his therapist better understand some of his obstacles toward continued growth.

Despair is more powerful when it is formulated out of focal awareness. At its most effective, despair is in marginal awareness. One lives by it uncritically. In situations when the self-system is not challenged, the despairing thought or perception "just is that way." The person doesn't really think about what "that way" is and isn't critically aware of it. Once it's exposed, it's open to criticism and available to change.

Despair is like an alarm which can go off when the status quo is challenged. It is "the watchdog of the self-system" (Pearce & Newton, 1963, p. 408). It can take the form of inner, unspoken beliefs that happiness, success, or any intense pleasure would be fatal. It brings back the feeling of imminent annihilation the infant experiences when it is in danger of losing continuity with the primary caretaker(s). While the infant cannot express that feeling in so many words, it can be inferred by observable behaviors.

Despair fueled by central paranoid assumptions is a major limiting factor of the human being's experience. In the adult, these assumptions arise when there is a threat to the self-system's structure. "Threat" is from the point of view of the restrictive aspects of personality. From the point of view of the integral personality[2]—the whole person—the "threat" is growth beyond perceived limitations. The antidote to despair lies in exposing and challenging the archaic nature of the central paranoid assumptions. They become less effective in restraining a person from satisfying newly emerging needs beyond their perceived limits.

The central paranoid assumptions fall loosely into three categories, forming the basis for how the adult has historically organized the limits of growth to prevent the experience of discontinuity from the primary caretaker(s) from happening again. They are the fear of disorganization, the fear of death, and the fear of loss of tenderness. The way in which each person handles these fears is specific to their history.

The Fear of Disorganization

The self-system develops through validation of the infant's needs and the functions required to satisfy them by the caretaker(s). The infant is dependent on validation to function. The self-system is internally consistent and contains the same limitations in satisfaction of needs as that of the primary validator(s). Later, if dissociated need intrudes into awareness, it disorganizes the structure of the self-system. The experience of disorganization in and of itself may not be painful, but it's painful when anxiety erupts and disorganization is coupled with the archaic threat of disconnection from a central, early caretaker(s) and the consequent fear of disruption of functioning, death, and of loss of love by that caretaker(s). If the self-system is challenged in a small way requiring minimal reorganization, it may be experienced with only slight discomfort or brief disorganization. It may hardly be noticed. In the case of severe anxiety, when major aspects of the self-system are being challenged, many of the functions and perceptions organized in the context of the original validator(s) feel shaky unless other validators are recognized.

The subjective experience of disorganization includes feelings of an inability to function, severe uncertainty and confusion, disorientation, and isolation, often associated with catatonia. The surrounding world feels unfamiliar and unreal. One feels unable to make decisions about even the most basic behavior, such as putting one foot in front of another. One feels insane.

This state of anxiety, including panic from the fear of death and loss of tenderness, is temporary. It resolves either through the incorporation of new perceptions of need and its satisfaction (toward growth) or a strengthening of restrictions of the self-system and rejection of those perceptions of what is possible (toward deterioration). If one realizes that they can survive the experience of anxiety and find new satisfaction—that they are no longer a helpless infant—the potential for growth increases.

The process of growth involves increased integration of new experience, expansion of function, punctuated by crises of anxiety in which more massive reorganization is required and the archaic feelings of despair are once again resurrected. These processes require new validation and support from alternate validators, including friends, authorities, the therapist, and even imaginary figures. It involves increasing recognition of the nature of one's own despair, and the ability to face and debunk it.

The Fear of Death

The emergence of the fear of death as an underpinning of adult despair takes various forms. One unfortunate way this is handled is via dissociation of the fear, which is expressed in continual risk-taking behavior, with risk increasing as potential expansion becomes more possible.

Another unfortunate method of handling it is to be constantly preoccupied with it by living with constant dread that seems to come from nowhere.

When a person is habitually in a depressed and frightened mood, it's possible that the original parenting figure(s) couldn't tolerate liveliness. The infant, empathically perceiving the parenting figure(s)' reaction, automatically attunes their own mood accordingly. The infant may adapt by becoming apathetic. For the adult, greater happiness may be experienced as a death sentence. The presence of a depressed or even fearful mood does not evoke the fear of death, but expanding one's mood toward liveliness may result in more massive terror or acting out to prove that looming change is dangerous, even fatal.

Self-medication through drugs or alcohol is a self-destructive way of handling the fear of death, effectively warding off potential opportunities for growth. The intoxicated state does not allow a person to develop an awareness of other people who might provide more relatedness, and so maintains isolation. It also lowers the ability to notice danger signals internally or externally. Paradoxically, such self-medication leads to health issues that hasten death.

Dissociation of the Need for Tenderness

In the case of the fear of loss of tenderness, a common pattern is to dissociate the need for it in varying ways using the human ability to selectively inattend relevant perceptions and needs. Here are some examples.

Preoccupation with Rejection

Rejection (real or imagined) is the miserable feeling in a person who unwittingly believes that the rejecting person is the only source of tenderness. In this case, the rejected person is reexperiencing the original rejection by the caretaker. This feeling of rejection is supported by the restrictive aspects of the self-system, specifically, by the self-revulsion built in earlier by the original primary caretaker and not sufficiently corrected by subsequent experience with others, often resulting in the experience of unrequited love. In addition, the "rejected" person often unwittingly organizes it.

> Laura and Bill start to date on a regular basis. They enjoy time together. However, when Bill wants to go camping with his buddies or Laura gets involved in a theater production, each partner becomes threatened by the enthusiasm of the other around an activity the two don't share. Each becomes jealous of the people the other will meet. There's a lot of attention to counting and comparing how much time they spend together. Each person feels "rejected" by the other because they no longer have exclusive rights to the other's time, as if they can't live without the other or get tenderness from any other source. Each is building their own case for why closeness always leads to disappointment, and that once a person becomes intimate with another person, they will lose them.

When mutual attraction doesn't happen and becomes a pattern of interaction, the rejected person has (once again) proved that love (tenderness) remains unavailable and that the mere search for it is too painful to endure. Being bitter is easier.

Fear of Being Alone Versus Loneliness

Another way one dissociates the need for tenderness is by making sure there are a lot of people around, but not relating to them.

An example would be groups of drug addicts engaged in getting high together or alcoholics drinking together. The activity is self-destructive. It clouds judgement, and the proximity of others doing the same thing provides a false sense of security, but in such circumstances, sharing anything productive is impossible.

In some circles, getting married may be considered necessary to prove one is "normal" or fulfilling parental and societal expectations by having a conventional family. In others, prestige or ownership concerns are more important than a tender relationship. In a dissatisfying relationship with someone, each person may hang onto the relationship, no matter how unpleasant, because each is afraid to "be alone." Each person feels no one would want them if they risked severing the unpleasant relationship. The fear of being alone helps to maintain the dissociation of the need for tenderness.

Genuine loneliness is longing for tender relatedness with people. Paradoxically, it can be experienced with great self-loathing and fear. If the need for tenderness has been dissociated, a person is initially likely to feel intense anxiety, including terror and self-loathing, when trying again. These feelings are signs that the need for tenderness is breaking out of its prison of dissociation. Drawing one's attention to these feelings in focal awareness can remove their power, giving a person the courage to reach out again for more tenderness.

SUMMARY

Despair depends largely on the particular history of the person experiencing it. It will contain a combination of three aspects of the central paranoid assumptions. The potential for new growth beyond the limitations of the self-system will provoke fears of the inability to function (disorganization), death, and loss of tenderness. If a person is unable to overcome their despair, they deteriorate, limiting their lives even more and rejecting new validation. Recognition of the fallacy of longstanding despairing assumptions by examining them in focal awareness, along with more hopeful validation, can debunk those assumptions and allow one's self-system to expand.

NOTES

1. Pearce and Newton (1963) first introduced the term and concept of the "central paranoia."

2. The integral personality is the sum total of all aspects of experience, dissociated and in awareness. Even those aspects of functioning that are forbidden by one's early experience, which one mostly dissociates, are contained in the integral personality. Because they are unmet needs, they continue to push for awareness. The degree to which they reach the borderline of one's awareness depends upon the intensity of need versus the strength of the security system.

Chapter Eleven

Cognitive Development, an Interpersonal Phenomenon

Cognitive functioning (thought, perception, communication, consciousness and memory) develops interpersonally within the self-system, which contains all conscious experience, productive and restrictive. Along with the self-system, it begins in utero (Goodrich, 2010) via proprioceptive sensations,[1] continuing in early infancy through the connection between the infant's internal biology and their primary caretaker(s) and later in interactions between them and their primary caretaker(s) and between them and the wider world.

AUDIENCE

The interaction between the infant and the primary parenting one(s) is initially non-verbal, visual, proprioceptive, and auditory. For example, in early infancy, before the child perceives a differentiated concept of "Mother," they perceive hunger, oneself crying, and satisfaction from nipple-in-lips. This chapter does not cover how neurological systems produce cognitive thought, a topic definitively covered by the neuroscientist Antonio Damasio and his associates (2018). Instead, it describes how human social interaction develops, creating its own processes that continue to elaborate into widening social realms and interacting reciprocally with both the neurological and the broader social world.

Through the last half of the 20th century, infant researchers, including Daniel Stern, Colwyn Trevarthen, and Andrew Meltzoff, studied repeated patterns of preverbal behavior in interactions between infants and their caretakers via videotape and other means and hypothetically describe early infancy subjective experience (Beebe et al., 2003). While their conclusions differ, they seem to agree that they now have empirical evidence using actual situations that infants begin to interact interpersonally with their caretaker(s) even as early as in utero (Goodrich, 2010). They also observed that crucial information is transmitted between infant and caretaker(s) via a multitude of means—motor, visual, auditory, olfactory, etc.—constituting empathic communication. Cognitive functioning begins with this interaction; the infant's initial primary caretaker(s) is their "audience."

An older child adds many more details to their cognitive understanding of the world. The child wants a cookie and has a concept of a particular cookie, which includes the caretaker(s)' response to wanting or having cookies. The communication "I want a cookie" is couched in terms tailor-made to the perceptual framework of the caretaker(s), still the audience in question.

People sometimes experience thoughts as a voice talking in their heads. The voice is talking to an eidetic or symbolic audience-person. The thought is not always verbal; it can be a gesture or a facial, tonal, or musical expression. In whatever form, thought takes place between the thinker and a personified other, the audience, past or present, real or imaginary. The person may not be aware of their audience itself (Pearce & Newton, 1963, p. 23).

Throughout life, levels of consciousness range from thoughts and perceptions in focal awareness to marginal, being barely in awareness. Communication of thought requires access to content and a perceived audience in or out of focal awareness. Consciousness, perception, memory, and communication are in constant dynamic interaction with each other.

THE INTERPERSONAL RELATIONSHIP IN EARLY DEVELOPMENT

In infancy, communication is preverbal, mediated through a still-maturing perceptual apparatus, and taking the form of empathy, tone of voice, smell, gesture, and touch. The ability to think develops over time in response to the mothering person's reaction to the infant's crying, cooing, gesturing, physiological reactions, and activity levels.

Trevarthen and his associates corroborate interpersonal theories: the neonate actively engages in relating to whatever interpersonal environment is available to meet its needs. The human infant "is an active and aware person" with the capacity to respond to the people in their life. "Photographic recordings of intimate and responsive exchanges with babies in the first hours after birth proved they do wish to imitate, and with astonishing discrimination and skill. Indeed, they are happy to negotiate exchanges of imitation, taking their turn and inventing new messages" (Trevarthen, 2019b, p. 1, summarizing Nagy & Molnár [2004]).[2] In short, perceptual-cognitive behavior is characterized as relationships between perceptions, which are organized in a hierarchy of increasing complexity.[3]

Trevarthen summarizes: "An infant who is only a few months old has a remarkable range of perceptual capacities that allows for imitative identification, emotional empathy and reciprocal communication that all humans possess" (Trevarthen, 2006, pp. 127–128). "The core of human consciousness is the potential for rapport of the self with an other's mind. This potential is immediate, unrational, unverbalized, conceptless, and atheoretical: A delicate and immediate with-the-other" (Trevarthen, 2006, p. 121). He is talking about empathy.

The concomitant inner experience can be hypothesized as mood. The infant's mood depends on the mood of the interacting primary caretaker(s). The patterns of interaction with the caretaker(s) form the basis for how the person sees oneself and the world:

> Picture a mother and a six-month-old infant in a stroller on a train. The baby is constantly exploring, touching, moving. The baby grasps the strap of a bag lying in reach. If repeated in varying situations, the mother's response creates a pattern of interaction that becomes part of the baby's expectation.

Here are three of an infinite variety of different possible scenarios:

1. The mother pulls the strap away or removes the baby's hand. The baby goes back to the strap and tries again. After this happens a few times, the situation escalates. The mother becomes annoyed and finally roughly removes the bag or smacks the baby's hand. The baby cries and the pair moves on to another scenario: mother's response to crying baby.
2. The mother ignores the baby's actions until the baby succeeds in pulling the bag out of the stroller and lets it fall on the ground. The mother becomes upset and struggles to scoop up the bag and its contents, disrupting her connection to the baby, who begins to cry.
3. The mother produces another toy, enticing the baby to play with it, while simultaneously removing the strap from view. The mother continues to play with the baby for the rest of the trip.

In each scenario a repetitive pattern of interaction between mother and infant sets up expectations in the infant about the experience of curiosity and visual-motor exploration, which can become a life pattern. If they remain similar over a multiplicity of interactions, they create a very powerful set of expectations derived from the primary caretaker's responses. It isn't verbal at first, but a verbal component develops, the icing on a cake. Underneath the words are sets of expectations based in non-verbal experiences.

Putting the non-verbal into verbal form for illustrative purposes, the thoughts are something like this:

1. If I try something new, I'm gonna get my hand slapped.
2. If I do anything on my own, I'll screw it up.
3. This is fun. I wonder where it leads.

Early interactions between the mothering figure(s) and developing person form the groundwork for the perceptual-cognitive framework in later years.

In infancy, thought is expressed in the form of experienced need and communicated via crying (when hungry, when cold, etc.). It's expressed physiologically in symptoms such as spit-up, colic, skin eruptions, and the like. It's also expressed gesturally via facial expressions and body movements. The audience's response shapes how the infant experiences any expression of need. If the need is not conceivable to the audience, i.e., is incompatible with the parental self-system, having the need is not experienced by the infant at all—it is inconceivable. To the totally dependent infant, experiencing such a need would be a dangerous rupture with the audience or mothering figure(s) responsible for their very existence. They must tailor their expression of need to fit with the mothering figure(s)' self-system requirements. Failing that, the infant experiences intense anxiety and terror in the presence of an anxious audience and develops ways to adapt by minimizing satisfaction, through the use of apathy or somnolent detachment,[4] to find a way to get needs met in an attenuated fashion that sidesteps the mothering one's anxiety. In the most extreme circumstances of continued unrelated caretaking, the infant will die (Spitz, 1945).

SYMBOLISM AND FORESIGHT

The infant gradually figures out the difference between mother when "good" and mother when forbidding or "bad" by grasping patterns that identify which one is present.[5] The process of grasping differentiating patterns and signals indicating satisfaction or disaster involves the development of symbolism and foresight, the basis for perception, thought, and communication (Sullivan, 1953, pp. 75–81).This smell, this pattern of movement, this tone of voice has happened before, and it turned out badly or went well. The process is not logical or thought out. However, grasping significant patterns of relatedness is accurate and tailor-made to responses of the caretaker(s). The following example illustrates an infant's adaptive responses to her mother. Note that her survival is partially due to the interaction with others acceptable to the mother.

Agatha had her only child, Sadie, at 25. She was very uncomfortable with her, feeling she wiggled too much. When Sadie was a few weeks old, Agatha accidently dropped her on her head. After that, Agatha was even more uncomfortable with being a parent. She didn't like picking Sadie up because she was afraid she might drop her again. When she cried, she ignored her, hoping that would teach her to be quiet. She also tended to forget she was around, leaving her by herself for long periods of time. Agatha's husband was more attentive, taking over some of the feeding and care.

Sadie was a "good baby," rarely crying and hardly moving, making it easier for Agatha. At three months, Sadie developed spinal meningitis and was hospitalized for two weeks on a respirator. Some nursing staff took a strong interest in her, spending time with her when Agatha was not present. Agatha watched her on the respirator and fantasized picking her up and cuddling her. She was sickly after recovery and still rarely cried. Agatha became more devoted to her, spending many nights up with her when she was sick. She freely cuddled her apathetic, silent baby and became skilled at perceiving what she needed since she rarely overtly expressed any demand for care.

SELECTIVE INATTENTION AND SUBSTITUTIVE OPERATIONS

The dissociated need doesn't go away. When the caretaker(s) can't relate to the need because of their own anxiety, the infant expresses the unacceptable need obscurely and indirectly in some form of avoidant behavior, accommodating to the limitations of the perceptual framework of their audience. Substitutive operations take myriad forms, but share certain characteristics, the most important of which is functioning to prevent emergence into awareness of a need unacceptable to the caretaker(s). Substitution is also reflective of the perceptual orientation of a parenting figure who cannot validate the need. At any developmental era, substitutive operations occur precisely when the forbidden need pushes for expression and can be identified by observing when they occur, which should be when one might expect certain functioning to emerge instead of the substitution.

Jimmy, four, was in daycare with children well acquainted with each other. They were learning to share and take turns. When a group was building a house of blocks, Jimmy would knock it over. If he wanted to be on the swings, he would push the other children off and take it for himself but then lose interest. If he wanted a toy, he would grab it from a child's hand and then destroy it. Attempts to help him find alternative behaviors got nowhere. While other children began to learn how to share toys, Jimmy couldn't catch on.

At a parent/teacher conference, Jimmy's mother proclaimed that Jimmy was "wicked." She had started early training him to not be a thief, keeping a close eye on him in stores and punishing him on the spot for touching anything. She explained that they didn't have much money, certainly not enough for toys. Jimmy destroyed toys he was given, so they gave up giving him anything, even when they could afford it. When she saw Jimmy with a toy, she usually took it away, assuming he would destroy it. The refrigerator was locked so Jimmy couldn't steal food. Jimmy was the youngest of four, so he lost most of the frequent fights over ownership of clothes, toys, and food. Children were essentially "wicked" and required strict discipline to prevent them from stealing or being destructive. They needed a "firm hand" to show them who was boss. Also, they needed someone to prepare them for the hard life ahead. It's a dog-eat-dog world, and they might as well get used to it now.

Enjoyment and exploration of a toy was unfathomable. Sharing was inconceivable. He substituted power and coercion, which matched the parental view of the world. Beyond the restriction on cherishing objects, these power operations also cut off the possibility of being able to relate with pleasure to other children, having fun playing together, an important next step in childhood development. Life was a constant power struggle for what he needed and wanted, often ending in the destruction of what he needed and wanted.

In another form of substitutive operation, paranoid preoccupations can be reliable substitutes for having fun with friends.

An adolescent, Ellen, accepts an invitation to go to a square dance with a friend. She does so despite her mother's constant mantra: *Don't trust other people. They will be quick to ridicule you.* At the dance, she joins in right away and is having a great time until someone asks her, "Where did you learn to dance?" She immediately experiences a severe drop in self-esteem and becomes self-conscious and awkward. She sits out the next couple of dances and begins to feel like a wallflower. She heard the question as ridicule, as her mother would see it, instead of a compliment. The paranoia fits the restrictive perceptual framework of her early audience. It would go on through life unless other experiences revised her paranoid assumption.

ALTERNATE VALIDATION AND EXPANDED AUDIENCES

As a person matures, more audiences become available, such as teachers, friends, friendly strangers, relatives, and people on the internet.

Molly, married with three children, was hospitalized for severe depression after a suicidal gesture. She had married young and been in an abusive relationship with her husband for 12 years. She was shy, rarely venturing out of her house. Her activities were confined to caring for the children and household duties.

During intake she avoided eye contact, was sullen and passive, and had her head bowed, making no attempt to communicate. During hospitalization, she began to talk to a counselor about the long-term abuse.

Over three months, according to the record, Molly's mood changed from depression and withdrawal to focused rage at her husband. On the ward she began to talk directly to staff and other patients. No longer passive and depressed, she was angry, lively, and hopeful. At her exit examination, she talked openly of leaving him with plans to retain a lawyer to ensure child support. She said that without counseling, the thought that she could file for divorce would never have occurred to her.

In contact with a broader audience, her counselor and her hospital ward culture, Molly could notice her resentment and desire for a better life. Molly's shift in mood is key: moving from thought to implementation, requiring a series of audience-supported (validating) steps in insight and learning.

Public icons with similar problems can also become the audience, along with imaginary, fictional ones. The person sees a movie or comes across a new point of view on social media that resonates intensely. The possibility of broader realities beyond their daily experience can make an impression, even be earthshaking. Real people as audience is usually more effective, but when the need is intense and the availability of support for a range of experience is limited, books, movies, television, and social media can provide very valuable additions.

Cultural heroes who may seem inexplicable to chronological adults can have a profound impact on children and adolescents. For generations *The Rocky Horror Picture Show* inspired teenagers to dress up like the unusual characters in the movie and perform in front of the screen. They probably found validation in the possibility of a much broader range of portrayed emotional, gender, and sexual expression. Widening the range of people as audience expands an individual's repertoire of behavior, often beyond the framework of what is conceivable to their parenting one(s).

A person's audience can be someone immediately involved in the interaction, but often, as with voices in their head (see above), it is someone else historically or currently important to them, real or imaginary, without the person necessarily being aware of the audience itself (Pearce & Newton, 1963, p. 23).

Nancy, a freshman in a large, urban college, grew up in a small town, never meeting people of different races or nationalities. She is white, of western European descent. Her parents are equally limited in their contact with people of different races and nationalities, regarding them as dangerous and strange. Nancy initially avoids students her parental audience would find objectionable. Her suitemate in the dorm shares her xenophobic views.

> She perceives any friendly overtures by such "undesirables" as hostile, aggressive, or pushy. She barely tolerates prolonged contact in group projects and spends much time and effort figuring out how to maintain distance.

Nancy's perceptions are out of awareness, even though her thoughts are solidly in focal awareness. She does not necessarily think, "Oh, Mom would hate these people," although, if asked, she would confirm her mother's attitudes. She assumes her opinions stem from her own experience, maybe using her suitemate's opinions to back her up. She would probably be insulted if anyone suggested she was simply parroting her mother: "I can think for myself!" Daily facetime calls with her mother buttress her viewpoint, but she barely notices how often they talk. The impact is lost on her, even if a friend were to point it out. "Doesn't everybody call home as often as possible?" Her failure to notice the degree to which she relies on her mother's opinions exemplifies how much she dissociates.

Nancy's reliance on her mother's opinions would exist even if her mother were not so available. The crucial audience controlling her perceptions is in her head, *eidetic*; the calls reinforce her existing attachment to her mother's perceptual framework.

A shift in audience could change this picture. It requires an expansion of people she trusts.

> When Nancy's suitemate withdraws from college, Jill moves in. She has many qualities Nancy's parents would approve of. She could bring her home to visit. They become fast friends. There is only one difference. Jill is dating a Black student, John.
>
> When Jill invites John to their suite to study, Nancy thinks, "If Jill likes him, he can't be all that bad." She tentatively decides to hang out and discovers he is also an archeology major and hates the same professor. Having expanded her audience to a suitemate with a broader view of life, she can accept a friendly interaction with someone inconceivable to her original audience. Also, John is a bit more "acceptable" because they think alike. The expansion to a wider range of acceptable peers is gradual. If John were not studying something Nancy cared about, she would have had a lot more trouble accepting him.

However, at first that audience must also be conceivable in some fashion to the original authorities. To the degree their original parenting figure(s) distorts the potential new audience, the person will as well. The process is gradual. With enough new experience, it is possible for the individual to ultimately be receptive to an audience that is, in fact, inconceivable to the original one.

DEVELOPMENT OF CONSCIOUSNESS

Physiology, including vision, mobility, and speech, is modified by interaction with the environment. Any organ, including the brain and sensory organs, requires use to develop. Therefore, as experience is accumulated, consciousness, mediated by a developing central nervous system and sensory organs, also develops (Trevarthen, 2007). As with any other function, consciousness develops in the context of interpersonal interaction within the limits of physiology and parental acceptance. Since perception, communication, memory, and thought depend on the brain and the sense organs, they in turn develop in response to experience.

Initial Infantile Experience

Recent photo and video observations of mother-infant interactions show the infant's eager and purposeful behavior (Trevarthen, 2019b, p. 1, summarizing Nagy and Molnár 2004]).

> This attentive aiming of the baby's sense organs is imaginative and creative using the wisdom of a body feeling its movements intentionally. It is not reflexive, triggered and "conditioned" by stimuli. Thus a blind baby can look, a deaf baby can listen, making the required movements "as if" they had sight or hearing, expecting new experience. Books for parents with eloquent photographs show how rich infant sociability normally is in intimate communication. (Trevarthen, 2019b, p. 2, summarizing Nagy and Molnár [2004]; Nugent and Morell [2011])

The mode of communication associated with early infantile experience is empathy, the capacity to feel what another is feeling. The results of research in the 20th century point to the importance of close interpersonal connection between the infant and person(s) oriented to its care (Spitz, 1945, 1946a, 1946b). Since then, empathy has been demonstrated empirically in the work of Trevarthen and his associates (1979, 1993a).[6] More recently, considerable research has demonstrated a physiological basis for the existence of empathy (Goldman, 2006, p. 134).[7]

Interpersonal theory also posits that empathy continues to function throughout life, remaining a useful mode of communication (Pearce & Newton, 1963, p. 53).

Research demonstrates that purely mechanical attention to the infant's needs without tender and consistent human empathic physical contact is insufficient for their survival (Ribble, 1965). At this early stage of development, it doesn't matter who the caretaker is at any given moment, as long as they are empathically connected to the infant. The events of the external and internal environment of the infant—e.g., temperature, sound, proprioception, touch—are all mediated through the caretaker. However, initially there is no identification of an individual mother generalized over all experiences. When the infant is hungry, they experience "crying-when-hungry." An accurate response by a caretaker to crying-when-hungry produces the infant's experience of "nipple-in-lips," which relieves the tension of hunger. The provider of the nipple can be Mommy, Daddy, or Great Aunt Harriet. Gradually the infant begins to develop attachment to a specific person(s), who becomes "mother(s)."

The infant can adapt to varying levels of care, ease of handling, and accessibility of satisfaction, but key to the organization of perception in early infancy is parental anxiety, a mixture of disorganization, terror, and rage in the caretaker when pushed beyond the limits of their self-system in relation to the infant's needs.

Clinically, a therapist can infer from the person's current moods, dreams, areas of functional difficulty, perceptual-cognitive patterning, and memories what might have happened when early functions were developing in infancy. The person might also utilize one's own current empathic reactions to identify with what it must have been like. As discussed throughout this volume, it's always necessary to keep in mind the potential of subsequent validated experience to modify patterns established earlier in life.

Mood-memory

Because experience in early infancy is related to survival and satisfaction of basic physiological, perceptual-cognitive, and emotional needs, or the thwarting of them, infants intensely feel pleasure, satisfaction, euphoria, terror, and anxiety. In adulthood, the memory of early infantile experience can reappear as if from nowhere and in powerful form as mood-memory. The mood-memory can be negative or positive, replicating the actual experience in infancy. They can also be dredged up from slightly later experiences (past the age of four or five months) in the parataxic[8] when there is still very limited capacity to verbalize and limited ability to have conscious memory. They are pervasive, felt with all the senses, including the proprioceptive or muscle receptors.

Mood-memories provide the backdrop of everyday experience after infancy. Current experiences are often seen chronically in the context of an overall mood that a person experiences as reality. These powerful moods dredged up from infantile preverbal memories are often assumed to be simply a reaction to a current experience. Instead, a current experience that is more hopeful than what they are used to, challenging their self-system's status quo, may be triggering the mood-memory.

> Maddie grew up with an extremely isolated, dramatic, and fearful mother. As an adult, she experiences terror whenever she faces new opportunities; the mood is familiar and always lurks in the background. It particularly overwhelms her as she prepares to take a road trip from Miami to Key West with her dormmates. On the way they cross a multitude of seemingly endless low-lying and exquisite bridges, and she becomes overcome with terror about tumbling into the open ocean. Her mood is not intensified because of crossing the "dangerous" bridges. She associates her intensified mood to the "real" threat, but actually her terror is connected to the excitement of a new road trip with friends, dredged up to dampen the fun.

Mood-memories can be symptomatic of either expansion or constriction of consciousness. They can be dredged up intensely at crucial times to poison enthusiasm about a new experience or to head off anxiety caused by growth moves, with sharply experienced despair at a crucial moment in the form of waking nightmare states or actual nightmares, which can include intense dread and the visceral fear of dying.[9]

How the negative mood is used is often a matter of perspective. The nightmare state can be seen as an evil omen, a sign to go back to the old restrictions, or as a sign that one's familiar bugaboos are showing their ugly faces again and one must be on the right track in pursuing new horizons. The exploration of personal history can sometimes provide relief for an adult suffering from a pervasive mood that limits their life. Understanding the root of the mood, the mood-memory, is the beginning of a relearning process. Their take-away insight is that their security system is conjuring up ways to maintain the status quo:

> Whenever Rachel approached a milestone, such as another academic success, getting her own apartment, or having a boyfriend, she became convinced that she would fail or some disaster would befall her. She would be overcome with intense, inchoate fears. She tried to pin the terror she felt on current issues, such as lack of preparedness, the possibility that she might get pregnant, evicted, etc. As each milestone was passed, she forgot about her previous accomplishment and focused on the next step with dread.
>
> When she began to explore her history in therapy, Rachel began understanding that the terror and dread she repeatedly felt might be connected to her early chaotic experience with a paranoid and envious primary caretaker who resented her moves toward independence and mobility during much of her early life.

If Rachel were to share her pervasive dread with a friend, it could lose strength. If her friend has similar problems, the reciprocal exchange might help her question the validity of her own negative, self-limiting feelings.

Mood-memories are expressed most easily in artistic form, such as music, art, or poetry, as in the song "I Think It's Going to Rain Today" by Randy Newman:

> Broken windows and empty hallways
> A pale dead moon in the sky streaked with gray

Artistic expression through music, art, or poetry can be used to get in touch with a powerful mood-memory and harness it productively in a consensually validated context as a way of communicating hope and encouragement to other people, if it resonates with their own inner moods. Music composed during social upheavals that resonates with the mood of masses of people gives them hope and courage.

HIERARCHY OF PERCEPTION

To understand how experiences develop perceptions, it is first necessary to understand how sensations are organized into *patterns that become perceptions*. A sensation of warmth in combination with a soft, fluffy feeling against the skin becomes a baby's perception of *blanket*. Additions to perceptions of temperature and touch are the smell of the blanket and the person holding the baby, the sound of the mothering figure's voice and other sounds from the surrounding area, and a feeling of motion and pressure produced by the mothering figure holding the baby or the movement of the crib or rocker. The actual process is much more complex because there are so many phenomena in any given situation. However, the idea is the same: Perceptions are the combination and arrangement of sensations impinging on the infant in an interpersonal context.

The combination of sensations becomes perception when experienced repetitively in a particular pattern. The perception of being held by the mother-when-angry is very different from being held by the mother-when-tender, although both perceptions have many of the same sensations. Physiology is also involved. Perception is always mediated by one's own physiology and tied to interpersonal interactions with the significant other(s). When the baby is sick, being held by the tender mother is different from when they are sleepy and held by the tender mother; when the baby is fully attentive, the experience is different yet again, and so on.

In addition, sensations are organized in a hierarchical pattern of levels of awareness. Sensations are sorted out in terms of their *importance* in any given context.

> An illustrative exercise of how this works is to sit quietly for 30 seconds and afterward quickly write down as much as you can remember of what you experienced. You will notice the feel of the seat under you; hear the sound of traffic outside, the hum of the air conditioner, the sound of a distant airplane; feel the temperature against your skin and any minor sensations, such as itching, muscle pain, etc. If there are other people there, you might hear them breathing and moving. You may see your surroundings more vividly and completely, including light level, stray movements, and extraneous objects in your periphery.

The effect is like a recording with ambient sound. With no one sensation more important than another, the result is chaotic, with limited ability to focus attention on any particular aspect of the experience.

Organization of levels of awareness is essential to the development of coherent perceptions. If all sensations have the same importance, it is impossible to focus attention, to make sense of any given experience. The capacity for organization of thought and perception is rooted in the perceptual-cognitive apparatus of the human infant. However, since the infant learns to use that apparatus in an interpersonal context in interaction with the mothering figure(s), a major determinant of the importance of any given sensation is the perceptual-cognitive orientation of the caretaker(s).

What the caretaker experiences as important is important to the infant. If the caretaker is focused on the developing needs of the infant, the infant will be able to focus on developing needs more appropriately. If the caretaker is distracted or disorganized with relation to the infant's needs, the infant will experience the same distraction and disorganization in its relationship to its own needs. There will be distress due to the deprivation, but there will not be a clear experience of what the distress is about, especially since the caretaker is not clear about it.

If there is negative focus on certain aspects of the infant's biological behavior, such as drooling or defecating, the infant will also experience distaste or self-disgust when they perform these bodily functions. For any aspect of behavior, such as mood or activity level, the infant's response mirrors the caretaker's perceptions.

If the caretaker is unable to conceive of the development of certain functions in the infant, those functions do not appear in the infant's awareness. The function and related needs are dissociated. A major example is the aforementioned studies of foundling homes by René Spitz (1946a) and Margaret

Ribble (1965). The need of the infants in the foundling home for cuddling was not considered important, and the results were fatal.

Obviously, the human race has survived, and an infant thrives when the primary caretaker(s) is aware of the importance of the needs and related functions necessary for survival and later functioning. However, there are a range of needs and functions that may be only dimly perceived by the primary caretaker(s) as important. To the degree that a primary caretaker is unaware of the importance of a function, to that degree it will be experienced as unimportant by the developing infant.

Parataxic Experience

Parataxic experience in late infancy is more differentiated than early infantile experience. In parataxic experience, sensation and perception are linked together by frequency of contiguity. There is no logical explanation for why things happen, but they have always been that way. There are patterns attributed to authority, but not logically connected. For example, when asked why people should be careful when crossing a street, a young child's answer may be, "Because Mommy says so" or "Because you're supposed to."

Meaning is private and understandable between the child and the significant people *who comprise the audience for any particular meaning* because they are associated with parental moods.

Frequently the parental one(s) must act as translator(s) for children just beginning to talk. Words initially also have private meaning, only understandable to the parenting one(s), not found in the dictionary.

In parataxic experience there is awareness of a self experiencing the world and awareness of time, but the are not tied to logic or current experience. Awareness is tied to the early experience with the parenting one(s) and applied to the current experience regardless of accuracy of fit. Parataxic perceptions and parataxic thought operate in adulthood as if they are part of reality, but they are not communicable to others in a logical way. They are dependent upon an expectation of the world learned early in life before independent judgment is developed. One may retain restrictive formulations originating in the parataxic mode that are not consensually shared by others.

> Susan could never hear someone whistling without wincing a little bit. It was their mother's favorite way of cutting off discussion or argument. Any further attempt to protest was dangerous. Whistling has no intrinsic harshness, but they remember it in the context of the mother-when-angry.

Adult parataxic perception often occurs with authority figures, a supervisor or boss. If the parenting figure(s) were rigid and unforgiving, a supervisor in adult life might be experienced the same way. Despite many indications to the contrary, a person may treat them with the same blind obedience and deference required by the parenting one(s) and see and think of the supervisor as also rigid and unforgiving. The situation is particularly difficult when the supervisor is in fact rigid and unforgiving. The person is accurate in their perception, but the degree to which the current interaction paralyzes them has more to do with the original parenting one(s).

In therapy, the person might perceive their therapist as having the same characteristics as the parenting one(s), i.e., transference. Part of therapy involves analyzing transference. However, since that parataxic distortion is always much more widespread, it's often easier for the person to begin noticing parataxic distortions about other people before they notice it with their therapist. As discussed in chapter fourteen, analyzing parataxic distortions outside the therapeutic relationship is usually more useful than analyzing therapist–analysand transference.

Racism is a common parataxic mode of perception. Seeing another human being as less than human based on early learned beliefs involves linking qualities that have no causal connection. They were experienced that way by the early parenting figure(s). As discussed above, without later corrective experience, they continue to be connected in a person's consciousness.

Dramatization

Starting at about six months, speech is still parataxic and words are private expressions shared with the mothering figure(s), but the primary mode of communication is dramatization, the weaving together of posture, gesture, motion, tone of voice, manipulation of objects, and shared emotion in order to communicate. The primary use of words to convey needs and perceptions is not yet developed. Words are used for dramatic effect in dramatization. It does not disappear with the development of speech but provides a backdrop for speech. It does not appeal to cause and effect but seeks to provoke an emotional response in the immediate audience.

LEVELS OF AWARENESS AND THE FORMATION OF THE SELF-SYSTEM

Based on the interaction between the caretaker(s) and the late infant, there is a continuum of level of awareness ranging from clear focal awareness to complete dissociation. Part of this is essential for the ability to focus attention and to develop perceptual and conceptual thought. Another aspect of the continuum, however, is based on the perceptual limitations governed by the restrictive apparatus of the caretaker(s). There are those aspects of human functions that are experienced as inconceivable to the primary caretaker(s) because they were forbidden in their own life. If functions considered "wicked" can be experienced at all, they appear in the awareness of the caretaker(s) and infant as "bad." Functions are available to consciousness in a continuum ranging from complete dissociation to focal awareness. In the continuum of consciousness, there are three basic personifications: "good-me," "bad-me" and "not-me." There is a range of experiencing the self engaged in various functions that goes like this:

- *Good-me:* in focal awareness and experienced with pleasure.
- *Bad-me:* also in focal awareness but experienced with negative emotions such as shame, disgust, and dread.
- *Not-me:* not experienced consciously at all. Not-me is the totally dissociated aspect of the self that emerges only in dreams. It represents what the person experiences as inconceivable to do.

The emergence of "not-me" experiences into awareness later in life constitutes a severe disruption of the perceptual-cognitive apparatus of the self-system accompanied by intense feelings of discomfort and disorientation. A thought that is very antagonistic to the parental view can presage a treasonous break from them, which is an impossible situation for the child and continues to be terrifying through adulthood (Pearce & Newton, 1963, p. 23).

As discussed above, such a rupture can only happen when there are new and important relationships with people with a broader range of experience of what is possible. They become an additional audience that makes the new thinking conceivable.

Latent Awareness

Functions learned and integrated into the conscious repertoire do not remain in focal awareness but move into "latent awareness"[10] and are only used as needed. Once they reach this level of consciousness, the functions are not dissociated. They can be called into focal awareness without anxiety in a high-stress situation or under changed circumstances (Pearce & Newton, 1963, p. 31).

> Edward, in his late 30s, was making a transition from Atlanta to New York. He was a bartender earning an adequate living. When he was a teenager, he played the flute and achieved soloist status in his 20s. He gave up his career as a solo flautist at 25 because he found it too stressful, opting for a more secure and less demanding job as a bartender. However, by his late 30s he was thoroughly bored

> and decided to look for a more fulfilling occupation. He moved to New York to finish his college degree so he could qualify for more interesting work.
>
> Because Edward had moved to a new location, he needed a way to find new friends. He finally decided to try out for a position in an amateur orchestra. Much to his "dismay," he found that in practicing for the audition he recaptured his ability to play almost effortlessly. Compared to his original learning experience, relearning the flute took only a fraction of the time. He was soon a full-fledged member of the orchestra.

For Edward, the function of playing the flute was never dissociated or forbidden. Maybe other issues prevented him from pursuing his career as a soloist, but his skill as a flautist had been thoroughly validated, so it was relatively easy for him to resurrect his playing and to use it in a new, more inviting social context.

SYNTAXIC MODE OF COMMUNICATION

Syntaxic language is consensually validated, more widely accepted, standardized speech that enables communication within a wider range of people. Perceptions are organized with consensual validation and related causally, occurring in conjunction with and modified by broader interpersonal experience. They are subject to logical scrutiny that can be shared with others.

To varying degrees, a child entering nursery school without alternate validation doesn't speak intelligibly. As they move from the parataxic to the syntaxic, consensually validated mode of communication based on interaction with other children and teachers, they learn to speak so others can understand them.

Patrick Mullahy (1949) describes syntaxic communication as follows: "Acquired from group activities, interpersonal activities, social experience . . . consensually validated symbol activity involves an appeal to principles, which are accepted as true by the hearer" (p. xxxi).

Development of syntaxic speech starts in school, in the juvenile era, where there is a range of social contacts broader than available at home. A child in this society normally has increased social contact with other children and adults through school, but also through leisure activities, such as sports and other games. In order to function within a wider, more varied set of social contexts, the child develops the political arts of compromise, cooperation, and competition. Concomitantly, the development of speech and thought must expand to fit a wider range of social situations.

Children in the early grades are very concerned with pronunciation and word usage. Not wanting to be a baby implies the need to understand and be understood in order to participate. Children may become distressed if they realize that a word they have been using reliably is a baby word only understandable by their primary caretaker(s).

The ability to read becomes an important focus in part because it is important to the surrounding adults, the parenting one(s) and teachers. In addition to other forms of communication (social media, music, TV, movies), reading connects the child to alternate validators not present, not real, or not even necessarily alive but who provide a broader range of experience.

More in general, consensually validated (widely agreed upon) rules of engagement are formulated in this period. These include concepts of cause and effect and fairness, rules of engagement necessary for functioning with peers and authorities. These rules are a combination of previously accepted notions of right and wrong based on parental dictates and the dictates of other authorities such as teachers, coaches, or religious authorities, on the one hand, and principles developed in the context of working out interactions with peers on the other hand.

> Catherine, Donna, and Barbara, all nine years old, decide to play Monopoly. They are very concerned about winning and the rules of the game, and they are very strict about cheating. Barbara tries to take an extra turn. The other two tell her that she's out of the game if she does. Catherine's younger brother, six years old, asks to play, too. The girls let him play for 15 minutes, and during that time they let him take extra turns and cheat a lot. Then they kick him out. Barbara objects. The other two tell her they let him cheat because he's too young to know any better. The three girls argue about the issue for half an hour since they have differences about what is fair.

THE RELATIONSHIP BETWEEN COMMUNICATION AND PERCEPTION

Modes of communication develop in conjunction with modes of perception. However, more primitive modes of communication and perception remain in the human repertoire and continue to be used productively or restrictively throughout life, even after new modes are learned. A habitual way of communicating can indicate a developmental point of fixation.

> Anna was raised by very rigid and competitive parents. They had very high academic standards and Anna was punished severely if she didn't get the highest grades in her class. She was not allowed to "talk back" or question her parents in any way. The only way she could communicate was through dramatic gestures, such as pouting or having a tantrum. She got very high grades in school, for which she was lavishly praised by her parents. Anna was not allowed to

> socialize with other children or engage in "frivolous" activities with them. She quietly accepted her parents' view: her goal was to achieve, but not to enjoy.
>
> Anna became editor of a prestigious magazine. She was very competent but preoccupied with maintaining her position as if everyone around her were out to get her job. She felt vulnerable. She related to close associates as either above her or below her, maintaining a haughty attitude toward those she considered beneath her. She was careful to impress her own boss with her competence and brilliance. If she made a mistake, she covered it up. She was secretive about her thoughts and feelings. Everything she said or did was designed to impress or intimidate. She developed a reputation for cutting people down with a sneer or a snarl. Known for her temper tantrums, she thought nothing of berating and insulting her supervisees. Privately, she had crushes on glamorous celebrities and fictional characters and had fantasies about them. She had bouts of extreme loneliness from time to time but dismissed these as signs of weakness that should be suppressed and never shared.

Maintaining her frame of reference from her childhood, Anna's orientation to the world is parataxic and childlike. Peers are seen as authorities or underlings, defined in the mode in which she learned about people. She has learned enough about syntaxic speech to be able to function technically as an editor, but much of her communication is dramatic, designed to intimidate or impress rather than explain or share in words. Consistent with her childlike view of the world, Anna has some ability to communicate, or she would not be able to function, but that ability is delimited by her bullying behavior. Some aspects of her dramatic style are productive because she has skill evoking an emotional response in others, but much of it is restrictive because it maintains her isolation and prevents her from learning how to interact cooperatively and with more pleasure with others.

The example of Anna is a snapshot of a person's life. There is always the possibility for change, given new experiences. However, it is an example of how perception and communication go hand in hand at particular levels of development.

MEMORY AS AN ASPECT OF CONSCIOUSNESS

Memory is dynamic and changes with the available audience, and it is subject to the same restrictions and distortions as consciousness in the present and modified by the restrictions of the self-system.

In therapy or in any new expansive relationship, a person explores not only what went wrong in one's life but also what went right, including what may have seemed impossible to work on until the new, more hopeful audience emerged. New memories surface from dissociation as needed.

As confidence in one's new potential expands, so do memories, often emerging as if they have always been there when the person's life has changed enough to make them accessible, which may coincide with a new therapeutic or life project or after integrating a new function.

> Katherine's presenting problem in therapy was her isolation. She grew up an "army brat" in bases all over the country and was never in the same school for more than a year, making it difficult for her to keep in consciousness the friendships she did make. Since her parents fought constantly and her mother was an alcoholic, she was also embarrassed to invite friends to her home. She didn't remember any close friends.
>
> During therapy, Katherine worked on making consistent friendships and began to engage in numerous social activities, which dramatically reduced her isolation. She began to remember that as a child she had in fact made friends with children who had more tolerance for her parents' problems since they had problems in their own homes. She also described more positive social group experiences from childhood and adolescence. She reported the more hopeful memories about friends as if she had always known them, which she did, but not consciously.

Memory can also become more restricted. An adult offspring may confront their parenting one with an early memory of them that they, because of their own upbringing and perhaps embarrassment, emphatically deny. With increased depression or emotional deterioration, memories and opportunities of happier times may fade. People can confabulate or change memory to fit current self-image.

Earliest Memories

Earliest memories of specific events of childhood are often confabulated, condensed, or otherwise modified. But they are still useful as symbolic expressions of one's current self-image. In legal interrogation, it is important to substantiate the factual reality of an event for various purposes. In psychotherapy, the person's view of oneself and one's interactions with others are central. The therapist is taking a history of the person's self-system, which includes how the person views the world. It is a given that the person's memory of their history will change as their current experience changes. If a person does not have a clear memory about an early event, it is sometimes useful to ask the person to "make it up." While not necessarily factually accurate, the person's imagining is likely to fit the reality of the history *as it seems* to the person.

SUMMARY

Cognition has many facets and develops in the context of the self-system. Human relationships are key to development of cognition in relation to an audience starting in early infancy, when the role of empathy is paramount. Anxiety occurs with disruption of the relationship between infant and primary caretaker(s), impacting cognition by selective inattention and substitution. Symbolism and foresight are involved in the process of learning; alternate validation is required for growth of perceptual development beyond the self-system of the parenting one(s).

Consciousness and communication progress from prototaxic to parataxic and finally to syntaxic mode. Mood-memory, originating in early infancy, is an ongoing aspect of personality that continues throughout life with varying degrees of impact dependent upon later experience.

Finally, throughout life the cognitive systems of perception, communication, memory, and consciousness continue to interact within an interpersonal context.

NOTES

1. Awareness of the position of one's body mediated by sensory neurons in the inner ear, muscles ,and ligaments.

2. Also see Nagy (2011).

3. For a comprehensive review of empirical research in infantile perceptual-cognitive development, see Cohen and Cashon (2003). For further elaboration of empirical research on infant cognition, see Trevarthen (2011a, 2011b, 2019a, 2019b) and Damasio (2018). Also see Buck (1984), Duncan & Fiske (1977), Eibl-Eibesfeldt (1989), Kendon (1980), Stern, D. N. (1994, 2018), and Trevarthen (2006).

4. "Somnolent detachment" in this context is a term introduced by Sullivan (1953, p. 57) for a type of security operation in which a person falls asleep when confronted by a highly threatening, anxiety-producing experience. The mechanism originates in infancy.

5. Sullivan (1953) uses the terminology "good mother" and "bad mother" to formulate in simple terms the infant's unverbalized or felt experience of whether a primary caretaker is satisfying or forbidding around a particular need (pp. 85–91). See also Pearce and Newton (1963, p. 82). These terms are not meant to denote the moral issue of "good" and "bad."

6. Trevarthen and his associates use the term "intersubjective sympathy" for empathy (personal correspondence, 2018).

7. See also Blakeslee (2006), Gallese (2005), and Rifkin (2010, p. 83).

8. In the parataxic experience of later infancy, sensation and perception are linked by frequency of contiguity. There is no logical explanation for why things happen as they do; they are expected because they have always been that way.

9. At that moment, the original fear of losing the vital connection with the primary caretaker(s) can be viscerally intense. See discussions of anxiety in chapters one, nine, and fourteen.

10. The use of the word "latent" is not the same as the Freudian concept of "latency," which describes, as a normal aspect of development in childhood, a period of reduced sexuality.

Chapter Twelve

The (Essential) Interpersonal Context of Learning

Functions are operations that satisfy needs. Learning is the process of developing functions, requiring validation in its initiation and progression. The quality of validation determines a function's proficiency to satisfy a need (Pearce & Newton, 1963, pp. 27–32).

Learning is popularly defined as the conscious cognitive integration of knowledge and skills. People learn cause and effect, language and motor skills, the three "Rs" (reading, 'riting, and 'rithmetic), memorizing, test-taking, advanced reasoning, artistic facility, and social skills, "how to behave" within the rules of a particular society. However, learning also occurs *not* in cognitive awareness starting from *at least* birth.[1] Every aspect of the neonate's and infant's development is dependent upon tender cooperation from primary caretaker(s).[2] Without cooperation and validation by the caretaker(s) responsible for the infant's very survival, they fail to learn and eventually can fail to thrive (Spitz, 1946a). Very early essential bodily capacities developing outside cognitive awareness require a comfortable, validating interpersonal environment to learn how to function smoothly. Organs learn what to do. A calm, attentive caretaker(s) during feeding along with comfortable patting and burping validate healthy development of the gastrointestinal system. Consistently uncomfortable feeding experiences can compromise development of the gastrointestinal system and manifest, for example, as chronic colic; the adult might develop stomach ulcers or chronic indigestion.[3]

Skin integrity is the capacity to respond effortlessly and accurately to tactile stimuli. The skin, also an organ, requires empathic cooperative primary caretaking to learn what it needs to do. It requires consistent tender caressing and cuddling, along with the caretaker(s)' capacity to respond appropriately when the infant's skin is too hot, too cold, or chafed. Skin can learn to function from consistently anxious cuddling but may respond to later physical intimacy with a rash or "the itches."[4] In periods of high anxiety, the person may be more vulnerable to skin-related conditions.

In addition to learning out of awareness, *conscious* learning beyond early infancy, defined as expansion of the self-system, requires validation by those who matter most. When they play "peek-a boo," the baby learns "permanency of object" (Piaget & Inhelder, 1969). Consistently enthusiastic response to the child's pleasure upon seeing another child or a tiny dog goes a long way in validating that the world is wonderful and friendly. Early playful exposure to colorful cloth books validates curiosity about artistic representations of things they see outside in the stroller.[5] The toddler also requires caretakers comfortable with exploration of what's around—for example, the manipulation of objects, such as playing with finger food—to learn how the physical world works. In a validating environment, the young child is the consummate experimental scientist and explorer.[6]

EXPANDING THE ROSTER OF VALIDATORS

When the earliest primary caretaker(s) approves others, siblings, an extended family member, close friends, godparent(s) and/or babysitters, the infant incorporates, to varying degrees of comfort, whatever that small circle of important people validates. If the primary caretaker(s) can validate comfort with people beyond this relatively small interpersonal circle in the child's very early life, the roster of important validators increases, even more learning can occur, and the self-system expands.

Especially during preschool years, original validators expand that roster of important people with, for example, a new babysitter, play dates, daycare, playground time, outings with friends and their children, chats with cashiers and neighbors, hosting a lunch (whether or not the other adults bring children, but better if they do), extended family gatherings (especially if other children are running around), or extension of the child's bedtime to hang with adults at an evening social gathering. To the extent that the original loved ones enjoy other adults and children, the child enjoys them as well. When they start school, they will be able to accept more validators. To the extent the primary caretaker(s) is isolated or suffers from social anxiety, they cannot effectively validate expansion of the child's roster of validators.

Accepting peer and adult validators beyond the immediate nuclear or extended family when the child enters school is crucial to expanding the roster and therefore also crucial to learning skills beyond those earlier validated. The child who has developed anxiety around carefree jumping and hopping before starting school might learn to have more fun with these skills in the schoolyard with others who are encouraging them. But this is not possible if capacity to experience comfort with people outside the nuclear or extended family was strenuously discouraged earlier. Nevertheless, peer pressure and/or a very empathic paraprofessional educator or teacher might win the child over and help them play more comfortably.

Validators are necessary in every developmental era to grow one's personality. They may be real people, on TV (even a cartoon character), on the internet, in books, in movies, or imagined (in fantasy, based on earlier experiences with validators), but children must be at least marginally open to them.

The bottom line: learning requires a positive or somewhat positive audience of significance to the learner. Beyond the first small circle of significant others, the child requires other "sponsors" who are "at least partially acceptable to the people who are *already important* to the individual" (Pearce & Newton, 1963, p. 33 [emphasis added]).

LEARNING BY IMITATION

Children also learn from modeling. The child responds to the primary caretaker(s)' mood. If the adult(s) enjoys hanging out, having friends feels good to the child. If they are excited about the child's pleasure playing with or alongside other children, playing in the presence of peers is fun. If the adult(s) enjoys learning new things (without strenuously pushing that "virtue" on the child), chances are the child enjoys it too. On the other hand, children can learn dysfunctional methods of solving problems, such as violence, drugs, or excessive eating. A close relative or an acceptable neighbor might validate another way to cope. In adulthood, it may take committed membership in a support group such as Alcoholics Anonymous, Narcotics Anonymous, or Overeaters Anonymous and a very validating relationship with a sponsor to shed the unfortunate influence of the original validator(s). It may take moving heaven and hell to get them to join such a group, but with enough encouragement from friends and/or a therapist, once they allow these new validators in, the learning shift can occur (usually not without intense reorganization of the self-system because the original validators are subject to being toppled from their stature or actually replaced).

The child also learns how to treat people. Corporal or verbal abuse teaches them to mimic that behavior, perhaps not against those they fear at home, but against a younger sibling or kids on the school bus. If the primary validator(s) consistently criticizes the child and/or others, the child may learn to demean themselves and others. If the child witnesses parental fights (even behind closed doors—children are much more empathic than adults realize) or one parenting one is contemptuous of the other (in mood or actual behaviors), they might learn that close adult relationships are supposed to be like that.

LEARNING BY COMPETITION, DESIRE TO BE ADMIRED, OR TO GET AHEAD

Competition starting in the juvenile era (or even earlier) can spur greater mastery of a skill. The work is attached to what others are doing and the desire to match or surpass them. In that sense the others are validators because they reside in the person's mind as mastery is practiced. In addition, people can be motivated by the desire for admiration by significant others: the team, coach, fans, colleagues, supervisors. Not unrelated is the desire to hone skills to secure a better job, promotion, or raise. Even if the conscious motivation to learn or master skills is to "beat out" the competition, debase a colleague, or prove a supervisor wrong, people might use previous and/or current positive validators to rise above perceived or actual negative interpersonal interactions in the present. Then there is "cutthroat" competition, seeing someone as the enemy who must be beaten instead of emulated. The cutthroat orientation still allows for learning, but it creates social distance and isolation instead of joy in matching one's skills with someone the person admires. There is no camaraderie.

ROTE LEARNING

Rote learning usually starts in the classroom, although preschool children are often taught, for example, to recognize colors and name things. Some already know how to recite the alphabet or how to read using flashcards, iPads, etc.

Learning essential skills via rote recitation or memorization is crucial. People cannot just depend upon logic to solve equations, for example. They must know basic algebraic rules. Likewise, metal sculptors create new forms when free from artistic "rules," but they require skills and safety precautions while soldering.[7] However, learning *simply* by rote potentially skips over steps of true understanding. Young children who master concepts of volumes and quantities in the sandbox by trial, error, and discovery are apt to have a deeper understanding of physics and mathematics later on (Piaget & Inhelder, 1969).[8]

BREAKING DOWN THE LEARNING PROCESS

Given an optimum interpersonal environment, learning useful skills takes place as follows.

People acquire information and experience in day-to-day life and engage in practice. It takes place in a relatively permissive and responsive environment, and with a sharpened level of awareness. It can include trial and error. Then the learning integrates, generally occurring outside of focal awareness, without distractions.

Expansion of an acquired capacity is exponential. A comfortable early integration of a capacity can build upon itself, the way a blastula doubles and then doubles again in the womb. "It spreads out over the course of a lifetime in a fanlike direction, to include more specific and more elaborate functions" (Pearce & Newton, 1963, p. 29).

If there is some interference with early leaning, a skew can manifest later. A child who develops a minor disability while learning to walk may have trouble when learning how to run (Pearce & Newton, 1963, p. 29).

Development of functions occurs in an orderly sequence. If a parenting one is determined that the child learn to walk before they are physiologically ready, the necessary mastering of crawling and pushing oneself up to stand may not become fully consolidated. Walking may develop with a skew, such as falling more frequently when learning how to run or not trusting oneself to learn bicycle riding. If a primary caretaker pushes the toddler to pronounce words correctly before they have muscles to skillfully articulate, talking later in the classroom might be accompanied with reticence and anxiety, even with stammering, especially under stress, when called upon to recite in front of the class.[9]

Earlier functions are not forgotten, although they may reside outside of conscious awareness, in marginal awareness. They can be called upon in specific situations. For example, early preverbal or partially verbal communication is achieved through dramatization. Most people are capable of resurrecting the dramatic when needed. This function is not less mature; it is appropriate for specific situations.

Once past early infancy, learning new functions takes place in three phases (Pearce & Newton 1963, pp. 30–31).

First, in marginal awareness, one prepares, figures out what other relevant functions are already learned and what might get in the way. An adult deciding to take a figure-drawing class might marginally think about earlier art classes, perhaps in elementary school. They might review previous comfort about learning alongside other people, including receiving and learning from criticism.

Then comes practice. Having decided to take the class, the adult, perhaps with some anxiety, but also perhaps with gusto, reworks a rudimentary skill until mastery, like a child learning to hop practices for days. The validator may disappear for a while, but practicing can go on with the memory of them.

The last phase involves insight. Reorganization outside of focal awareness has occurred, after which they consciously recognize that they have learned the function, even if only rudiments have been mastered. Validation from a significant other, an "immediate audience" (not necessarily the original one), is required to firmly place the function in focal awareness. (Pearce & Newton, 1963, pp. 31–32).

Since the final phase of learning involves consciousness and a validator of importance, the self-system's acceptance of the learning is limited by what is conceivable to the validator. A very young child's roster of significant validators is usually small. If the child who finally learns how to hop tries to show off this new skill to a fearful or envious significant adult, the function, at whatever level of proficiency they attained while practicing, might not stick, might stick with intense anxiety, or may be relegated to the integral personality to wait for more favorable validators later. Acceptance may occur later in the schoolyard, where the original validators are temporarily replaced, or in adulthood, when they "risk" taking a dance class because of medical necessity, inspiration, curiosity, and/or peer pressure.

Once a function is learned, the elaboration of that function does not require further *direct* validation. The original validator, consciously remembered or not, generally powers the elaboration (Pearce & Newton, 1963, p. 32). If the child's parenting one(s) enjoys taking them to fun art galleries or posts their first scribbles on Instagram or on the refrigerator, a love of art (perhaps even pursuing art as a career), learned though the empathic connection with the parenting one(s)' self-systems and through imitation, continues into adulthood whether or not the parenting one(s) is present. If a primary caretaker enjoys a particular skill but has been frustrated from pursuing it, parental envy[10] can muddle the child's comfortable elaboration of that skill. For example, a parent is a very talented and exquisite vocalist, but they only sing in the shower and in the church choir. For economic and other extenuating circumstances (possibly including their own upbringing), they end up becoming a struggling single parent making a living in an unsatisfying, low-paying job unrelated to music. The child hones the skill of singing, loving it just like their parent, but has trouble pursuing a career in it.

> An adolescent with a promising voice is discovered by his high school music teacher, who encourages him to apply for a scholarship to a music conservatory in another city. The mother, having never fulfilled her own dreams, unconsciously finds it difficult to approve this opportunity. She even criticizes the teen when he solos in the senior play. The teen ends up commuting from home to the local college and drops singing altogether.[11]

A person can learn a function and misuse it to limit life; the self-system uses the function in the service of security operations (Pearce & Newton, 1963, p. 28). For example, the early infancy function of ingestion is essential, but overeating can seriously impede growth, socially and physiologically. Childen learn to sort objects into categories, and mastery of that skill is useful thoughout life, but over-preoccupation with making sure everything is put neatly in its proper place can interfere with everyday living.

LEARNING WHILE ANXIOUS

When the significant validator(s) is not comfortable with the child's learning projects in a given developmental era, that learning occurs with a skew, leaning in one direction or another (much like a tree that leans this way and that depending upon the quality and quantity of sunlight, water, etc.). The degree of skew depends upon the degree of anxiety at the time of learning in the presence of the significant other(s).

For example, an infant begins exploring their body by touching their genitals, to the anxious horror of their primary caretaker. They may continue to touch, but clandestinely and with anxiety. (Such an unfortunate interaction must be repeated for the baby to learn that exploration of its body should be secret and with misgivings.) Later, they might still be anxious around touching themself or another. Their pleasure might be fraught with guilt.

If the primary caretaker's anxiety is very intense, the baby may eventually avoid such exploration altogether. The need for self-exploration and exchange of tenderness involved in cuddling with and touching someone else doesn't go away but presses for satisfaction—in this case, often emerging in puberty with tremendous anxiety couched as guilt, self-revulsion, or disgust at and/or fear of another person's need for tenderness.

Integration of pleasurable peer interaction is closely tied to the comfort of the primary validators with their own and the child's peers, in addition to the child's access to situations allowing for such interactions. If primary validators allow access to others, but tend to interact with suspicion, the child may also be suspicious. In adulthood their interactions in the workplace might be tinged to varying degrees by inaccurate suspicions of colleagues, hampering or skewing interaction. This skew might be mitigated if the child observes alternate validators relating more freely with others.

As the person matures, more people can become important additions to their audience; the original validators can have less influence over comfortably learning a new function. The learning projects of each developmental era and how validators help or hinder the consolidation of such learning are discussed in relevant chapters.

Finally, the repeated use of a previously integrated function occurs when the next level of functioning has not been comfortably learned. The person perseverates on the last validated function. For example, a person has difficulty getting thoughts into words understandable by the world beyond their primary audience. They may, instead, heavily rely on dramatization of needs, a mode of communication developed during late infancy. As adults, they may use words dramatically, but not precisely, to communicate ideas.

ACADEMIC LEARNING

Validation required for comfortable and successful learning must occur well before the child's first day in school. In addition, they need to feel somewhat comfortable spending extended periods of time outside the purview of their significant parenting one(s) and to be somewhat comfortable with peers and alternative adult authority figures. They also must have some confidence that learning new skills is possible. A toddler, for example, whose exploration of their environment evokes a response of, "No! Don't touch that!" because of poor toddler-proofing may be fearful exploring nursery school blocks. A child dutifully trained to never touch things belonging to others may have difficulty playing with nursery school toys. New learning experiences can be fraught with apprehension.

In short, when the self-system goes to school, it welcomes opportunities to the extent that it is prepared to make use of them. In a new validating environment, the self-system has the possibility of expanding, even if it stumbles with anxiety along the way. But comfort with people beyond the parenting one(s) is crucial. The worst-case scenario is homeschooling, unless it includes significant interactions with other peers and adults.

Outcomes are varied when a parenting one helps with homework. Learning a particular topic is less relevant than the helper's attitude or mood, regardless of how much the adult knows about the topic. In the best of interpersonal homework help, the adult is curious and encouraging; if the adult does not know a skill, they learn with the child. Positive validation of the child's capacity to master skills promotes the possibility of learning and consolidating them. Hard-hitting criticism, frustration, emphasis on "being the best," rage, threats, apathy, etc., do not carry the day.

Parental envy that is out of awareness and not deliberate hampers the learning experience. If adults experienced discouragement in their own homework years or other deleterious situations such as economic hardship or strenuous household distractions, it can become more difficult to validate positive academic learning. They might be extremely motivated to ensure their child never has to endure similar obstacles. But since envy is out of awareness, the outward parental preoccupation that the child achieve only top grades can have the opposite effect. If they are punished for less-than-perfect grades, they can become fearful in school, hide or change report cards, bury a test that scores a 98 instead of 100, cheat on tests, or plagiarize from the internet, rather than face parental wrath. They might think, "What's the use? I get punished, no matter how hard I try," and simply give up. Another form of parental envy is manifested in comments such as, "I didn't have it as easy as you do" or "I always did poorly in school." The hidden envious message can be, "Don't outdo me; I'll feel inadequate." If a child performs much better in school than the parenting one(s) did, responses might be "Don't boast," "Who else in your class got an A?" or "Who got an A-plus, and why didn't you?" All come at the expense of comfortable learning.

The overly strenuous push for the child to excel in school might not originate from parental envy, but simply from parenting one(s) desperately wanting their child to be the best in an overly competitive, classist, and racist society. The fallout might be that the child becomes isolated, a "geek," or a "bookworm" ("You can't go out and play with the others; you have to do your homework right now") and does not acquire adequate interpersonal skills. Or the child rebels altogether, forever a source of embarrassment to, say, academically and professionally successful parenting one(s).

Sometimes household children are compared to each other. Ranking children can profoundly affect comfortable learning. As discussed below, sometimes children assigned male at birth (AMAB) are favored and encouraged more than those assigned female (AFAB).

Optimally, older children in the household can validate the learning of younger ones, not only by enthusiastically paving the way for them to start school, but by generously helping with homework. It's up to the adults to provide a physical and emotional atmosphere for all this to occur.

SEXISM, CLASSISM, AND RACISM: THE LARGER INTERPERSONAL SPHERE

Although attitudes have changed regarding female academic, professional, and vocational achievement, sexism can still play a significant role in the quality of validation within a household and community. The parenting one(s) might even unwittingly choose toys, activities, afterschool classes, computer games, and books for their children based on gender. Boys might be groomed for the breadwinner role, girls for keeping house and raising children. When young girls attend school, sexist attitudes about what should be emphasized and validated still persist in some communities; high school and college students are potentially influenced about what courses to take, where they should apply to college (or even if they should go to college), and what major to choose based on attitudes of teachers and guidance counselors toward gender, class, and race. As with classism and racism, the availability of role models is essential. If a woman-identified parenting one has put aside her own aspirations, there may be unconscious envy if her AFAB offspring strives for more than she was able to allow for herself.

Other biased attitudes at home, in the community and school can also adversely affect how people learn and what they aspire to, including those who are silently or overtly LGBTQIA+. Furthermore, people learn at different rates and in different ways. Their skills might be overlooked if they are, for example, poor test-takers or have disabilities. Parenting ones, teachers, and administrators must validate all under their charge.

During enslavement in the United States, it was dangerous, if not lethal, for enslaved people to learn how to read. Now classism and racism, but primarily racism, are responsible for excruciatingly substandard housing, homelessness, and woefully underfunded schools, severely compromising successful academic learning. When social conditions change for the better, overall academic learning tends to improve.[12] Even if a person does overcome strenuous odds and succeeds academically, opportunities for well-paying jobs (or for jobs at all) are increasingly limited.[13] This topic is beyond the scope of this book, except to say that more people are managing to develop political perspectives, harnessing their intelligence (not necessarily and not always expanded though traditional schooling) to push past the current society's limitations.

The SEEK (Search for Education, Elevation and Knowledge) program and the study group that grew out of it at the City College of New York are an example of how people pushed past those social limitations. During the 1960s Civil Rights Movement, people struggled to win more academic opportunities. The SEEK program was developed for youth whose high school averages didn't qualify them for admission to college (Malloy, 2016). It was organized around awareness that young people whose intelligence had not been recognized and encouraged for whatever reasons (including racism and classism), in school and/or at home, required validation from counselors, teachers, and peers. In addition to receiving stipends for attending, the program opened dorms for students requiring a different interpersonal living environment.

The SEEK English department developed a curriculum for students in the first-level "pre-baccalaureate" writing course that recognized the need for on-the-spot interpersonal validation. The classes were longer than usual; no one brought homework home (mainly because some home environments, particularly those that were crowded and demanding of the students' attention, were not conducive to concentrated learning); student tutors and a teacher circulated through the class to help students with writing; they taught students to trust their thinking and to write freely first and edit later using classroom lessons. Students completing this persistently validating one-semester course performed significantly better on final writing exams than students who completed two semesters of traditional freshman composition (Malloy, 2016, pp. 243–244, 508).

Out of this paradigm came the study group (Malloy, 2016, p. 511), a kind of "failure anonymous" group for students (SEEK and non-SEEK) on "academic probation." Students met in small clusters with a teacher/counselor trained to run support groups. They were taught three types of study, all of which assumed that validation was required for success:

- *Parallel Study:* The students studied silently in the same non-distracting environment with other peers (similar to childhood parallel play). They took breaks together and exchanged ideas. They also found ways to replicate parallel studying outside the group, such as in the library, the cafeteria, or a coffee shop, checking in by phone with a "study partner."
- *Supportive Study:* If a student had to study alone, they checked in by phone with a peer to report how it was going, even if that peer was not studying.
- *Cooperative Study:* To complete a writing assignment, two (or more) students asked the writer questions about their topic, writing or recording their answers to produce a rough draft. During the "talking it out" phase, the writer was encouraged not to worry about organization, grammar, or "saying it right"—just to think out loud. Then the writer rewrote the rough draft, perhaps with tutorial assistance.

For other kinds of studying, say, for an exam, the student gave another student a list of questions—often from study questions at the end of a chapter. The other did not need to know the topic, just to be there with questions, providing a positive audience for formulating correct answers. Another scenario: students studied in a group for the same exam, each becoming an "expert" on a chapter or topic and teaching the others, who asked questions and discussed. Peer pressure forced them to be prepared. Graduate students preparing for comprehensive exams often use this tried-and-true method.[14]

Students on academic probation experienced validation for the learning process. Students who were used to getting Ds and Fs were suddenly getting As and Bs (Malloy, 2016, p. 511).

Leaders of the study groups for students on academic probation were trained and aware of what happens to people when their self-systems are challenged.[15] Some students become extremely anxious as the process succeeds. Individual and group counseling is required to help them understand where their anxiety is coming from. They learn to combat the "undertow" when things are going right and, to reduce anxiety, they are inclined to return to old ways. They do not need to know the technical intricacies of how the self-system operates, but they do need to understand about pushing boundaries beyond their "comfort zone." Students may need to be gently guided though explorations of their childhood histories and current living situations.[16] When the study group model was first getting off the ground, some group leaders were not aware of what can happen when the self-system is challenged too quickly. One student, just about to fail out of college, earned an A on a paper using validation methods described above. One day he was jubilant, having never earned higher than a D or F. The next day his self-system repudiated, his "undertow" took over: he quit college to join the army and was ultimately shipped out to Vietnam. It was urgent that the group leaders understood the degree of anxiety such a leap in accomplishment can create and how to include that insight in their groupwork.

SUMMARY

Interpersonal validation is essential for learning. The embryo, neonate, and infant require validation in order to thrive. The individual's self-system incorporates learning under the influence of their primary caretaker(s)' self-system(s). Expansion of the roster of important validators is essential if the individual is to recognize and use opportunities to integrate functions beyond the purview of the original primary caretaker(s)' own self-systems. Since quality of validation is on a continuum, the learning process is extremely complex. In addition to environmental (including natural and human-made) catastrophes and physiological and genetic issues faced by people with disabilities, the interpersonal milieu contributes to the quality of learning: the immediate and extended family, the school, the playground, the neighborhood, the community, books, movies, TV, the internet, social media, famous people, socio-economic conditions, racism, classism, wars, displacement, holocausts/diasporas, pandemics—the list is infinite. The learning and the ever-changing brain is not "hardwired." Given validating opportunities, "late bloomers" do bloom. People revisit and hone poorly consolidated skills if opportunities for alternate positive validators arise later in life—but only to the extent that they are open to those alternate validators.

NOTES

1. The physiological and concomitant emotional environment within the womb along with stimulation such as music from outside the womb are responsible for how the fetus develops. Smoking or alcohol during pregnancy are examples of chemical interference.

2. People can also be born with organic weaknesses such as susceptibility to digestive dysfunction. Primary caretaker responses can exacerbate or mitigate innate or genetic physiological weaknesses. When a caretaker is upset, worried, and exhausted in response to a chronically colicky infant who incessantly cries, unfortunate interactions can occur. These interactions can be synergistic. Some infants are born with serious and debilitating physiological dysfunctions, such as cerebral palsy or blindness. Caretaker empathic, cherishing support of the infant and their struggles is crucial in helping them grow, thrive, and successfully navigate life in spite of limitations. A classic example is the interaction between Helen Keller and her educator, Anne Sullivan (Keller, 1903).

3. Validation and the infant's learned response to it are on a continuum. From the beginning, the *quality* of validation determines the relative comfort of unconscious learning, from total expansion of function to its not being able to expand at all. For learning to occur, validation must consist of accurate and timely responses to the infant's need for tenderness.

4. The problem could be further exacerbated if no alternative, more comfortable validator for cuddling is available.

5. "Enriched environments differ from the normal environment of a rat cage by providing the animal with playthings and opportunities for increased social interaction. As a result of the increased cognitive stimulation, the brains of animals raised in enriched environments are slightly larger. The implications for early childhood experience on human brain development are obvious" (Fields, 2009, loc. 4595, 2nd par.). "MRI scans show that the corpus callosum area is decreased 17 percent in children who suffered childhood neglect" (Fields, 2009, loc. 4633).

6. Some neurological research examines underlying chemistry in learning. Fields (2009) provides fascinating physiological substantiation: "By regulating the flow of information across a synapse, circuits can be strengthened or weakened, in effect allowing the circuits to change their behavior from experience—that is, *to learn*. Our memories are not bottled up inside neurons, but rather they are stored in the connections between neurons linked by synapses. With new experiences, new connections are made between neurons and others are lost" (loc. 416). "[B]rain wiring is directed by environmental experience, not simply defined by a genetic imprint" (loc. 3735). "[M]icroglia help us rewire our neural circuits to enable us to learn" (loc. 4329, 1st par). (Microglia are infection-fighting brain cells that Fields posits also function to help learning.)

7. Optimal learning occurs through a mixture of self-discovery and taught skills. A budding artist required to strictly follow the rules of "good" or "proper" art or behavior for the particular era they live in might not truly blossom, or they do so with significant struggle. Van Gogh studied the fundamentals before he broke with

tradition to develop his masterpieces. Unfortunately, his father disapproved of his son's "immoral" ways; ultimately he succumbed to his primary validator and committed suicide.

8. In an optimal learning environment, such as the Montessori classroom, the "teacher" validates spontaneity and provides guidance. See also Fields (2009, loc. 4595, last par.).

9. In discussing how one function is a prerequisite for the next, such as crawling is essential before walking, it is necessary to keep in mind how and to what extent the child's needs are met. A caretaker of a deaf child or a child born with cerebral palsy would benefit from an understanding of what all children need. Figuring out how to provide appropriate opportunities for the satisfaction of the needs of a child with disabilities or one born under the most unfortunate conditions, in most instances, depends mainly on who the caretakers are and what opportunities are or could be made available in a particular community or society.

10. Not consciously deliberate. See chapter thirteen.

11. This phenomenon is often characterized as "fear of failure," but it is usually "fear of success," i.e., fear of going beyond what is conceivable to the person's self-system, which has been constricted by parental envy.

12. For example, along with social improvements that were made in Cuba after the revolution, there was a comcomitant improvement in literacy and a much larger percentage of graduations from institutions of higher learning. Starting with the literacy program shortly after the revolution, which reduced illiteracy by 95 percent throughout the country, there are now so many doctors per capita that Cuba can send their doctors abroad to help others in crisis (Mercer, 2017).

In 1969, the Black Panthers, recognizing the need for children to have a healthy breakfast before going to school, organized the Free Breakfast for School Children Program, which was later replicated (with varying degrees of success and longevity) by federally funded programs. A person cannot learn on an empty stomach.

13. See, for example, Goldstein's *Capitalism at a Dead End* (2012).

14. The armed forces and NASA make excellent use of the collaborative process in crucial circumstances. See, for example, Noe et al. (2011). Writers of TV shows (particularly situation comedies) commonly brainstorm script development (Johnson & Stevens, 2003). While each member of the collaborative team brings expertise to the effort, the group experience can create an atmosphere that enhances everyone's skills. The product is better than if each person had submitted a proposal or script.

15. See chapter nine.

16. In the SEEK program, students had counselors and role models to help them with this struggle, which accounts for why that combination of validations succeeded as well as it did. See Malloy's in-depth discussion of the program, including myriad examples of how counseling and validation were crucial in its success (2016).

Chapter Thirteen

The Interpersonal Theory of Envy

Envy has its roots in the unsatisfied and often unconscious (unrecognized) needs of the envious person. For example, the envious person may unconsciously assume that liveliness, friends, competence, and/or intelligence are unobtainable. The envious person typically behaves unwittingly with some form of rejection of the other's behavior, such as disapproval, disparagement, discouragement, disgust, or dismissal. Or by not noticing, as Sullivan (1954) explains, by selectively "inattending" (p. 270) to the other person (or some particular aspect thereof).

> Nancy says to her co-worker Cora, "I had a great date last night!" Cora, seemingly spontaneously, responds, "Where should we have lunch today?"

Nancy's need for Cora to take pleasure in her experience and be curious about it is apparently ignored by Cora. Selective inattention was at work. Nancy's excitement was not ignored, but targeted. Cora was envious of Nancy and unconsciously intent on communicating to her what envy attempts to communicate: "If my need cannot be satisfied, then neither can yours." Envy is not experienced as envy. The experience is one of loathing, distaste, rejection, ridicule, or even indifference for the satisfaction the other has, or it isn't noticed at all. If confronted with wanting to undermine the other person's satisfaction, the envious person will deny it. Envy that is unchecked and largely unconscious is a powerful and disruptive force in all relationships. It moves against one's own personality growth and intimacy by further dissociating a need, thus severely interfering with the satisfaction of it. Possibly it moves against the satisfaction of the envied person's need, particularly when the other person requires validation in order to consolidate it.

A particularly damaging example of envy is *parental envy* of the infant or child because it occurs in the earliest stages of development and learning. The very young, vulnerable person is most susceptible to the influence of significant caretakers during this time when choices of people to relate to are severely limited and emotional patterning is developing. The child's experience is fundamentally negatively impacted. A depressed caretaker, for example, may experience the curiosity of an active, exploring two-year-old as threatening and annoying. The adult's own restrictive self-system does not allow for open curiosity, and therefore they cannot take pleasure in—i.e., validate—the child's investigation of the world. That would be too disruptive to the organization of the parenting one's personality. Instead, they may, for example, prohibit the infant's exploration of its body or discourage the child's friendliness toward strangers or interfere with the child's pleasure in mastering a project. The parental experience, unconscious, and not actually recognized, is, "I am being threatened." The restrictive aspect of the parenting one's self-system is, indeed, under attack by the *potential* awareness of dissociated need(s) stimulated by the behavior of the child and the anxiety that would accompany that newfound awareness.

Learning and development are synonymous in the earliest years of a child's life. Humans are a social species, dependent on the goodwill of significant adults to satisfy their innate needs of survival and growth. Therefore, the degree of parental envy directed at the child who is curious will significantly affect that child's learning/development.

If a parenting one is envious of a child's spontaneity and liveliness, they may respond with anger. For example, the toddler jumps into a muddy puddle while wearing new sneakers. As the parent abruptly yanks the playful child from the puddle, the child, sensing the parent's rage, learns that enjoying splashing around is "bad" and (if not corrected by alternate validation) may come to believe, "I am bad. Don't be playful and curious." Not only muddying the sneakers, but the overall spontaneity and liveliness of the child are perceived as bad. The adult caretaker(s)' envy of the child's needs seriously compromises their capacity to provide caring validation. They also lose the opportunity to learn from the child about needs of their own that were previously stunted. All adults have adapted to a mix of validating and prohibiting responses from their own early significant caretaker(s). Those prohibitive responses may have been based on parental envy they themselves experienced as children.

> Kay's mother was intolerant (unconsciously envious) of intense pleasure. With the help of her therapist, she recalls her aversion to her own child's intense pleasure when petting a dog for the first time, and how that stemmed from her own fear of intense pleasure, originating from her own mother's fear, resulting in her envious response to her child's pleasure.

To prevent a rupture in connectedness to a significant caretaker(s), the developing young person confronted with envy must dissociate the attacked need and the specific functions related to it. A very young person's life literally depends upon maintaining the relationship with a primary caretaker at all costs, even if they're envious. Later, with newfound validation, they may expand their self-system to include the satisfaction of that dissociated need. When that fortunate experience occurs, they become anxious and may reexperience prohibition from earlier envy: "This is wrong; this is embarrassing. I'm bad"—some form of repudiation of the need. If the person gives in, the need will retreat back into dissociation. However, a validating audience (friend, partner, or therapist) may make it possible for the need to remain in awareness and get satisfied, expanding the productive aspects of their self-system.

Needs colliding with parental envy will, until corrected through the expansion of experience and relatedness to a wider audience, continue to push for satisfaction from their dissociated state. Part of the very definition of a need is that it is ineradicable. It pushes into awareness for belated satisfaction, along with its related functions. The self-system expands. The satisfaction of a dissociated need is a struggle no matter when it occurs in life. That struggle is likely to unconsciously evoke the earlier threat of disconnectedness from the parenting one(s) along with the very unsettling, uncanny experiences of anxiety: personality disorganization and often dread.

Meaningful independence from parental control and restriction of growth of the self-system are, in large part, indicative of the increasingly independent and interdependent (with other peer adults) person moving to make up for the deficits rooted in early restrictions to growth, including those resulting from parental envy.

JEALOUSY VS. ENVY

Jealousy and envy are often used interchangeably in Western culture and perhaps in others.

Envy conceals extreme vulnerability to anxiety related to the envious person's unfulfilled need. The envious person is confronted with someone who has or does something they cannot consciously conceive of. They do not have the conscious thought that they want what the other has. The sole motive for envy is that the other person is satisfying a need of their own that the envious person has dissociated.

Jealousy is not about dissociated needs. It is a very complex and painful process usually involving a group of three or more persons, one or more of whom may be illusory (Sullivan, 1953, p. 348). The jealous person has a deep *conscious* conviction of their own inadequacy, which is painfully felt when, for example, a third person is perceived to be preferred by one's partner. This frequently occurs in adolescence involving real or imagined sexual activity, but jealousy may occur at any age from late infancy on.

> Eleven-year-old Claire believes that Sarah, her friend since first grade, is deliberately trying to upset her by sitting next to Sally in the lunchroom. Claire becomes jealous and stops speaking to Sarah, keeping secret her deep-seated belief that Sarah likes Sally better and that it was just a matter of time until Sarah "dumped" her.

A person can be jealous of another person because the other owns or is able to do something the jealous person consciously feels unable to attain. It could be anything: a new electronic device, an article of clothing, a trip, a new career, a life-partner.

The outcome is on a continuum from inspiration to have what the other one has to overt rage expressed in, for example, revenge or destruction of what the other person has. In some circumstances, jealousy becomes delusional and leads to violent behavior, such as a "crime of passion."

When jealousy becomes a source of inspiration, it is an opportunity to move past the feeling of something being unattainable. When a jealous person moves past their despair, anything is possible if they organize it: "If I want that badly enough, I'll figure out how to make it happen."

PART III

Practical Applications

Chapter Fourteen

Interpersonal Theory and Psychotherapy

> One achieves mental health to the extent that one becomes aware of one's interpersonal relations. (Sullivan, 1966, p. 207)[1]

Interpersonal psychotherapy's[2] goal is to reduce a person's difficulties in living that block need satisfaction, ensuring continued evolution and expansion of productive functioning via a therapeutic relationship (Pearce & Newton, 1963, pp. 439–440; Sullivan, 1953, p. 175).[3]

For Frieda Fromm-Reichmann (1960), the goal is

> alleviation of the patients' emotional difficulties in living and the elimination of the symptomatology, this goal to be reached by gaining insight into and understanding of the unconscious roots of patients' problems, the genetics and dynamics, on the part of both patient and psychiatrist, whereby such understanding and insight may frequently promote change in the dynamic structure of the patient's personality. (p. x)[4]

This process involves expanding awareness of one's needs and the limitations one has placed on satisfying them based on heretofore unexplored restrictive assumptions. It includes assessment of one's current functioning in light of their history, particularly their developmental interpersonal history. It involves learning how to deepen and expand one's interpersonal relationships for greater intimacy and satisfaction.

THE THERAPEUTIC ALLIANCE

No matter why a person initiates therapy, their therapist becomes a particularly safe and positive audience for growth, allying with their integral personality,[5] where unmet needs push for recognition. The therapeutic relationship is a very significant primary integration[6] in the person's life.[7] While different from others in its organization into discrete sessions without social interaction in between, it is nevertheless a loving one.[8] The therapeutic relationship establishes a positive audience, validating ever-expanding and deepening primary and near-primary integrations. When treatment terminates, the therapist usually continues to reside, without structured sessions, in the background as a positive audience. If the person later bumps into a particularly stubborn area of emerging need that painfully challenges their self-system, they might resume therapy for "booster shots" or for some assistance with a new project.

WHY THERAPY?

From the interpersonal point of view, many decide to pursue therapy because they are undergoing a powerful, often conflicting struggle about the possibilities for growth and change toward a more gratifying life. Their self-system is being impacted by their integral personality's push for change and their central paranoia's effort to maintain the status quo, both vying for influence over their self-system.[9] Pearce and Newton describe this battle as if there were two voices competing to be heard over one phone line. By the time the voices reach the self-system, some sort of compromise may occur so the self-system can handle, without too much reorganization, the dissociated needs pushing for change (Pearce & Newton, 1963, p. 426). How much compromise—which voice is more dominant when all is said and done—determines how much the integral personality has succeeded in moving the need into awareness in the self-system, as opposed to how much the central paranoia has mustered the self-system's security apparatus to weaken and lose (partially or entirely) this round of struggle. If the self-system's protective wall of security apparatus has been breached, the self-system can become unraveled while it struggles to reorganize itself to either partially or fully accept the new learning or shove it all back out of awareness to await another opportunity. The "unraveling" is experienced as anxiety, including disorganization plus some form of dread.

Many people seek therapy because they are or have recently been painfully experiencing the struggle and resultant disorganization of their self-system. They often fear they are going "crazy" because of the self-system's disorganization. Their lives might have changed in such a way that they are now aware (or partially aware) of issues they haven't addressed and want to confront. Self-system upheaval can occur during life changes, such as leaving home, getting a promotion, meeting new people, or reevaluating current relationships. It can be instigated by a person's hopeful action or thought but can be perceived as negative because of the anxiety that arises while trying to expand.

A person may also seek therapy under pressure from family, friends, or colleagues dismayed by their behavior, as a result of a court order, or because their spouse or partner threatens separation unless they seek professional help. Perhaps the person's behavior prompts others to notice their cry for help, including suicidal statements or attempts.

Sometimes an event motivates them to deal with a long-standing problem in living such as a phobia, recurring panic attacks, debilitating obsessive-compulsive behavior, chronic bouts of mania and depression, etc. Perhaps they finally have mental health insurance.

They might have recently come out or are about to initiate gender transition and need help dealing with people's actual or anticipated reactions.[10]

Even if a devastating crisis has motivated a person to look for a therapist, the purpose of therapy is to help them find ways to expand their personality to cope with the issue. The crisis might be bereavement, a frightening medical diagnosis of oneself or a loved one, a serious accident, rape, job loss, an imminent or actual break-up of a long-term relationship, recurring nightmares after returning, say, from a war zone, one too many alcoholic blackouts or almost overdosing from drugs—wake-up calls for help. The therapist addresses the impact of the crisis and helps them reorganize their life to continue with, initiate, or reinitiate their process of growing.

INITIAL SESSIONS

In the initial sessions,[11] the therapist strives to understand why the person has come. Their presenting problems are, to varying degrees of clarity and confusion, expressions of how they perceive what is going on and what they need help with. The person consciously views their problems through the lens of their self-system. The first order of business is to elicit that perception in words, if possible: "What brings you here?" Listening requires curiosity, which involves asking for elaboration of the issues and empathically listening "with the third ear" (Reik, 1949). There is also much to be gleaned from the emotional atmosphere in the room, including non-verbal cues. Despite the popularity (or necessity) of teletherapy, in-person interaction is optimal.

During this initial phase the therapist assesses the person's "mental status." There may be a need for immediate intervention, such as hospitalization for a person in clear and present danger of suicide or harming another.

The therapist forms initial hypotheses about the person's needs. For example, are the person's dissociated needs becoming more conscious? What resistance is evidenced in how the person wards off awareness of those needs? If the person encounters the forbidden/dissociated needs during a session, what is their reaction? Once the self-system has been breached, are they in a panic, terrified to allow anything to shift beyond the tiny whiff of possible change instigated by needs now pushing forward from the integral personality? Are they in a dread state, having been terrified by the self-system's disorganization as it tries to integrate a positive change? Are they convinced they will die if they don't get everything under control? Has their self-system become so unraveled, so disorganized that they have forgotten how to cross the street? Are they afraid their disorganization is so obvious that they'll become ostracized and isolated, lose their job, or be unable to take care of their children? Has a reaction to meeting a need emerging from the integral personality so flooded their self-system that their central paranoia's formulations have moved from a sleeping nightmare to a waking psychotic episode in which the person feels that aliens are invading their brain? Have they become listless, unmotivated, and, in essence, "on strike" in life, paralyzed with terror?

> John, 20, is a cashier in a fast-food restaurant. It's a dead-end job, but the only one he could find. He had managed to finish high school, but his grades were so poor that college was out of the question. One day, he woke up "in a fog" and felt as if his feet were made of lead. He managed to survive his workday, but on the way home, he realized he had missed his bus stop. Then, to his dismay, he took the next bus going in the same direction. These "blank-outs" had been going on for a while, but this time he decided he had a brain tumor or early onset dementia. After several medical evaluations came back negative, he decided to seek therapy.[12] He is hesitant but finally "confesses" these incidents to this stranger-therapist. Will he be hospitalized for insanity?

During the first several sessions, the therapist learned that John's "blank-outs" started after a colleague praised one of his doodles. Then he divulged that he had secretly concealed cartons of sketchbooks with his doodles, portraits, cartoons, and designs since middle school for fear of being teased and ostracized. After further inquiry, the therapist and John uncovered layers of despair about never amounting to anything. As far back as he could remember, older siblings and an overly strict father derogated him. His mother was coping with many medical and emotional issues, along with raising a large family and dissociating her husband's derogation of her and the children. Drawing in secret became his way of coping. By the time he started school, his secret method of coping had already been well established. The therapist started asking into various unmet needs. Simply by probing for specific incidents, the therapist was validating John's unmet need for his competence to be recognized by those in his childhood household.

The therapist formed a hypothesis that his unmet need to be recognized for his endeavors had pushed forward from his integral personality, disrupting his self-system, because his need was inadvertently satisfied by his colleague's enthusiasm. This "threatened" to open a significant opportunity to expand his potential and be recognized by his peers as a "person of worth."

> Larry, 34, is a successful creative property rights attorney in a prestigious law firm. He is unusually distracted at work, unmotivated, isolated from colleagues and friends and riddled with nightmares. His husband complains that they don't socialize anymore, and he doesn't respond to him, even in bed. At his husband's insistence, he recently consulted a psychiatrist and was diagnosed with depression. He decided not to take medication because he didn't want to be on Prozac forever, like his mother. He should just "shape up," thank his blessings, and get on with the next stage in his life: buying a house and adopting a child. Maybe a few sessions with a therapist would help him feel thankful and happy about his successful life.

In inquiring further into Larry's presenting problems, the therapist learned that the "depression" started soon after he and his husband began discussing future plans. They're financially comfortable, and most of their friends, of various gender identifications and sexualities, are settling down and starting families. They had endured hurdles around their families' reactions to their gender identification and sexuality, including his father refusing to attend their wedding, but now, several years later, they seem to have moved past all that. Larry's mother, after struggling with their "most unusual and unnatural" relationship, would be pleased to be a grandmother for the first time, even if the child were adopted and "motherless."

The therapist formulated an initial hypothesis that there might be unmet needs pushing for satisfaction now that the marriage was shifting into more permanency and responsibility. What else has the person been thinking about? What else had he been hoping to do with his life? Describe the nightmares. Describe his relationship. Why can't he share what's going on with his husband? The therapist still had no clue about what's really cooking, but in obtaining more information, it turns out that Larry studied law at his father's insistence, having abandoned his real interest, theater arts, to pursue a safe, "respectable," well-paying career. Although he had challenged his family's traditional values, he is unhappy and bored with his job, and his husband is pushing for the same kind of lifestyle he had fled from. In addition, his clients are embroiled in creative rights suits, and he is drawn to the details of their craft. Finally, his mother would be disappointed if he didn't settle down and have a child, especially since her own life had been full of disappointments—why she was on Prozac. Perhaps, he says, his depression is hereditary, and he should just learn to cope.

These examples illustrate how the therapeutic process uncovers the person's dissociated needs, residing in the integral personality, push for a place in the sun and how the self-system reacts to that push, ranging from devastating disorganization to simply a vague, uncomfortable and disconcerting feeling that something is wrong, along with expression of the person's particular security operations, mobilized by the central paranoia. To varying degrees of intensity and success, the security operations strive to camouflage and distort the integral personality's push for acceptance. Mustered to protect the self-system from changing the status quo—the way things always were—security operations are striving to push those needs back into the bottle.

Based on early sessions, the therapist forms hypotheses about what might be added to the person's list of presenting problems, including experiences and needs not in the person's focal awareness.

During the initial encounter the therapist also discerns the person's comfort level with allowing this stranger-therapist to learn more about them. The therapist observes an important aspect of their security operations, the degree to which they can allow an empathic, curious listener to be on the side of the person's integral personality. This reveals the kind of resistance the person mounts against the potential for emotional intimacy with another human being. All depends on the person's experiences in life from birth onward—the degree to which the security apparatus of the self-system will allow the person to get on with the integral personality's need to be clear with the therapist in order to derive therapeutic benefit.[13] Not that it would be simply "healthy" if a person suddenly trusted this stranger. But if they have come for help and then present a rosy life (to take this point to its extreme), the therapist gently returns to the business at hand: Why have they decided to spend time and (usually) money on this process? And why now?

The therapist also begins assessing the person's capacity to tolerate anxiety. What rationalizations have they maintained to sustain the status quo? How difficult is it for the therapist to obtain more than vague generalizations? What topics in the initial inquiry seem to ring the person's alarm bells?

It is also useful at this initial phase to obtain a brief sense of the person's current and past interpersonal life, starting with a description of current relationships. Where does the person live? Alone or with one or more other people? How do they spend each day, evening, weekends? What do they do for fun?[14] Who are the primary people in their life? What are they like? What goes on between them?

The questions are also indications of what is relevant, communicating a point of view in addition to seeking information. "Who are your friends?" as opposed to "Do you have friends?"[15] is crucial because it immediately establishes the assumption that people have friends. The therapist asks for elaboration. Close friends, if a person has them, are possible sources of continued validation and support. For some, friendships need to deepen or be rekindled. If there's a long list, it is therapeutic to ask who the "go-to" people are. If their mother is their "best friend," the therapist can privately form a hypothesis that the person might not have emotionally (sometimes not physically) moved very far from the original family orbit. If the person does not have friends, but says they do, the therapist can notice they do not want to "admit" their isolation at this time, while they observe that the therapist considers friendships important. If the person says, "I don't really have any," "I don't need friends," or some formulation about people being untrustworthy, etc., the therapist privately adds[16] social isolation to the problems the person cannot yet acknowledge. As discussed below, people require an ever-expanding and deepening audience of people who validate the expansion of their self-system beyond whatever has been limiting their life so far.

To begin understanding the person's problems in the context of how things got to be this way, the therapist also inquires, in broad strokes, into the person's history. After establishing the person's age and where they were born, the therapist asks about their original parenting one(s), siblings (including the person's place in the order), other children living with them, and others consistently around the person during the formative years (approximately the first 10), including people who lived with them or nearby. When asking about their parenting one(s), Sullivan (1954) suggests determining what they did for a living and if there were dramatic changes in their economic situation, and if so, the age of the person. Then he suggests asking what sort of a person their father was. Then, if there was a marriage, "Were they happily married?" Then, "Describe your mother" (pp. 73–75).[17] Now, with a more contemporary understanding of the various configurations people grow up within, there can be no assumptions. The biological parents might not be married, might never have been around, or were hardly there. The primary caretaker(s) might be a grandparent, an older sibling, a relative, or a foster or adoptive parent; the parenting one(s) might not be heterosexual. The significant caretaker(s) are those who interacted most intimately with the person from birth.

In addition, the therapist asks for a single-incident earliest memory. As discussed in chapter four, one's earliest memory is a rudimentary formulation of the child's perception of the world, their place in it, and the nature of their significant relationships. It unwittingly serves as a template for later experience. Recalling and examining it in adulthood is often useful in clarifying significant aspects of current problems in living. For example, the earliest memory of an isolated young woman was of an empty swing in an empty playground. Later discussions of this memory and related historical experiences of isolation enabled the woman to notice how and why she organized her life to emotionally mimic the desolation of that earliest memory.

One often recalls ongoing early memories prefaced by "we used to" or "I always." While useful, a *single-incident* earliest memory can yield that all-important template for later experience. If the person doesn't remember how old they were, the therapist asks them to guess. The therapist then helps the person elaborate: "What happened next?" "What did you feel?" "What did you think?"[18] It is not concerning if the person initially recalls an incident that happened even as late as adolescence, although the therapist can push for an earlier one. As therapy progresses, they often uncover earlier ones.

In developing the historical timeline, the therapist inquires about each developmental era, starting with stories about pregnancy. Of interest is the person's memories, not what they can obtain by interviewing anyone in the present.[19] Stories and incidents they can remember on their own reside in their consciousness. Later, in ongoing therapy, they might be encouraged to interview appropriate people. This can be helpful in the effort to fill in the gaps and to understand more about their parenting one(s): how they were brought up and how, given their own history, they viewed and treated the person at birth and growing up.

If a memory is a story, when were they told? What was the context? Little by little, bits of other developmental eras are beginning to be filled in. For example, if their mother had a very difficult pregnancy, unlike when she carried the other siblings, when did this story first come up? How old was the person when it was told? What did the person feel and think at the time?

It is also useful to know about times away from the familial orbit, such as sleepovers with friends, sleep-away camp, overnight class or team trips, and summers with friends or relatives. Children can learn a lot simply by having dinner or a play date at a friend's house, including other parenting styles.

Useful questions for each developmental area can be gleaned from pertinent chapters in this volume and *The Psychiatric Interview* (Sullivan, 1954). Of course, answers to questions bring up more questions; there is no formula for how the inquiry is conducted.

If the person insists they just want to work on current problems, the therapist explains that they can't work in a vacuum. They need to collaborate to understand how the person developed into who they are. To focus just on the present is to sidestep the interpersonal origins of the issues. People are brought up by people.

For example, if the person complains of "anger issues," techniques of anger control are usually superficial and transitory. The goal is to understand what needs are not being met in order to make changes in one's life that will make them less angry. In that context, it is helpful to examine their formative years: how those same needs were not met, and what had prevented them from recognizing and/or satisfying those needs. Recognizing how their rage developed can help form insight about how, in the organization of their current life, they might be repeating history. Because rage does not dissipate overnight, a useful tool in "controlling" the rage during this period of analysis is for the person to recognize the feeling or mood that precedes the rage and use some techniques to mitigate it or nip it in the bud. But as they gain more insight, they can recognize incidents in the present that bring up moods from the formative years.[20] Unlike when they were a dependent child, they can make substantive changes in the organization of their current life so that those incidents happen less frequently.[21]

If the person is dismayed that they don't have all the answers to these historical questions, the therapist explains that no one has all the information. Whatever is available in the person's "memory bank" is helpful at the moment. More will be remembered as the process unfolds. There is no such thing as a "good patient."

When generalizations come up, the therapist asks for details. For example, the therapist asks the person to describe a specific incident to illustrate how their father was "always irritated." Whenever relevant, it is important to ask for specific examples. Details can stimulate memories of feelings, moods, desires for unsatisfied need satisfaction, and the parental forbidding gestures[22] associated with them. These new memories provide the bases for insight about how needs were originally dissociated. Additionally, the therapist cannot assume they know what the person is talking about. They ask for clarification: "Say more." "Can you give me an example?" "I don't understand." Vividness of memory expands awareness and provokes new insights. The more the person can describe specific incidents, the richer the content and therapeutic benefit. Sometimes a person's memory is jogged by describing in detail their childhood home, holidays and birthdays, arriving home from school (or how homeschooling was organized), doing homework, dinnertime (or how they coped with no one caring about where or when they ate or if they ate at all), and bedtime routine.

It is also essential to learn when significant changes took place during the formative years, such as parental separation, a radical shift in financial circumstances, foster placement or being sent to live with relatives, relocation and/or a change in schools, opportunities for alternate validators, close peer interactions, deaths, illnesses, war, migration, earthquakes, etc. Functions developing in a certain era can be significantly affected by dramatic changes in a child's life at the time that function needed to develop.

Even if the therapist does not comment, the person hearing themself recount memories, perhaps for the first time, can be a very crucial, insightful emotional experience.

ORGANIZING AND USING A HISTORICAL INTERPERSONAL DEVELOPMENTAL TIMELINE

After several sessions of this "broad strokes" phase of inquiry (the number of sessions determined by how much information is forthcoming), the therapist's homework is to organize a working timeline of pertinent historical events in the person's life, from in utero (if stories are available) to the present. Most important are the formative years. The therapist looks for enduring interpersonal patterns, the contiguity of certain events, and significant changes in the person's life. Also important are opportunities and experiences that have been positive or partially positive in the development of the person's self-system. Depending on their own self-systems, the original caretaker(s) provide positives, or the analysand wouldn't be here at all.

The therapist is also formulating a more comprehensive list of the person's current problems in living, extrapolated from their presenting problems. How are those problems related to what has gone on in each developmental era? Putting the information in perspective in the context of developmental eras helps the therapist hypothesize about where things might have gone awry, what important developmental experiences are missing or skewed, in the effort to determine the point of fixation[23] and to develop a therapeutic strategy.

The therapist uses what they have garnered so far to prepare a summary, worded and timed so their analysand can make use of it.[24]

In the summary, the therapist relates the current problems in living to the historical information they have gathered. It is also geared to restating and adding, in interpersonal terms, to the list of issues that might be tackled therapeutically. The therapist might gently outline opportunities the person might organize for themself in order to grow, for things to change in their life. They might, if appropriate, ask the person to come up with possibilities. All is open to correction. Maybe, for example, an incident didn't exactly go down the way the therapist heard. The collaboration sets the stage for further collaboration. As treatment proceeds, therapeutic hypotheses and strategies are open to revision.

The summary is likely to make the person anxious and hopeful. The person needs to hear, as best they can, that they can derive benefit from examining how their problems originated instead of simply labeling themselves as, for example, a panicky or "codependent" person or suffering from a particular popular diagnosis[25] such as "bipolar disorder," "depression," or "ADHD."[26] Instead, change is possible, involving adjusting their significant audience and organizing opportunities to make up for insufficiently validated areas of functioning, even if the endeavors involve some anxiety.

The therapist must be mindful of how much anxiety the person can stand. If the summary is not based on what the person has already articulated or is already beginning to understand, it can alert the self-system's restrictive apparatus and make them more defensive against change. If the summary throws them into massive anxiety, they might repudiate everything and bolt out of therapy.

Sometimes the person comes to insightful conclusions based on hearing themselves tell their own history, articulated out loud to this receptive audience. This is the most effective summary.

As therapy proceeds, they will figure out what learned patterns to keep, what to alter, and what to reevaluate and perhaps replace because they are thwarting further growth. The therapist forms more hypotheses, usually shared as short summaries, other times filed away until later. Optimally, the analysand comes up with hypotheses as well.

The therapeutic collaboration is an uneven process, often with disagreements, clarifications, and reassessments. The therapist pushes against misperceived or accurately perceived resistances, and the person pushes, usefully or defensively, for the therapist to get the story straight.

ONGOING THERAPY

The next stage is the meat and potatoes of interpersonal psychotherapy. After the initial summary or summaries,[27] ongoing therapy focuses on the present and the past, cultivating a deepening understanding of current issues and how they relate to the past. Pushing for more memories helps build insight about what the person brings into sessions. When they bring up a strongly felt experience in the present, the therapist asks if it feels familiar. There is likely a historic antecedent to a strongly felt current experience that, if remembered, will help the person notice previously unnoticed themes in their life.[28] The therapist also validates useful projects in the present, such as joining a group, developing and deepening friendships, going back to school, rekindling or initiating a hobby, or changing career path.

This is not to suggest that current feelings are only understandable by examining the past. People do go through various degrees of emotionally charged experiences, positive and negative, in their lifetimes that are just that—emotionally charged experiences.

In focusing on a historical interpersonal timeline, several therapeutic processes have been put in motion to be utilized in ongoing therapy.

Detailed Historical Inquiry

The very act of going over one's own history brings up dissociated needs that can then push for acceptance into the self-system. The person can get in touch with unsatisfied needs and what they need to do to get them satisfied.

The other advantage of going over various misfortunes in their upbringing is that they can understand current problems in the context of their developmental interpersonal history, not because they have a hereditary defect. They begin to realize, for example, they were not "born" with a propensity, say, for self-debasement, but grew up in an interpersonal environment in which their primary caretaker(s) abased them. There is no self-debasement gene. With the therapist's assistance (perhaps through an understated but pointed comment), the person is more able to hear that their lowly self-image was "trained" or "programmed," and that what was learned can be unlearned. What was not learned can be learned. They are not stuck with their low self-esteem. A person who wards off physical intimacy with another human being because touching is so disconcerting is not stuck with a "phobia"; they might realize that cuddling with a pet can be a developmental step toward more comfortable physical experiences with a person.

In addition, the person is apt to notice the therapist cares enough to learn this much about who they are and how they came to be. Perhaps no one ever cared to know that much about them. That the therapist is that curious, that interested, can be extremely therapeutic—although they might try to repudiate the experience (and might succeed) by a formulation such as, "No one needs to know my business" or "What's my therapist's ulterior motive?"

In the collaboration, moving back and forth from the interpersonal present to the interpersonal past is the dynamic essence of the therapeutic process. The person can come to realize that certain assumptions well learned in childhood are now illogical credos and obstacles in living: If they buy something they like, enroll in a class, or travel, they're "spoiled" or selfish." "If you are proud of an accomplishment, people will think you are boasting." "If you ask a question, people will think you are stupid." "If you talk at a meeting or at happy hour, people will discover how stupid you are." "If you try talking to someone at a party or on social media, they'll think you are desperate for friendship." "If you question your friend's behavior, you'll be demeaned, abandoned, or punched."

For example, a person who, for their very survival, wisely complied with the demands of their abusive parenting one(s) can realize that disagreeing with a friend or suggesting alternate solutions in a business meeting will (in almost all cases) not evoke parental-like wrath. They are no longer helpless, dependent children. Avoiding saying what they're thinking has long outlived its usefulness. Or the person realizes they are drawn to abusive relationships because they knew no other kind of relationship growing up. Sometimes avoiding dangerous confrontation with a current abuser might be the wisest course of action; reassessing the origins of their choosing abusive relationships and doing something about it (such as finding a safe way out of the relationship) might be safer than a direct confrontation. Optimally the person comes to the insight themself; a brief formulation by the therapist may be of use, but only if it is bolstered by what has already been on the table, preferably from historical incidents.

The person also learns not to toss out everything they absorbed growing up, just those aspects that are now obstacles. Nor do they need to be angry at their early primary caretaker(s).[29] Everyone, including their parenting one(s), comes by their attitudes and behaviors honestly, from their own interpersonal histories. No need to cast blame. They need to understand how unfortunate attitudes and behaviors of those close to them have had an unfortunate *effect*. The goal is to keep useful patterns of living and reevaluate and change those that obstruct.

The original primary audience is not the only one that influences a person's personality development. Subsequent experiences impact the self-system positively or negatively. For example, a neighborhood and school can present alternate assumptions and behaviors from those formulated in the earlier years. On the other hand, if the neighborhood and school environment happen to reinforce what has transpired in the earlier years, there are fewer opportunities for the self-system to expand. Negative experiences outside the original interpersonal milieu can in fact reinforce unfortunate interpersonal patterns in living. In addition, hardships during those years, such as war, famine, racism, diasporas, im/migrations, pogroms, earthquakes, or hurricanes, have profound effects. Although primary caretaker(s) and hardships are usually the most influential, at least until preadolescence, a reciprocally beneficial relationship with a best friend can decrease negative impacts.

Since the formative years are usually just that, formative, the person's internal audience, even in adulthood, tends to be primarily the one(s) most influential during those years. A major part of the therapeutic project is to emphasize the need to question one's original internal audience: to kindle and rekindle friendships that can provide alternate attitudes and assumptions that validate other ways of seeing oneself and the world. If a person has grown up very isolated and with a limited primary audience, perhaps one suspicious of those outside the immediate interpersonal orbit, making friends was probably very difficult, and it might continue to be difficult during therapeutic work.[30] Until they can adjust their audience to include others outside the therapeutic office, the therapist might be the only person, or one of the only people, in alliance with their struggle to reshape and expand their self-system as they reevaluate and shed obstacles.

Most often, people live with a lifetime of unfortunate assumptions thwarting growth and creating "symptoms" such as those found in the *DSM*.[31] Therefore the work is not accomplished in a few sessions, nor does it take another lifetime. As people gain perspective, symptoms can fall away or become less frequent, less debilitating, and shorter in duration. Insights beget insights; when the therapeutic collaboration is working, the expansion of the self-system can snowball. It may take longer than the person intellectually wants but quicker than they emotionally feel they can handle, since change involves anxiety and dread.

Establishing Point of Fixation

Over time, consolidation of the functions pertinent in one developmental era prepares the person to work on functions of the next era. The point of fixation is often reached because needs evolve based on the nature of the integration of previous needs—i.e., there is not adequate preparation to move on.

For example, were they unable to feel like a true member of a group among juveniles in school, or are they still, in adulthood, interacting with peers in the uncooperative, self-centered mode of childhood? In this example, the person's point of fixation is at the start of the juvenile era. If they are ultimately going to forge meaningful intimate relationships, they first need to experience a strong bond with a group, where the group matters more than individual prestige, where cooperation, competition, and compromise without the loss of self-esteem are achieved for the sake of the group. The person needs to organize opportunities (through encouragement in therapy and/or other helpful experiences) in which they can practice learning true group membership. Caring about the group prepares one for the next developmental stage, the ability to care about another individual as much as one cares about oneself. It is a causally related process; each new function is built on previous abilities.

Pushing the Point of Fixation Forward

The therapist might directly suggest projects to make up for under- or undeveloped developmental functions. Or, during inquiry, the person may come up with the insight that certain developmental milestones need to be addressed.[32] With therapeutic validation, they can start to work on making up for unfinished business, say, by joining a group or noticing how they denigrate current group experiences.

Or the person may not have had the opportunity in childhood for parallel play with peers. A current project might be enrolling in a painting class or learning how to comfortably attend a concert or sports event. If the person's infancy experience lacked sufficient cuddling, a project might include adopting a pet.

Dreams in Therapy

Ongoing therapy also makes use of dreams that emanate from the integral personality. Dreams might point to areas that are now pushing for further exploration; expose the central paranoia's deepest fears, manifesting as despairing assumptions, dread states, and mood-memories; clarify current and historical detrimental patterns of living; and reveal distortions and paranoid formulations about what the dreamer thinks about people. Without a historical context for analysis, the richness of dream communication—to both the person and the therapist—is lost.[33]

The person usually leads sessions with incidents, worries, marginal thoughts,[34] major and minor emotional crises, dreams, memories, despair, hope, security operations, insights, gains, and setbacks in particular therapeutic projects. In addition to asking for elaboration, it is most often useful to understand and interpret this content in the context of the person's interpersonal history, peeling away deepening layers of the historical onion. Through this collaboration, the person's enduring and fondly held assumptions can emerge in consciousness. Are they helping or thwarting the project of growing?

Sometimes the therapist helps solve specific current concerns, such as dealing with a work crisis, appealing a grade or finding assistance with Medicaid or a housing issue. If sessions devolve into solving crises and problems, however, interpersonal analytic work can get lost. Or the person may bring in concerns that take up therapeutic time, but something else might really deserve more attention.

INTERPERSONAL PSYCHOTHERAPY AND ANXIETY

Anxiety[35] is central in therapeutic work. Expanding the person's functioning to promote growth involves some reorientation and, to varying degrees, an emotional separation from a person's original validator(s). That separation produces anxiety, a combination of the original fears with a new disorientation because of changes in one's perceptual world view. Anxiety accompanies the disorganization and reorganization of the self-system, often along with an uncanny sense of dread, with the introduction of possibilities beyond original limitations set by the parenting one(s).

Since the therapist's job is to help the person expand functioning, the person usually becomes anxious when expansion is anticipated or occurs. They will grow, resist, or some combination thereof, depending upon their ability to tolerate some disorientation, versus becoming overwhelmed by fear and other uncanny emotions.[36] Their fear, triggered by the central paranoia's protection of the self-system, is caused by the reexperiencing of the original emotions associated with the anxious parental response(s) to the emergence of the need, which over time became fully or partially forbidden.

Security operations, fueled by the central paranoia, emerge to maintain the original integrity of the self-system and reinforce restrictions. To the extent their security operations succeed, a person is no longer anxious. Examples of security operations might be formulations such as: "If I get too close to someone, I will be betrayed." "I'm too [fat, skinny, tall, short, ugly, old, young, etc.] to join an exercise class." "No one will want to hear what I have so say." They will repudiate the new insight to the extent that they comply with the security operations. The self-system is to that extent fully or partially protected from changing.

A simple definition of anxiety is disorganization plus terror. It can take many forms. Usually the person emerges from the anxious feeling salvaging some of the new functioning they have learned, but also reasserting some or all of the old restrictions. These can be lessened or increased, depending on whether the resolution is in a more hopeful or restrictive direction.

Anxiety arouses the uncanny emotions one avoids as if their life depended on it. It can involve disorganization, disorientation, and dysphoria.[37] It can be vaguely disconcerting, or it can induce unnerving dread, fear of death, or fear of insanity. These uncanny emotions might be, for example, particular "mood-memories" stemming back to infancy when the emotional and/or physical disconnection with the original primary caretaker(s) provoked abject visceral terror at a time when a need was pushing for satisfaction.[38] The person might break out in a sweat or feel like they're having a heart attack.[39] Adulthood competencies, such as navigating from point A to point B in a familiar neighborhood, driving, or saving a document, are suddenly difficult or impossible. It can involve a physiological breakdown, such as imbalance or eczema. Since no one wants to experience anxiety, people very rapidly move into rage, despair, or dissociation. They might try to dull it with alcohol or drugs. They might have nightmares. In its extreme, the anxiety may be so extensive the person's cognitive apparatus stops functioning and they lapse into a psychotic state for a time, usually brief.[40] Or they might struggle with insomnia, afraid of disconcerting dreams or nightmares that might shed some clarity on the situation. They might become suicidal.

Unfortunately, anxiety accompanies the process of the self-system's reorganization and expansion. While conducting the therapeutic inquiry and formulating interpretations, the therapist must be aware of the amount of anxiety that might get evoked. On the one hand the therapist cannot be afraid of the person's anxiety; on the other, therapy must not move so quickly that the person completely falls apart. The therapist always has one foot on the brake, the other on the gas. Because the self-system is devoted to maintaining the status quo, it is usually quite protective of its integrity. The security operations protecting it from taking in too much at one time are very efficient, so growth usually happens in starts and stops. It sputters, slowly and then quickly. Or it goes very slowly, seeping in little by little until the person's self-system can take in the rest. The therapist is always assessing the relative strength of the security operations versus the push of dissociated needs, as well as the availability of validating social structures in the person's life, such as friends, organizations, and groups, to provide support should the person become extremely anxious.

One of the contradictions facing early stages of the therapeutic process is that the person often feels more rattled as they recall their history and/or begin to move in the direction of growth. The person came into therapy to feel better, and they just feel worse! If this complaint comes up, the therapist tries to help them understand the role of anxiety. A corollary to this situation is when the person in the early stages of therapy suddenly believes and acts as if they are cured. This "flight into health," a sudden conscious or out-of-awareness spontaneous "recovery" from a problem without insight in order to avoid dealing with a particularly anxiety-provoking analysis of the problem, is a maneuver to avoid anxiety altogether. They may be moving into areas of growth too quickly and are in danger of crashing. With nuanced interpretations and management, the therapist and analysand can find a delicate balance between speeding up and slowing down.

If the person makes a major push forward and their self-system becomes so severely disorganized that they can't function, or a person is suicidal, they may need to have supportive friends (if they have them) to monitor them and create a safe haven. In the most severe situations of disorganization or suicidal ideation, the person might need hospitalization for their own safety, which, depending upon the quality of inpatient care, may or may not lead to the person developing a useful perspective of their current situation. Given that so many psychiatric facilities, at least in the United States, are primarily focused on *DSM* diagnosis and psychotropic solutions, many people are discharged within a few days or weeks with inadequate or no after-care treatment, except perhaps for medication management.

> Ronald, 53, has been unemployed for five years, having been terminated because of difficulties with his supervisor. Sputtering attempts yielded only a few interviews, and temp assignments have not resulted in a full-time position. He feels that life is slipping by. Although his fiancée has not complained about it, he worries about having very little to contribute financially to their small apartment. This will be his fourth marriage, and so far (he says with hesitation), his fiancée is not emotionally abusive like the others. Before he called for an appointment, he was offered a position at minimum wage. He is loath to take

it, certain he will again find himself in a job he hates, overworked, underpaid, fighting with his employer, and ultimately fired. He takes it because it will bring in some income. He denies suicidal plans, but the thought has occasionally crossed his mind. Maybe he should try therapy once more, now that he finally has insurance to pay for it.

Ronald's "symptoms" of "depression" and the fear of life continuing on the same track drove him into therapy. Now that he has forged a more productive relationship, he was free to explore new possibilities and did not want his career pattern to repeat. But he assumed it would and felt trapped in the pattern. During therapy, he resurrected old talents and skills set aside because of an extremely chaotic childhood that derogated and thwarted his interpersonal and intellectual growth; he recalled the repetition of those childhood patterns in several abrasive marriages. This time, after exploring his attitude about the job, he decided not to fight with his new employer, even though he accurately perceived that he was exploited and underpaid. He would bide his time while developing old skills and seeking better employment. The first time he entertained the idea in therapy that he could work on his need for friends by taking some adult-education courses in art history, he had several repeating nightmares (the same childhood ones) and panic attacks on his way to work. For a while it would take heaven and hell to push him to enroll in one of these courses. But at least he entertained that it was possible.

The therapist gradually helped him learn that moving a bit out of his self-system's "comfort zone" can evoke anxiety. The storm, however it manifests, is now more manageable, and the good news is that his anxiety indicates that things are moving in a positive direction, as contradictory as that might sound. Ultimately, he needed to become less fearful of anxiety and learn to weather the storm, understanding that he was on a productive road. He was integrating new learning and fulfilling heretofore unfulfilled or partially unfulfilled needs. Because people usually feel the storm will never end, he also needed to know that it's temporary, and that anxiety comes with the territory of change.[41]

To understand the timing of anxiety, it is important that the person have insight into how their self-system has been organized. After the initial sessions and then during the more detailed inquiry into the person's developmental history, there can be, over time, insight about why certain new opportunities and experiences provoke anxiety in the present. For example,

Ronald's parents were in constant destructive turmoil within the household. They were friendly with their neighbors but avoided forging close friendships. Because of their own upbringing, they taught their children that the only people who could really be trusted were family members and selected members of their extended family. Ronald remembered that his attempts to make friends in the neighborhood and at school were discouraged: the little boy across the street

> only wanted to be friends because Ronald had a tricycle; the only reason he was invited to a schoolmate's birthday party was because the schoolmate's mother wanted her child to have a lot of presents. When people seem friendly, they always have "ulterior motives."

The more Ronald delved into his history, the more he discovered the etiology of his discomfort with forging potential friendships. The insight was his when he was ready to see it, but not without a few nightmares and a few more panic attacks. This time his therapist helped him understand that the insight represented an emotional step away from the original primary caretaker(s), with the inevitable accompanying anxiety.

Additionally, by becoming clearer on their upbringing, people move into emotional territory that they probably haven't entered before. That creates anxiety because it threatens the accustomed connection with the parenting one(s) and family.

Another example:

> Walter, 26, seeks out therapy after a northern California wildfire destroys his childhood home, where he had been living with his alcoholic, widower father, who just committed suicide.
>
> Since Walter's mother died in childbirth, he was primarily raised by a father who was rarely available because of alcoholism. When he was available, he derogated Walter's aspirations and opinions. The neighborhood he grew up in and the schools he attended offered almost no alternate validation because they essentially mimicked what went on at home. In older adolescence he began to meet people who held other world views. He started fighting with his father but not without guilt and remorse.
>
> Before the fire, Walter had been spending his evenings and weekends performing in poetry slams and hanging out in small cafes. Occasionally he landed part-time jobs, and he had been trying to save money to move out of his father's home. Now homeless and traumatized by his father's suicide, he has been couch-surfing with friends and occasionally with his sister, 10 years older, and her husband, who both strenuously disapprove of his refusal to get a "real" job and forget his "pipe dream" writing aspirations. Like his father had been, they are particularly critical of his left-leaning politics and cross-dressing. Except for his best friend, his crowd in his hometown is also very homophobic and conservative. Like his father, sister, brother-in-law, and most of his friends, he frequently drinks to oblivion. His best friend suggests therapy, and his sister wholeheartedly approves because it will "finally set him straight." Walter's presenting problem is that he is in mourning and feels extremely guilty for not preventing the suicide by coming to his father's financial rescue by obtaining a full-time, respectable job.

As the therapist delved into the details of Walter's history, it was important to repeatedly assert that uncovering and divulging his father's problems is not equivalent to blaming him. In exploring his father's history, he began to understand that everyone is brought up by people, that everyone comes by their problems honestly. The work is to determine the *effects* of the upbringing on the developing child, retaining the positive and reevaluating the negative. They can ultimately reject those obstacles to growth and live differently without judging themselves or the ones who brought them up. To avoid the anxiety of clearly understanding his father's problems in living, and how his upbringing and surrounding environment were thwarting his growth, Walter had turned to alcohol, the solution of choice for his family and those he hung with. Walter's participation in Alcoholics Anonymous and finding a living arrangement away from his family were crucial, along with understanding that he could survive the anxiety kicked up by making those external changes.

As one evolves, experiences of upheaval continue to occur periodically. The ancillary goal of therapy, then, is that one becomes accustomed to anxiety and is increasingly familiar with their styles of self-limitation to avoid it. They learn that weathering the storm without drowning can, in increments, improve their quality of life. Usually, once a person understands the process, upheavals are expected and temporary, and experienced less painfully and with less dread.

MEMORIES AND MOOD-MEMORIES

Positive and negative feelings evoked by memories and mood-memories are central to the therapeutic process. They are reexperienced in current interpersonal interactions, in dreams, and in recalling the past. A major part of the therapeutic process is for the analysand to get in touch with early memories, how they felt, and how they can now understand them through the lens of current reflection in a safe atmosphere that validates reevaluation of earlier assumptions interfering with their life. Although they might not want to "relive" upsetting moods from the past, getting in touch with these feelings is extremely important because they present opportunities for the therapist to reiterate that they are no longer a helpless, dependent child, unable to extricate from those responsible for their basic needs.

Mood-memories are usually from infancy, before there are actual remembered incidents.[42] The mood-memory may be a background sense of sadness or irritability, barely noticed but shaping one's perception of how the world is. The therapist can suggest that the mood-memory, although probably triggered by current experiences, is lying in the background, "waiting" for something to give it potent "validity." There will probably be a lot of strenuous denial and rationalization, but part of therapy is putting background mood into perspective.

For example, if a person is chronically concerned with whether others are abandoning them, analyzing the person's background mood can reveal how the person tries to create consistency with the mood-memory from infancy.

In the following example, the person's early recurring nightmare provides a symbolic expression of how their chronic mood is connected to early experiences with the parenting figures.

> Alice, in her mid-20s, sought therapy because she was constantly besieged with sudden feelings of abandonment in social situations, regardless of what was really going on. In therapy, she recalled a recurring nightmare in late infancy. Even though in real life she was already walking, in the nightmare she is crawling up a steep hill. She is scooting here and there in a panic because cars are jumping onto the sidewalk to run her over. Her parents are walking way ahead, holding hands, oblivious to her crisis. Since the nightmare is recurring, she knows the candy store across the street is safe because it has steps going down to the entrance that cars can't follow. She also knows that once she tries scooting across the street, a car will inevitably run her over. She always ends up trying because she is too exhausted to keep scooting out of harm's way. She wakes up as the black underbelly of a car rolls on top of her.

The work in therapy is to understand how Alice's mood is not consistent with what is going on in the present.[43] The analysis of her mood-memory and relevant history is crucial. Now when the mood-memory surfaces, she can work on noticing it for what it is and shove it aside. The goal is to make it less frequent, of shorter duration, and less strenuous. It will take practice because change happens little by little.

A mood-memory can also be evoked by the senses. It can be a fragment of music or a smell that recalls a strong feeling, positive or negative.

RESISTANCE

Interpersonal therapists are skilled specialists trained to be "experts" in interpersonal relationships. If necessary, they help their analysand recognize that their therapist is also a peer, albeit with particular expertise and particular blind spots, not an undisputed despot. Although the person may distort their therapist, analytic interpretations are not articulated from on high. The interactions are collaborations. The analysand is an expert on their history; the therapist on making connections and helping them organize and understand their history to promote growth. If the therapist does not act like an absolute authority, the process of peer collaboration is facilitated. Interpretations are hypotheses, even if the therapist is convinced of their accuracy, always subject to correction. An archeologist finds a fragment which seems to be part of an ancient pot. They look for more fragments and put them together to see if they fit. Even if the therapist feels the person is resisting an interpretation, they must keep an open mind, allowing them both to see if it fits. An accurate interpretation might be resisted, but it is best if the analysand eventually owns it as theirs, even if it has been on the table for a while from previous summaries or interpretations.

The work is a delicate and difficult balance. A person's security operations to maintain the self-system's status quo are varied and well oiled. The therapist navigates the collaboration with that struggle in mind but cannot assume the person is simply "resisting."[44]

HOPE AND DESPAIR

By keeping in mind that "despair is the watchdog of the self-system" (Pearce & Newton, 1963, p. 408), the analysand and the therapist can manage the ebbs and flows of the therapeutic process. The person's hopeful insight, eloquently articulated in one session, might be followed by several bouts of despair organized by their defense processes to keep the self-system intact. Or a disorienting shake-up of their self-system kicks up despair. They may mount an "airtight" argument that change is simply a "pipe dream," that their problems are so insurmountable that whatever hope they entertained for a nanosecond is miniscule when faced with the enormity of the task at hand. "Yes, but . . . " is a common refrain in response to an interpretation (their therapist's and/or their own) that might threaten their self-system's integrity. Growth is not a linear process; it is more like a sine curve, with the crests rising a bit higher each time. Sometimes the higher the crest, the more strenuous the gravitational pull downward is likely to be. It is always a tug-of-war between hope and despair. The work for the therapist and analysand is to understand the role of despair, find positive validators to join their side of the tug-of-war rope, and win the struggle. Otherwise, despair wins.

Striving for a hopeful outcome is akin to attempting to walk up a down escalator. Although it is hard work and involves anxiety, one must climb up faster than the escalator moves down, or one moves down as well. Not moving at all is also tantamount to moving down. The climb is much easier with a support system of people, that positive audience to assist with the climb. For a very isolated person, it is crucial to help them find others to maximize validation for growth. If the person asks how long this whole process will take, a useful reply is "little by little," as long as despair gets challenged when it pops up.

THE WELL-DEFENDED SELF-SYSTEM: STOPS, STARTS, AND SPUTTERS

A person's self-system ranges from porous to tightly constructed, depending upon the person's interpersonal history. While it is not an exact scientific equation, the more they have been taught early on to be available to influences outside the original primary integrations, the more their self-system accepts change. Whether promoted by therapy or not, the ability to relate to other people and obtain validation from them is key to growing and continuing to grow.[45]

Therapists rarely run across a self-system that welcomes change with open arms. Many people who come into therapy possess a relatively tightly constructed self-system. They may be in psychiatric trouble because their self-system has reacted with strenuous disorganization to a brief encounter with an emergent need. Also, if their self-system is relatively rigid, the person most likely has few, if any, current positive interpersonal integrations to use as support for change in their current lives, replacing the original one(s) who historically organized the person's self-system to be so rigid. Often a possible new supportive friend or partner, who might become that all-important new integration in the person's life, is summarily rejected as the person flees to more familiar integrations, either the original one(s) or ones similar to them. Their self-system remains fairly rigid or even makes more paranoid formulations, just in case. The arduous task in therapy is to loosen up the self-system's rigidity.

The task is not accomplished by short-term intervention. It took years to build this person's particular self-system. However, it need not take the same number of years to loosen it, to allow unmet needs to enter and rearrange things. But the reorganization of the self-system generally cannot be accomplished in, say, 12 sessions (as some short-term therapy interventions recommend). The amount of time varies, with no clear estimate. Sometimes the person moves very quickly; other times painfully slowly; other times they retreat. Change can snowball, but it will take time and patience to get it rolling.[46]

When therapy has proceeded relatively successfully, change takes off on its own. Structured sessions are no longer needed when the person can continue growing with their friends and primary integrations, knowing that growth with accompanying anxiety never stops. They also know that occasionally old mood-memories, dread states, or assumptions originating from the central paranoia can pop up. These reside just at the margin of awareness, in the stream of consciousness. But now, with the benefit of therapeutic understanding, they are recognized for what they are: temporary lapses, usually when more growth is threatening to happen or is happening. They are in continuity with the person they have always been, but their newer primary integrations (including the therapeutic one) can lower the volume of the original one(s). The therapeutic primary integration continues to influence them after the structured sessions have stopped.

THE IMPORTANCE OF REPETITION: THE USEFULNESS OF DISSOCIATION IN THERAPY

Often the therapist comes upon an insight that the person is not ready to accept. The therapist might try it out but cannot be discouraged if the person just can't "hear" it yet. The insight has been relegated to the integral personality, temporarily dissociated. It may take many repetitions using different words and examples before their self-system finally accepts it. If all goes well, the person eventually brings the insight into a session, as if they just came up with it. Until then, the self-system has protected its integrity until ready to hear the "new" thought without major upheaval. They may never remember that the therapist has been saying it repeatedly for the last year or so, but that's fine, as it should be. The therapist might simply say: "Good to notice."

TAKING NOTES

Taking notes during sessions is extremely useful. Once the person notices that the therapist is attentive and curious, notetaking usually is not distracting. On the contrary, the therapist cares enough to make sure they remember pertinent facts. The person notices that the therapist refers back to incidents in the person's life to ask more questions or to illustrate an analytic interpretation. The therapist has done their homework.

Taking notes also keeps the therapist on track during a session, especially if a topic is threatening to the therapist.[47] The therapist is their own seismic indicator, registering when the topic makes them antsy. They can make a marginal note for supervision. Or in reviewing their notes, they discover they fled from a topic without adequate exploration. Especially during initial organization of historical data, they find gaps in the timeline. The analysand is usually comforted when their therapist returns to a notebook page to clarify a point, registering that the therapist cares enough to review between sessions. Sometimes, it is prudent to leave a topic because it is making the person too anxious. The therapist stars the issue in the margin, returning to it at a more appropriate time.

Finally, notes assist the therapist in formulating initial and subsequent summaries.

SYMPTOMS AND DIAGNOSES

People usually seek mental health treatment because they want relief from debilitating symptoms. Most practitioners are trained to form diagnoses based on the symptoms neatly packaged in the *Diagnostic and Statistical Manual of Mental Disorders* (American Psychiatric Association, 2013). But while convenient for filling out insurance documents and social service applications, diagnoses are of little therapeutic value. People might be comforted by their diagnosis. But the diagnosis can also vaguely validate despair: they are "damaged." They have a chronic "disease" that must be medicated[48] and/or treated with short-term therapy packages or behavior modification. Convenient short-cuts. No need for expensive time-consuming insight-oriented psychotherapy.

However, "cure" does not involve landing on a diagnosis based on symptoms. For example, a person does not suffer from a "disease" called "obsessive-compulsive disorder"; rather, they have developed over time, generally from childhood, a way of coping with their interpersonal situation. They are over-relying on a rather productive function (the ability to organize entities) to obscure what else is going on around them, to protect their self-system from noticing dissociated unfulfilled needs. As a youngster, if they were to truly get in touch with how much certain needs were not being met by their loved one(s), it would be too terrifying; they might not have been able to cope with that perception. But in adulthood, obsessive-compulsive behavior, as with any security operation, is a well-oiled practice whose purpose is to keep the self-system from making use of current experience to challenge the self-system's status quo. The person remains securely unaware of dissociated needs. Instead, life has become consumed with that security operation. There are as many flavors of security operations as there are atoms in the universe, all of which can be understood in the context of how and why they were originally formed.

Pearce and Newton organize symptoms into two trends of classification (Pearce & Newton, 1963, pp. 240–243). As discussed above, one trend consists of the myriad ways a person curtails their life with security operations, that is, modes to maintain dissociation, for example, obsessional or hysterical. The other refers to what happens if the barrier between dissociation and the self-system is broken, the dissociated needs breaking into awareness and the security system failing, activating reorganization and potential expansion of consciousness. Brief self-system lapses may be scarcely noticed, a moment of confusion or memory lapse. Longer, more extensive reorganization may present as catatonia (involving paralysis and muteness) and resolve into either expanded functioning or a "paranoid resolution," restricting needs more tightly.

THE THERAPEUTIC INTERPERSONAL FIELD

The interpersonal relationship between a therapist and their analysand is not one-way. To be effective, the relationship must be one in which both derive satisfaction. The focus in the relationship is the analysand's life problems. Satisfaction comes from solving those problems. For the therapist, the relationship provides an opportunity to learn more about a new person and about human beings in general, and to become emotionally intimate with a wider circle of people. This involves being curious and caring as well as the ability to think in the presence of the person's anxiety and forbidding gestures, and to increase one's feeling of competence. To do so, the therapist must recognize the limits of their own self-system and how to move past them. Both people need to grow from the experience. Because of their own therapy, training, and practice experience, the therapist becomes, little by little, an expert in understanding internal battles and interpreting historical content and dreams. But the other person comes with a whole new set of experiences and skills, including creative and, most often, quite devious ways for their self-system to expand or resist its growth. Most or all content is often new for the therapist to learn from and untangle. That challenge in and of itself can promote the therapist's growth. In addition, the person's perception or misperception of the therapist, if handled therapeutically, can promote growth in both participants.

As a participant-observer, the therapist must understand their own security apparatus, their own self-system's resistances to changes. They come into each therapeutic relationship with their own baggage of creative and devious ways to promote or undermine their own growth and the growth of the person they are collaborating with. For example, a new therapist might find it difficult to believe that, given their own upbringing, they could actually have a positive therapeutic effect on another human being. Or they may, during the therapeutic interaction, become envious of the person's push toward an area of experience inconceivable to themselves. They may focus too heavily on the person's resistance to change in order to prove the "truth" of their own low self-esteem; or they may use a person's growth spurt as proof of their own professional worth. Even the experienced therapist needs supervision and therapy to catch those maneuvers. It is useful for them to continue their own therapy to grow beyond whatever originally brought them into therapy, even if it had been to undertake "didactic psychoanalysis." Whether or not they continue in therapy, they need to expand their self-system in their personal life, to continue to explore realms of experience beyond their own comfortable status quo. They need to continue expanding and deepening their friendships and sources of pleasure. If a therapist stops growing, eventually their analysands will stop growing. In the best scenario, the therapist also derives some inspiration from their analysands' growth moves. Inspiration could come from a particular experience a person describes that is far afield from what the therapist can conceive of, or the therapist may notice that a person is braver than they are in traveling down new, seemingly perilous experiential roads and surviving to tell the tale.

While the therapeutic interpersonal relationship has all those hallmarks, it is not a traditional reciprocal friendship. The therapist tries to keep abreast of and work on their own limitations, their own stumbling blocks in their private internal battles. However, it's generally not useful for an analysand to know about their therapist's internal struggles; they can use the information to decelerate the therapeutic process ("My therapist has trouble forging close friendships, so I don't need to try." "If my therapist is so troubled, how can they be of help to me?"). Likewise, it is counterproductive, and usually unlawful, to socialize outside the office. In the office, the therapist needs to be approachable, not a stiff, blank slate.[49] Sometimes, a brief, well-timed glimpse into a therapist's personal story might be useful. For example, the person considering taking up a long-lost hobby to rekindle and broaden satisfaction (and meet new people along the way) might be inspired to learn that their therapist, with some trepidation, did the same thing.

WHAT ABOUT "TRANSFERENCE" AND "COUNTERTRANSFERENCE"?

Transference and countertransference are, in Sullivan's terminology, distorted perceptions[50] of who the other person is in an interpersonal interaction. He discourages overt analysis of transference with the therapist in favor of analyzing how it plays out in other relationships in the person's life (Havens, 1976, 1977; Kvarnes & Parloff, 1976; Lionells et al., 2015, p. 618).

Analysis of analysand-therapist transference and countertransference should not be the primary treatment focus.[51] It tends to become obsessive and loses the focus of growth for the person in the world they live in. As the person gains insight into how they distort their perceptions of others, they may begin noticing how they might be distorting their therapist. The therapist can notice and remark on the therapeutic distortion, but, under most circumstances, it is better to bring it back to how distortion plays out with peers, authorities, etc., in the person's lifetime experiences. How the person relates to the therapist is probably how the person relates in interpersonal fields in day-to-day life. Distortions of their therapist's personality based on interpersonal, historical assumptions can become a launching point for discussing distortions outside the relationship. The therapist notices how behaviors borne from distortions keep the person isolated and not easy to be with in the short term or over time. For example, the person might perceive the therapist as an authority, possibly making them into their original parenting one(s). This might also be played out in the workplace with their supervisor, perhaps with unfortunate consequences. It is more useful for the therapist to focus on the workplace and privately notice transference in the therapeutic relationship.

However, the therapist must recognize their own role in the participant-observer interaction. To that end, therapists, even seasoned ones, should undergo their own personal psychoanalysis and remain under supervision. "As we set out to investigate and clarify the principles of intensive psychotherapy, we must study, therefore, not only the therapeutic process as such, or the patient's personality in terms of his interpersonal processes, but also the personality of the participant observer, the psychiatrist, in terms of his interpersonal relationships" (Fromm-Reichmann, 1960, p. xv).[52]

Issues the analysand brings up about the therapist's personality should be taken seriously. The therapist must self-examine and discuss the perceptions in a manner useful to the therapeutic relationship. Even if the person does not bring these issues up, the therapist must always be mindful of how their own problems might be interfering with the process (are they acting too authoritative, controlling, dismissive, impatient?). Depending upon the capacity of the analysand and therapist to look squarely at their relationship, frank discussions, including therapist apologies and restatements for better clarity, can be productive and come as a relief. The person needs to have their perceptions validated; otherwise, the integrity of the relationship is threatened.

Finally, bringing the analysand-therapist relationship too much into focus can be embarrassing to the analysand and make them self-conscious during sessions, harming their self-esteem, provoking unnecessary anxiety, and perhaps causing them to censor. It is better if they, through discussion of outside interactions, can privately adjust their distortions of their therapist over time. Protecting the person's self-esteem and avoiding excessive anxiety are essential.

SUMMARY

Sullivan's underlying assumptions are profound in their simplicity: people are brought up by people and "we are all much more simply human than otherwise"[53] (Sullivan, 1953, p. 18). The therapeutic goal is to increase "a patient's skill in living" (Sullivan, 1953, p. 175).

The therapist's driving paradigm is to forge an alliance with their analysands' integral personalities, understand their problems in living in relation to their interpersonal histories, challenge their own and the others' security operations, ward off their own and the others' despair, and be unafraid of their own and the others' anxiety. Therapeutic practice involves a lifelong commitment to growing the self-systems of both themselves and their analysands. This means struggling to be open to self-evaluation and change, learning genuine humility and patience, and finding satisfaction in their chosen career, even if some of their analysands are decidedly uncooperative in the therapeutic collaboration. The therapist needs to respect their analysands and their struggles,[54] no matter how they present themselves, even if they seem impossibly stuck. This implies developing the same amount of respect for themselves in their own struggles.

NOTES

1. Sullivan, H. S. (1966). *Conceptions of modern psychiatry.* W. W. Norton & Company.
2. This chapter is a summary of interpersonal psychotherapy. The reader is urged to study the references cited in the chapter to learn more.
3. Psychotherapy within interpersonal theory is distinguished from currently popular short-term "Interpersonal Therapy" that borrows the word "interpersonal" but is different from the approach in this chapter. See the introduction.
4. Fromm-Reichmann does not mean "genetics" as in inherited genes; she means the genesis from living within interpersonal milieus.
5. See chapter one for definitions of terminology.
6. See the chapters on developmental eras.
7. Although this discussion is not about child therapy, the dynamic is essentially the same. The therapist can become a new primary integration in the child's life and a part of the child's interpersonal developmental history. For example, simply having fun with a six-year-old, enjoying being in the same room with the child, and attentively listening to the child's' perceptions are all therapeutic for a child used to abusive, punitive adults.
8. "Loving" as in mutually cherishing and respecting.
9. See definitions of the terms, self-system, central paranoia, integral personality, dissociated needs, and security operations/processes in chapter one.
10. Two particularly helpful books for practitioners working with transgender issues are *Counseling Transgender and Non-Binary Youth: The Essential Guide* (Krieger 2017), and *Sex, Sexuality and Trans Identities: Clinical Guidance for Psychotherapists and Counselors* (Jacobson et al., 2020). Also see chapter sixteen.

11. Sullivan (1954) refers to this phase as "The Reconnaissance." (pp. 72–93). In his germinal book, *The Psychiatric Interview*, Sullivan (1954) cogently details the structure of these sessions, from the "Formal Inception" and "Reconnaissance" to "The Detailed Inquiry." It is not only basic reading for the beginning psychotherapist but also remains the seasoned interpersonal practitioner's bible. It includes a discussion of anxiety and the self-system. Although dated, the importance of this book cannot be overemphasized.

12. Just because doctors have ruled out physiological causes does not necessarily mean it's "all in the patient's head." The patient needs to make sure that ALL tests have been administered and an underlying medical condition has not been missed. However, mind and body are inseparable; no matter what, a person in physiological crisis can derive psychotherapeutic benefit.

13. Since therapy is a collaboration between therapist and the person, benefit also depends upon the therapist's capacity to be an attentive participant/observer.

14. Sometimes, it is useful to obtain an hour-by-hour accounting of weekdays and weekends, noticing in particular what goes on between the individual and other people.

15. In general, it is best to avoid "yes/no" questions. Open-ended questions yield more information.

16. To share in an initial summary (see below) if the person is ready to accept that addition to their list of presenting problems.

17. The reader is urged to study *The Psychiatric Interview*, particularly "The Early Stages of the Interview" (Sullivan, 1954, 59–93).

18. Asking what the person felt *and* thought at the time might yield more information.

19. For example, if the person were to ask their mother for a story, it might be different from what is in the person's consciousness, rather than what the person has assumed was the "truth" up to the present.

20. This is not to suggest that rage is an emotion to be avoided. There are plenty of experiences that legitimately will make a person angry. However, blind, unmitigated rage is usually unproductive.

21. Often an adolescent begins to see what is not going well because they have more experience outside the home and/or away from their immediate interpersonal environment. Their rage is generally legitimate, but they are usually not emotionally well equipped to find solutions because one foot is still at home, and one foot is leaving home. Because the interpersonal environment they are trying to leave still consists of their primary audience, they end up in a fight, often with the goal of trying to change the minds of the people they are closest to. As adults, they can instead work to change their primary audience, so they are no longer in a fight for the right to have their perceptions validated and their needs met. In therapy, the adolescent can work to change the audience and get their perceptions validated with the help of therapy. Adulthood may not come if the audience doesn't change.

22. A forbidding gesture is a non-verbal mode of communication that expresses dissatisfaction or disgust with what another is doing or saying. A person cannot remember the actual gestured message of disgust from infancy, but now, as an adult,

they might be able to get in touch with the mood-memory of self-disgust and connect that mood-memory to stories about their infancy.

23. The developmental era in the person's life in which growth has stumbled. See chapter one.

24. There may be more than one summary during this initial phase, the first after a few sessions, and one or more comprehensive ones after more information has been gleaned. There are no rules. How brief and how comprehensive they are depend upon the therapist's intuitive or more conscious assessment of what the person can hear at the moment.

25. With the current popularity of diagnostic terminology, it is easy for a person to settle with the notion that they have a psychiatric "disease" that must be endured and/or medicated away, rather than believe that change is possible. Simply labeling their problems will not pose a challenge to their self-system, which needs to open up to new interpersonal experiences and expand.

26. Attention deficit hyperactivity disorder.

27. Sometimes the therapist has been thinking and puzzling for a while, reading and rereading notes, and, without planning it, formulates a summary on the spur of the moment during a session. Some therapists find it more useful if they write several points ahead of time (some therapists even read their summary to the person); there is no formula for how this all transpires. Interpersonal theory in the back of the therapist's mind navigates the way.

28. Also see the discussion of mood-memories below.

29. Sometimes the person continues to harbor anger at those who brought them up as a way of keeping the fight going with them.

30. Understanding the person's point of fixation is crucial in this process. If a person has not yet integrated parallel play, they are probably not going to easily jump into making close friendships. Getting comfortable going to an exercise class, watching a game at a sports bar, or finding a cozy corner to read or work on their computer in a coffeeshop might be the way to start the project.

31. The list of symptoms in the *Diagnostic and Statistical Manual of Mental Disorders* (2013) includes obsessive-compulsive behavior, bulimia, depression, etc. But there are also many restrictive patterns in living not listed there. See below on symptoms and diagnoses.

32. The initial broad-strokes inquiry might result in this insight. Usually it can happen later, in ongoing therapy.

33. See chapter fifteen.

34. See chapter one.

35. Anxiety and stress are different. See chapter one.

36. Sullivan (1953) defines "uncanny emotions" as akin to awe, like the first glimpse of the Grand Canyon, along with dread, a sense of "horror and loathing," all of which have "a sort of shuddery, not-of-this earth component" stemming from the emotional experience of early infancy (p. 10).

37. An overwhelming, uneasy feeling accompanied by strenuous dissatisfaction with one's life.

38. In addition to unpleasant ones, such as sad and rageful, mood-memories can also be pleasant, such as exuberant and blissful.

39. The *DSM* (2013) refers to these symptoms as "panic attacks."

40. If the psychotic episode is handled poorly, that is, simply medicated without insight into its origins, the person might become "chronic" over time.

41. The beginning therapist also needs to be less afraid of their own and their analysands' anxiety.

42. See chapter two.

43. However, if the person, out of awareness, chronically organizes to be surrounded by people who do tend to reject them, they reinforce the validity of the mood-memory. The actual rejection is not as potent as it was during the person's early years, although it may feel that way.

44. Occasionally the therapist offers solicited or unsolicited advice. While not the major focus of the work, they might have more experience and training in certain areas of living and can help the person avoid serious pitfalls, navigate a thorny issue, or locate resources. The dynamics discussed above apply here as well.

45. While it sounds as if there is simple cause and effect, actual lives are, of course, very complex. There are so many variables that an equation or formula is not possible. But general interpersonal theoretical principles still hold: people are social animals that are forever, from in utero onward, impacted by interpersonal interactions.

46. This formulation usually is in opposition to the structured criteria most insurance gatekeepers use to authorize sessions. For example, if the person has been in therapy twice a week and is making improvement in small, bumpy increments, authorization to continue this "level of care" may be denied. The gatekeeper might argue that the person now needs medication if twice a week is still necessary, or that once a week is good enough in spite of the gains achieved by the current "level of care."

47. For example, the therapist might also have had a very disjunctive alcoholic parent, and the similarities are too close to home.

48. This is not to suggest that medications should never be prescribed. However, if the work can be accomplished without *long-term* dependency on them, the person has a better chance of gaining insight into the etiology of debilitating issues, has a better chance of growing and changing, and is more likely not to relapse. Because medications can feel like a "cure," a person might terminate insight-oriented therapy. Fearful that the symptoms will return, they then deal with the side effects of medications over the long term.

49. See below for how the therapist can productively make use of the person's distortions of who the therapist really is.

50. He uses the term "parataxic distortions."

51. Many contemporary interpersonalists posit that analysis of transference and countertransference should be a major focus, essential in the therapeutic process (Lionells et al., 2015). While extremely aware of the therapeutic dyad and the role of the therapist as a participant-observer, the theory posited in this chapter advocates that the therapist primarily focus on analyzing distortions in the person's interpersonal relationships outside the therapeutic dyad, particularly with current significant others,

and how those distortions were formed through early and subsequent interpersonal experience.

52. Fromm-Reichmann (1960) advocates more intense analysis of transference-countertransference during sessions than is advocated here.

53. With this principle, radical for his time, Sullivan was emphasizing that "homosexuals" and people diagnosed schizophrenic must not be placed in a category of "other" and treated as such. In the current social climate, not only must his one-genus postulate be reasserted, it must particularly call attention to "recently acknowledged complexities in gender identity, development, and both the vulnerability and resilience of transgender communities; in other words, a greater understanding of the diversity in the human condition" (Taffel, 2020, p. 17). This applies to all peoples who are oppressed and whose common humanity must be emphasized.

54. Fromm-Reichmann (1960) provides an eloquent and invaluable description of how a therapist respects the person they are working with, even in the most dramatic, seemingly impossible inpatient scenarios. In a companion autobiographical book, *I Never Promised You a Rose Garden*, Hannah Green (1964) describes her own inpatient treatment by "Dr. Fried."

Chapter Fifteen

Dreams

Their Origin, Development, and Use in Therapy

COMMON VIEWS ABOUT DREAMS

People have used dreams in various ways since the beginning of recorded history, and probably before (Mullahy, 1948, pp. 72–73): to predict the future of battles and individual fortunes, to communicate with deities and the dead, or as ceremonial rites of passage, such as dreams that tell adolescents their future role as adults. Artists and inventors write of going to sleep, dreaming, and waking with new inspiration. There is probably something to all of this, as well as some misperception.

Dreams and the Brain

In the 1970s, many neuroscientists concluded dreams are effluvia, sensory reactions to different levels of brain activity (Hobson, 1977), that dreams are responses to chemical activity in the brain stem "rationalized" by the cerebrum, with no significance beyond that. However, Solms (2021) countered that dreaming has a strong relationship with the brain structures controlling motivation and emotion.

Blechner (2013) lists the many ways the function of dreams has been described, concluding that "there need be no single function of dreaming, any more than there is a single function of waking thought" (pp. 259–260).

Newer brain studies suggest that dreams may relate to the exploration of previously unnoticed connections in one's experience (Zadra & Stickgold, 2021).

In an intriguing TED Talk, Stickgold (2021) outlines how the brain changes waking thought to dream thought, allowing us to "sift through the neural networks that encode all of our memories, all of our ideas." There are "15 billion nerve cells and 125 trillion connections between them." The brain goes through these connections, even ones weakly related to significant events, searching for those that might help us understand them better. In sleep, the brain shuts down the hippocampus and frontal lobes, removing logic, reasoning, and impulse control as well as detailed recent memory. It decreases noradrenaline flow, "creating a bias for finding weaker associations," and finally increases in the limbic system, intensifying emotional responses. The result of these changes in the brain while asleep creates "dream thought," which allows the brain to "identify, explore and strengthen previously unexplored associations that might help us understand what has happened to us in the past and what might happen in the future" (Stickgold, 2021). The work by Zadra and Stickgold (2021) supports most closely the interpersonal approach to dreaming.

THE INTERPERSONAL VIEW OF DREAMS

The interpersonal approach to dreams is rooted in the classical psychoanalytic work of Freud (1913). It utilizes Freud's concepts of the unconscious and symbolism in sleep to express troublesome issues in one's life but departs significantly from the Freudian model to build on an approach suggested by Pearce and Newton (1963, p. 349). In their model, a dream is a poetic formulation of the current push for satisfaction of dissociated needs as they conflict with central paranoid assumptions and security operations.[1] The dream can present either the need, resistance to admitting the need into awareness, or both. When awake, the dreamer can repudiate the need or recognize the irrationality of paranoid assumptions blocking need satisfaction. A dream might also illustrate one's level of interpersonal development.

Dreaming is thinking and feeling while asleep. According to Sullivan, "Remembered dreams are to be regarded as experience as valid as any other" (quoted in Lippman, 1996, p. 285). Dreaming can be a tool providing important sources of data, allowing the dreamer to more fully understand obstacles to their growth and development.

Dreaming is activity of the integral personality[2] outside restrictions of the conscious self-system, used as messages in sleep (from the integral personality) to the waking self, the self-system.

Interpersonally, dreams express a range of thoughts and feelings about current and past relationships' effect on current experience. They illuminate how the dreamer restricts relationships and obstructs needs.

Dreams are timely, emerging when someone is concerned about a problem and symbolically grappling with it in sleep. They tend to clarify obstacles to a more fulfilling life, illuminating what is problematic in current living.

The same kind of material comes up in other ways and can be interpreted from a person's creative activity or from psychotic content. Dreams, creative activity, and psychotic ideation use symbolism to convey a message not necessarily acceptable as conscious, "rational" thought. Like artistic symbolism and psychotic ideation, "dream code" is designed to get past the restrictions of the self-system via poetic expression of the dreamer's problems in living. Because it uses imagery that specifically fits the dreamer's history, it has a particular impact on the dreamer, transcending logic and making it hard to argue away.

If a person is a frequent dreamer, data about the person's most pressing current concerns and their historical contexts are more readily understandable. Yet not all dreams are dramatic or even clear in their communication. Much depends on how much the dreamer is in some way hopeful enough (or less defended) to listen to the messages.

As with other forms of thought, a dream has an audience.[3] Usually the level of one's hopefulness depends on the audience for their dream, if there is someone in their life who can be perceived as available to understand their needs. A therapist can become that audience.

Dreams can refer to the dreamer's history, their relationship with a current significant person, real or imagined, or their most pressing current life project(s). Usually, they are about all three.

Dream interpretation is a collaborative process. Because dreams carry symbols representing meanings not acceptable to consciousness, it is somewhat difficult, if not often impossible, for dreamers to interpret their own dreams without the assistance of somebody else, preferably somebody who has a grasp of the dreamer's history and current life issues.

Dreams are not always remembered. However, remembered or not, the effects have an impact on the dreamer's waking mood. Something is formulated, although out of awareness. If remembered, the dreamer usually has the potential to clarify what is being communicated. Usually, it's about one's waking behavior or what the dreamer, outside of conscious awareness, is working on about life. Often, if a person has not been remembering their dreams, they begin to recall them when they start therapy. In a productive therapeutic relationship, the therapist increasingly becomes the audience for their dreams. The dreamer literally tailors them to the therapist; the dreams become less and less obscure to both as they get to know one another in the therapeutic collaboration.

Interpersonal theory infers that unremembered dreams can have an impact, but more obscurely. The audience is there, but it is more obscure to the dreamer. Even if they do not remember the dream, people may often wake up in a strong mood. It is posited that this is because they *have* formulated something out of awareness, to an audience not consciously acknowledged.

As the therapist becomes a more significant figure in their life, the dreamer intensifies using the therapist as the audience. The dream communications are in part *to* the therapist, to the extent that there's a collaborative effort, enhancing the likelihood that both will even more fully understand the messages and the needs that prompted them. Sharing dreams promotes the goal of therapy: to help the dreamer, through insight, achieve maximum satisfaction in life, with fewer and fewer unnoticed obstacles. Those obstacles can be brought into conscious awareness through dream interpretation. In the following example, the obstacle is despair.

> Alex, a young woman in therapy who had extricated herself from an oppressive home situation but moved into an almost equally oppressive marriage, had a nightmare about her dilemma: a giant hammer was descending from the sky to crush her. She ran to the other side of the world and there, too, another hammer came down to crush her. She awoke screaming and brought the dream to her therapist, who suggested that she believed her parents were all-powerful and could follow her anywhere. Her despair was that she could never escape her fate, no matter where she turned. This coldblooded look at her own despair was a relief to Alex, freeing her to set about planning for a divorce and a job.

The following example illustrates how a dreamer's misinterpretation of their dream can be destructive because without the alternative interpretation by a therapist, they emphasize the despairing aspects.

> Stephanie became severely panicked after recurrent dreams that she would be locked up in a psychiatric hospital. After dramatic, repeated claims that her dreams foretold the future, she was indeed locked up. The scary symbolism evoked by the unwanted power to predict imminent disaster and make it come true can be seen from a broader perspective. Stephanie had recently come home after two years abroad teaching English. She returned to her parents, who had very low expectations for Stephanie; she squeezed back into a familiar dependent and infantilized role within the family structure. She had been raised to see herself as incapable of independence.
>
> Her need to leave home continued to press with greater and greater urgency, but establishing her own living arrangement would have required more independence than she had. Her desire to leave home and connect with peers was inconceivable, but very powerful, and the conflict was tearing her apart.
>
> Seen through the lens of her history and level of development, Stephanie's dreams are expressions of her despair about leaving home, probably with her parents as her only audience. Stephanie and the most important people in her life could only consider her idea of leaving home as insane. If she had had a

therapist or positive group experience, she might have been able to regard her assumption as an obstacle to be questioned and challenged.

Dream interpretation is dialectic. While dreams illuminate the dreamer's misperceptions and security operations, they come from strategic thinking occurring when the dreamer has moved in a more hopeful direction. So when a person dreams about anticipating a pleasurable experience, their security system turns it into something that might go wrong. It's the therapist's job to clarify that, pointing out the habitual distortion.

Nightmares

Nightmares are extremes of the same paradox. Most dreams contain a formulation of the central paranoia or paranoid assumptions outlining how dreamers assume they are stuck and, when analyzed, how those assumptions, when clarified, stop growth. Nightmares differ from ordinary dreams because they are formulations of the dreamer's *most* despairing assumptions. Because they lay bare the worst things one can feel about oneself, they evoke emotions like dread, terror, and self-loathing. They include the negative mood-memories[4] from early in a person's life that form the basis for central paranoid assumptions and are very powerful. In a nightmare these early primitive moods are encased in current symbolism, reinforcing the dreamer's notion that their fragility and dependence in infancy continue to be real.

Nightmares are symbolic formulations of those assumptions: the fear of death, disorganization, and loss of tenderness, usually waking the dreamer. Harvey (2009) treats the scary nightmare as a sign the dreamer had made some expansive choices.

The nightmare results from a breakdown of the defenses guarding the integrity of the self-system, which then activates the central paranoid assumptions. The dreamer's integral personality is challenging their own assumptions, poetically illuminating them, potentially holding them up for critical examination.

> If you remember that the dream's basic formulations are always the most connected to illuminating the central paranoia, then, when a person's made some, more than one, baby steps in some direction antagonistic to the structure, the integral personality holds the restrictive structure away a bit enough to be able to view it, to view that part of the structure which they count on, believe in and have always used. But that's the formulation of the dream, what it is that they have always believed. Coming back almost to bite them in the ass, pull them into the old, restrictive way of thinking. But the reason the dream isn't true at the point the dreamer's dreaming it is that the dreamer has made that step away

enough to be brave enough to view how the person sees the world or that part of the world, that conviction. (Harvey, 2009)

Nightmares and Psychotic Experience

[B]y doing something that challenges my long cherished central paranoid assumptions, I can shatter the structure of consciousness abruptly. That can be experienced in a continuum from a nightmare, absent-mindedness, disorientation and dizziness, or even a psychotic break for a brief period, which is not experienced as odd in the moment—only looking back on it. However, there is no difference between that experience and any other human experience. The new challenge can be repudiated by paranoid reformulation, for example in a nightmare, or it can be validated by a more hopeful audience. Much depends on what sources of validation exist. (Harvey, 2009)

Fugue States

A fugue state is another form of altered consciousness, like a dream or waking nightmare. It may be accompanied by pleasure, paranoid, despairing thoughts, or both. It may be artificially brought on by alcohol or drugs, but also may occur in sleepwalking or an intense emotional emergency. Someone who is in such a state, with or without the aid of alcohol or drugs, might interact in a way quite different from when fully conscious. They might be more friendly or affectionate or more openly angry. The point is that the behavior in the fugue state is dissociated and the person, when fully conscious, could not conceive of doing it.

As Sullivan (1953) describes it, a person in a state of sleep who does not appear to be asleep is doing something they have dissociated that they would never do in waking life. He also discusses the "deliberate fugue state," in which "the person braces himself [*sic*] with an attitude of 'well, hell, let's take a chance on anything once. . . . ' and then plunges into some situation, with a sort of tightening up of everything, often keeping his eye on something irrelevant—that is, preoccupying himself with things really tangential to what he is after" (p. 323). According to Sullivan the fugue state may signal the reintegration of a previously dissociated experience or an impending psychotic break. It often occurs in adolescence.

Automatic Writing as a Kind of Fugue State

In a home for runaway youth, two residents brought a new girl into the counselor's office because they thought she was "acting strange." She had already told them she didn't know why she had left her aunt's house, but as she was talking, she began to get very drowsy, put her head on her arm and spontaneously went to sleep. Her other hand rested on the desk. The residents quickly suggested that the counselor put a pencil and paper under her hand. While she slept, the girl took up the pencil and began to sketch a stylized drawing of a wild-looking, scary lady with a knife and someone running away yelling, "Get me out of here!"

The Developmental Process of Dreams

As far as can be observed, dreaming begins around the end of the first year and becomes more complex as the capacity for symbolic thinking develops. Recent research in infantile development suggests that the infant is capable of observation in utero.[5] When the repetitive appearance of certain objects (such as a nipple or a bottle) coincides with a certain satisfaction, the infant begins to see the object as a signal that satisfaction is on the way. (The same process works with negative or dangerous repetitive patterns.) This process of expectation (or foresight) enables the beginning of symbolism. As the ability to symbolize, to have one thing stand for another, develops, so do dreams, which require the use of symbolism.

Dreaming is more easily identified a few years later when the child begins to verbalize the nightmare. While it is possible to infer the presence of dreaming even in an infant (giggling, grimacing), the nightmare that occurs two or three years later is more easily reported and memorable.

When young children talk about dreaming, the content is symbolic even if it resembles waking behavior since it is reported as a dream and has been screened by the child's defenses.

Dreams in Childhood

Dreams make use of current experience, and they comment in some way on the current context in a person's life. In childhood, for example, there is often the expression of the need to get away, to fly, to leave the current context. Or there is perhaps the expression of terror about the intrusion of the outsider, or the dangers of the subterranean moods of the significant people in one's life, or fear of their abandonment. As a person grows, the subject of dreams expands to a wider range of significant people and experience, consistent with the person's life experience. However, perhaps even before articulation of speech, dream content usually does contain historical referents and moods that are indeed very early, from early infancy.

How Dreams Are Used in Therapy

> If you ask, how are dreams important to therapy? The answer is: it's data, and as such is helpful in doing a long-range study of a person when we have that opportunity. If you're looking for data to fill in, to help the person fill in, so the person can understand more and therefore change more, then, it's part and parcel of therapy. . . . And often because it takes away the layers of obscurity that we would use to cover ourselves, who we are, it gets through the obscurity because it's symbolic, so it's hidden a bit from the patient for a while (long enough to make use of it in an analytic study). Dream study is useful in putting personality development together, locating the point of fixation,[6] the functions that got stopped; the functions the person's still needing to explore; how best and in what small ways to [find] memories that are not easily accessed; and how to find little experiences in daily living that can add enough to disrupt the rest of the self-system. (Harvey, 2009)

Implied here is the notion that the purpose of therapy is, in fact, to disrupt the self-system enough so that the most pressing developmental needs and functions can poke through a person's defenses and get some time on the air. Dreams are extremely important in that effort.

The point of fixation for a dreamer can be identified by the kinds of interactions they describe in their dreams. For instance, is the person involved in a struggle with a powerful figures or in a large group or engaged in collaborative efforts with people?

Listening to Dreams

When the person recounts a dream in therapy, the therapist listens to their wording, their tone of voice, as a subjective, empathically experienced process. If a dreamer states that the experience of a dream is a certain way, it is that way, no matter how seemingly irrational or impossible it seems. It's important to keep in mind that it is the dreamer's dream.

As Harvey (2009) describes it, a therapist needs to be relaxed, not focused on details or what the dream should logically be about, noticing one's own reactions to the dream, as if listening to poetry. A therapeutic response should be simple, echoing the symbolism of the dream: "Like answering a poem with a poem."

Likewise, the logic of dream thought transcends linear sequence. With multilayered symbolism, the contradictions are all true because they reflect the uncensored commentary of the dreamer. Contradictions of all kinds can appear in a dream, but the contradictions in themselves can represent a reality for the dreamer. Knowledge of the dreamer's history also helps make sense of the dream, to understand the meaning of the contradictions.

Symbols in Dreams

Symbols a dreamer uses need to be understood in the context of their personal history and their current associations. A person can't dream something they haven't experienced, but they can symbolize something they experienced at a much younger age. For example, a small wave to an adult may seem huge to a young child. A tidal wave can also be symbolic of the power of a mood.

The experiences in dreams are idiosyncratic creations based on the particular history of the dreamer. They may use common symbols (especially children who haven't developed more sophisticated defenses yet), but each one is unique to the dreamer.

Associations in Therapeutic Dream Interpretation

One can think of obtaining a person's dream associations as exploring the path from their integral personality to their self-system, or conscious mind. It's not linear. The process of exploration needs to follow the person's path in that same circuitous way. Asking for associations in an open-ended fashion allows the person to explore their own thoughts more freely in response to the content of the dream. Despite its vagueness, the person usually answers the question, "Your associations?" without hesitation.

The dreamer's associations to a dream provide a link to the symbolic meaning the dreamer is using, as well as the historical and current contexts in which to view the dream. However, rather than asking specific questions about each potential symbol, the therapist needs to give the dreamer more room to make connections allowing for richer exploration of the dream. By asking for associations in an open-ended fashion, they allow the dreamer to explore more freely the dream-message from the integral personality to the self-system, to go where it leads them. The dream may not even be mentioned again, but the person may continue to talk about the dream in the context of associating to it. That may be more enlightening than anything else. There does not have to be a formal interpretation.

Sometimes a dream is connected to something or someone the patient unconsciously needs to share with the therapist.

According to Harvey (2009), immediately asking for associations to every detail in the dream is less useful than letting the person associate more freely. The person needs room and time to let the thoughts come. It's OK if there are silences.

In the process, a person may tell the therapist what the dream means, but they may also just want to talk about someone in the dream, but that's the association to the dream, what it provokes inside them. After obtaining a person's associations it may be helpful for the therapist to ask about some of the details in the dream that seem of interest. Even if the dream doesn't come up again in a session, the telling of the dream and the therapist's response may lead to more helpful associations in the session that clarify the therapist's and/or the person's thinking.

Again, it's not always necessary for the therapist to come up with an interpretation, to come up with something "important." Most important is the sharing.

Dreams tend to refer to history, current problems of interest to the dreamer, and the relationship with the therapist. It's useful to tackle just one of the three aspects. It's part of the therapist's job to decide which area of life—historical, current, or analytic—to discuss with the person in the moment.

Like Sullivan, Harvey takes the position that it is usually not advisable to discuss dreams in relation to the transference, especially if the analysand is new. The attempt to discuss the analyst–analysand relationship can be a distraction from what brought the person to therapy: their needs. It would be more helpful to direct the discussion to history by asking when the dreamer has felt that way before. However, if the mood in the dream about the therapist is particularly intrusive and the person is a long-time analysand, it might be possible, for example, to ask what they are angry about. "I may have done something that I didn't think was important, but it may have been important to the patient, taking up a night of the person's life to dream about it" (Harvey, 2009).

SUMMARY

Dreams are data for the therapist and the person in the long-term study of their life. They are symbolic communications to some audience, real or imagined. They happen in context because they express the developmental level of the dreamer; they utilize historical experiences as well as the current experiences of the day. They can be utilized in therapy to delineate aspects of therapeutic analysis that warrant further exploration, help dreamers recognize their dissociated needs and how they create obstacles to meeting those needs, and formulate a summary of where the person has evolved in their interpersonal development.

NOTES

1. The person's restrictive defenses are the formulations derived from an organized, complex system of despair (the central paranoia) about what is possible; they form the basis of a security system designed to ward off learning from new experiences

that would threaten the tender connection with the original primary caretaker(s). The self-system's security operations, forged by the despairing system, determine whether to allow those thoughts in or keep them out. See chapters two and eleven.

2. The integral personality is the total of all aspects of experience, both dissociated and in awareness. See chapter one.

3. As discussed in chapters eleven and twelve, every thought has an inner audience.

4. As discussed in chapter two, in adulthood the memory of infantile experiences such as pleasure, satisfaction, euphoria, terror, and anxiety are intensely felt and can reappear later in life as if from nowhere and in powerful form as *mood-memory*. The mood-memory can be negative or positive, reflecting the actual experience in infancy. Such mood-memories can also be dredged up from slightly later experiences (past the age of four or five months) at a time when there is still very limited capacity to verbalize and limited ability to orient oneself enough to have conscious memory.

5. See chapter two.

6. The point of fixation is a zone of experience not yet consolidated, which would be the individual's expected next area of development. See chapter one.

PART IV

Issues

Chapter Sixteen

LGBTQIA+ Issues and Interpersonal Theory

> To talk about homosexuality's being a problem really means as much as to talk about humanity's being a problem. (Sullivan, 1972, p. 196n)[1]

Interpersonal theory maintains that the development of the capacity for adult peer intimacy[2] is crucial, not a person's gender identity and/or sexuality. If, willy-nilly, young people learn, despite whatever has gone wrong in their lives, to incorporate the experience of love,[3] they can do so with any other human being, depending on how much the capacity to love has been developed as they were growing up.

Sullivan's (1953) one-genus postulate that "everyone is much more simply human than otherwise"[4] (p. 32) probably provides the best starting point for discussing LGBTQIA+ (lesbian, gay, bi, trans, questioning/queer, intersex, asexual/agender/asexual/ally, and others[5]) issues in the context of interpersonal theory and practice. People *are* more human than otherwise and therefore confront a problem that most other species probably do not share with us: the majority of people in most contemporary cultures, not necessarily always in prehistoric or so-called primitive cultures (McCubbin, 1979, pp. 10–11), bump into taboos about sensual pleasures with someone of the same gender. (Of course, taboos still exist about sensual pleasures, period.) Surely most species (including most plants) require some kind of heterosexual contact to procreate and sustain themselves.[6] But sensual experience is sensual experience, and many species would not turn their noses up at a good sensual roll in the hay without consideration of gender (Blechner, 2009, p. 11; Schrefer, 2022).

But humans have a problem: various societies or cultures. Currently, in the "electronic age," Googling "therapy and lesbian" or "therapy and homosexual," for example, would yield debates about whether or not to "cure" "wrong" sexual orientation and discussions about whether therapeutic "redirection" or "conversion therapy" works.[7] Of course, within the "redirection" or "conversion therapy" interventions is a presumption that LGBTQIA+ people are psychiatrically impaired, that true intimacy is a heterosexual phenomenon.

It took until 1987 for the *Diagnostic and Statistical Manual of Mental Disorders* to completely remove "homosexuality" as a mental illness. Faderman (2015, pp. 279–297) dramatically chronicles the struggle to push against the American Psychiatric Association. Even after 1987, it took years for training institutes, even among the most liberal, to allow practitioners other than heterosexual to assume training and supervisory positions. The William Alanson White Institute of Psychiatry, Psychoanalysis and Psychology, founded in 1943, finally has an LGBT Psychotherapy Service.

Sullivan (1953), ironically one of the founders of the institute, refused to consider "homosexuality" a psychiatric "problem." "[T]o think that one can remedy personality warp by tinkering with the sex life is a mistake, even though it is a very convenient doctrine for psychiatrists who are chronic juveniles" (p. 295).

Interpersonal theorists maintain that "curing" non-heterosexuality should not be a therapeutic issue. A person's ability to relate intimately is key, not the person's gender identity and/or sexuality.

Although Sullivan never explicitly came out (nor could he without committing professional suicide), some of his biographers and colleagues contend he identified with gay people. Unlike most of his colleagues, he insisted that gay people were not to be treated as crazy or as criminals. However, he also theorized that gay men may have identified with a caring mother in the face of an unavailable or distant father. Sullivan was revolutionary in his attitudes toward LGBTQIA+ people, but he still assumed that gay people (perhaps including himself) experienced deficiencies in their early interpersonal lives. But, although he alluded to the notion that heterosexuality was more "mature" in a few places, he also said the opposite more often. Sullivan was probably not convinced that heterosexual relationships were more mature, but that he was, in the course of his career, bowing to social pressure. Being heterosexual was clearly more convenient.

At least out of context, some individual passages contain implicit or explicit assumptions that heterosexual relationships are the most "mature" relationships, or even that the most fulfilling and unrepressed sexual act is with a person of the "opposite sex."

Most simply, either because of professional pressure at the time he wrote, or because he, for whatever reasons, bent to that pressure, those passages are from a heterosexual point of view. His point of view can be interpreted thusly: people make healthy adjustments when they have unfortunate histories, and whatever an individual finds most sexually satisfying is okay, as long as it doesn't harm themselves or others.

The problem here is placing relationships and sexual satisfaction on a maturity (or any other kind of) scale. Mutual caring and growth are mutual caring and growth, no matter what the interpersonal configuration. Sexual satisfaction is sexual satisfaction, and over the millennia people have found a multitude of ways to achieve it when they are brave (if the culture demands such bravery) and creative—including people who identify as heterosexual. Sullivan (1953) quips:

> Since I have set up three classifications of intimacy, four classifications of the general interpersonal objective of the integration of lust and six classifications of genital relationship, this results in seventy-two theoretical patterns of sexual behavior in situations involving two real partners, As a matter of fact, there are only forty-five patterns of sexual behavior that are reasonable probable; six are very highly improbable, and the rest just aren't possible. (p. 294)

In many states in the United States sodomy is still against the law. It took until June 26, 2015, for the United States to legalize same-sex marriage (*Obergefell v. Hodges*; Supreme Court Opinion on Same-sex Marriage, 2015), making it the 17th nation to do so.

Furthermore, there has probably not been an experiment in which early developmental historical synopses (from birth to late adolescence) are presented to therapists, who are then asked to determine if the adults turned out to be LGBTQIA+ people. Probably even therapists well-trained in interpersonal development would not be able to reliably predict the eventual gender identity and/or sexuality in adulthood, at least not with statistical significance. In other words, they would not be able to come up with a universally predictive set of developmental events that cause someone's gender identity and/or sexuality. In comparison, interpersonalists can, for example, posit that the lack of parallel play opportunities in childhood makes it more difficult for a child to move into the juvenile era of cooperation, competition, and compromise without the loss of self-esteem, and that as an adult that person might have difficulty, therefore, working comfortably in a team or even in a cubicle next to other cubicles.

> What "causes" homosexuality is an issue of importance only to societies which regard gay people as bizarre or anomalous. Most people do not wonder what "causes" statistically ordinary characteristics, like heterosexual desire or right-handedness; "causes" are sought only for personal attributes which are assumed to be outside the ordinary pattern of life. (Boswell, 1980, as cited by Blechner [2009, p. 49])

"The problem is that almost any attempt to question why someone becomes homosexual turns into an exercise in covert hatred, when the unconscious motivation behind the asking is unaccepting and pathologizing" (Blechner, 2009, p. 55).

Most likely the therapist "subjects" would suggest possible adult issues worthy of therapeutic intervention—problems in living, to various degrees, depending upon the developmental residuals—and even those would be hypothetical because experiences, particularly in preadolescence and adolescence, can and do challenge the self-system to change. The issue is simply about growing up, leaving home, and trying on new social roles. This makes predictions about adult personalities solely on the basis of very early developmental experience impossible.

Freud, among others, was friendlier toward gay people than many of his contemporaries and followers. Although he was privately prejudiced (Blechner, 2009, p. 33fn, citing Wortis [1954]), he nevertheless wrote to a mother of a gay man:

> Homosexuality is assuredly no advantage, but it is nothing to be ashamed of, no vice, no degradation, it cannot be classified as an illness; we consider it to be a variation of the sexual function produced by a certain arrest of sexual development. Many highly respectable individuals of ancient and modern times have been homosexuals, several of the greatest men among them (Plato, Michelangelo, Leonardo da Vinci, etc.). It is a great injustice to persecute homosexuality as a crime and cruelty too. (Freud, 1951, pp. 786–787)

In 1930, Freud joined his signature to a statement calling for the repeal of the law against relations between "consenting adult males" that read, in part, that "homosexuality . . . [had] been present throughout history and among all peoples." The law which penalized it represented an "extreme violation of human rights" (Blechner, 2009, p. 33).

Sullivan also moved vigorously against mainstream psychiatric prejudices. "As a psychiatrist for the military forces, [he] attempted to remove homosexuality as a disqualifying factor for admission to military service, although he was eventually overruled by the military establishment" (Blechner, 2009, p. 26, citing Bérubé [1990]).

INTERPERSONAL THERAPY

Sullivan is credited with around an 86 percent "cure" rate on an inpatient unit of schizophrenic males (who happened to be gay men) without psychotropic or electroconvulsive therapy interventions (Blechner, 2009, p. 110). Sullivan

(1962) reported on the "cure" of schizophrenia, not of "homosexuality": the inpatients experienced positive resolutions of their psychoses, a mental health state more readily available for growth-provoking interpersonal relatedness. For many reasons, Sullivan's approach to schizophrenia and to gay people was revolutionary for his time (and even for the 21st century) because he didn't think of schizophrenics as "sick" any more than he thought of gay people as perverse or criminal. He staffed his unit, established in 1930 at Sheppard and Enoch Pratt Hospital, primarily with gay men and people comfortable with gay people in order to create a loving, caring, non-judgmental, non-homophobic atmosphere, required for a positive resolution from a schizophrenic break. Gay people could not begin to work on their problems in living in an environment that *also* looked askance at their gender identification and/or sexuality. Being a gay man was not their dysfunctional symptom, their "problem" in living. Coming out to themselves, enjoying sex the way they wanted to, or even a having a fantasy about such forbidden desires might have *triggered* the psychotic episode because the idea was so abhorrent to their families and society that it threw their self-systems into disarray.

But being an LGBTQIA+ person doesn't cause them to be "crazy." A loving, safe, and supportive environment is a prerequisite for any possibility of a positive resolution of a schizophrenic episode regardless of a person's gender identity and/or sexuality. People cannot grow and change without a cherishing interpersonal environment. It seems self-evident, but Sullivan's work was groundbreaking. Unfortunately, with exceptions, his inpatient model is not generally accepted or practiced today.

So it is understandable that LGBTQIA+ people often seek out self-identified LGBTQIA+ therapists. They don't want the added issue of their gender identity and/or sexuality (burgeoning or otherwise) to stand in the way of having a positive therapeutic relationship. The issues they present are no different from anyone else's: a pattern of failed relationships, staying too long in a dysfunctional relationship, noticing how isolated they are, depression, obsessions, "panic attacks," "anger control," fear of going crazy, failing out of college, hallucinations, death of a parenting one, the crisis of reaching retirement age, and so on. An LGBTQIA+ individual might add to the list how, if, and when to come out to their parenting one(s), spouse, children, boss, straight friends, and/or themselves, or how to navigate gender transition. It is similar to someone figuring out how to deal with an interracial or inter-religious relationship, depending upon the interpersonal milieu they identify with or feel alienated from. Of course, this is not to suggest that it is a prerequisite that an LGBTQIA+ individual work with an LGBTQIA+ therapist any more than a man should work with a male therapist, a Catholic should work with a Catholic, or a person of color should work with a person of color. No rules here. Bottom line: there needs to be a positive therapeutic relationship.

Being an LGBTQIA+ person is not a problem. The therapist and/or the individual assuming that being an LGBTQIA+ person is a problem *is*. The person seeking therapy may have found themselves, often with great struggle, and they may need to finally talk to someone about it. Their human issues are also of importance: Are they fulfilled? Are they maximizing their potential to lead happy, productive lives? By whose standards? How can their personal demons and obstacles to growth be cleared away so that they can, little by little, organize their interpersonal infrastructure for making the most out of the time they have on this planet? For example, if a loving, productive relationship happens to be a lesbian one, why would anyone shun it or criticize it?

As with anyone, therapists need to take a detailed history. They need to constantly return to a person's history throughout the course of therapy. That's the whole point. How did a person come to be who the person is, and what obstacles stand in the way of becoming what the person might become? But the purpose of conducting a historical interpersonal analysis should not be to find out why a person gender identifies as they do and/or why they are or are not attracted to one or more persons sexually, romantically, and/or emotionally.[8] Understanding a person's self-system is crucial. Understanding the person's security operations that prevent challenges to the self-system is crucial. Understanding that anxiety comes with the territory of changing the self-system is crucial. Knowing that there are no reported deaths from experiencing anxiety is crucial.[9] (Dissociation of needs is more likely to cause accidents, disease, and destructive or self-destructive behaviors.) A stagnant or debilitating LGBTQIA+ relationship is as problematic as a stagnant or debilitating heterosexual relationship. The approach is the same. The therapeutic projects uncover the historical developmental interpersonal etiology of how one ended up in that unfortunate relationship (no matter the configuration), and help one make better choices in the future based on insights gleaned from the inquiry and analysis and the willingness to try new experiences.

So when an LGBTQIA+ person, usually after a positive therapeutic relationship has been forged, finally comes into the office ready to "confess" their most "awful and repulsive secret," the therapist must simply listen. After hesitating and going off on tangents, the person finally blurts out the "awful truth" and waits with the utmost dread for the therapist to run for the hills. After a moment or two of silence, the therapist finally says, "So I'm still waiting for this awful secret of yours. What's the punch line?" Having established that expression of their true self is not the problem, they can get to work on the real stuff.

It may indeed turn out that a person is really denying desires for same-gender exploration, and is so stuck in parental and/or societal values that they need therapy to clear the decks. The same is true in reverse. Perhaps a lesbian is lesbian because they are defying strict parental taboos, not because they are really into it. They need to feel comfortable with whatever they do, including, if they need to, acknowledging that their true self is heterosexual without worrying that they are now simply conforming, or risking people saying, "I told you so" or "You finally came to your senses." Perhaps they are bisexual. They need to clear away the historical obstacles, try new experiences without worrying about alienating their original primary caretaker(s).

This same orientation to exploring sexual experiences is relevant to understanding adolescent behavior. Safe sexual experiences are not "promiscuous"; adolescents are simply garnering experience. And people do not need to be adolescents to do so. People never outgrow their need for new experiences.

Of course, the literature is still replete with all sorts of theories and professional preoccupations about sexuality or whom a person sleeps with (or wants to sleep with): Is a person born predisposed to a particular sexuality? Is it in the genes? Is there any gender at all, or do family and society "gender" a child from birth according to the child's genitalia? Are we born simply sensual and get pushed or not pushed into a gender and/or sexuality? There are also lengthy discussions about how LGBTQIA+ people have such and such different developmental histories from straight ones.

But, to reiterate, one does not need to construct a developmental interpersonal theory (or any theory, for that matter) about how someone *becomes* an LGBTQIA+ person. It doesn't matter. Ultimately the answers are not as important as what a person does with their life to maximize satisfaction of needs, sexual and otherwise.

CHANGING ONE'S GENDER IDENTITY AND/OR SEXUALITY

People who can express themselves in the ways they are most comfortable generally report a much happier and fulfilling existence (depending upon where they live geographically and culturally). But like everything else, some problems in living usually don't just disappear because of a shift in gender identity and/or sexuality. Those who are questioning and perhaps changing their identified gender, whether or not they opt for a sex or gender confirmation procedure, can come into therapy with the same interpersonal issues as everyone else.

Deciding to change one's gender identity is difficult, whether or not the person opts for a sex or gender confirmation procedure. The process is usually accompanied with a great deal of reflection and the need for significant interpersonal support.[10] Given the transphobic climate in the United States (and in many other countries), it would be unusual if the person didn't need help with that issue.[11] Again, for a person who is thinking of, anticipating, or completing a sex or gender confirmation procedure, the therapeutic project may still include confronting interpersonal obstacles to a fulfilling and productive life.

Asexuality

As discussed in chapter seven, asexuality is a sexual orientation, "just like being bi, gay, lesbian, pan, or straight" (The Trevor Project, 2021). For asexual people, sexual attraction is on a continuum from no sexual urgings to sexual attraction once the person forms a strong emotional connection with someone else. It cannot be assumed that asexuality is a problem requiring treatment. Likewise, it cannot be assumed that not feeling romantically attracted to anyone (a-rom) is a problem requiring treatment.

Pronouns

Finally, people have the right to their pronouns; they still might be forced to struggle to assert and maintain that right depending upon where they live and whom they interact with. It is essential that practitioners who work with LGBTQIA+ people ask their analysands for their pronouns (not their "preferred" pronouns—people are who they are, not who they "prefer" to be). If therapists are new to respecting people's pronouns, they need to apologize if they slip.

SUMMARY

We live in a racist, sexist, ageist, classist, homophobic, transphobic, misogynist society. There have been advancements since 1968, fueled by the resistance of people of color and their allies. However, women are still objectified, despite all the gains. They are still seen as sex objects and are coerced implicitly and explicitly into acquiescing to cis men. Sexually graphic pornography, most of which depicts masculine power and control over women, is more or less allowable. But until the first decades of the 21st century, even a semi-passionate kiss between two women on TV or in the movies was abhorrent. The movie *The Kids Are All Right* (with all its problems about how it depicts a lesbian relationship) was avant-garde in 2010. There has not been much advancement in the acceptance of same-gender partnership either, although same-gender marriage is now legal. And Rachel Maddow is a lesbian news anchor on MSNBC. In 2019, Lori Lightfoot was sworn in as Chicago's first Black and openly LGBTQIA+ mayor. As of this writing, LGBTQIA+ people now hold governmental positions in the United

States. Little by little they are at least being recognized as legitimate people. Nevertheless, the airwaves are full of propaganda that continues to promote divisions and demonizing of all kinds. People are still being murdered because of who they are.

Homophobia, transphobia, and other issues of gender identity and sexuality in the United States have been and continue to be major problems. For LGBTQIA+ people, and especially for people of color, expressing one's true self continues to be extremely dangerous.[12] Therefore individuals might seek therapy precisely because the society they live in, to varying degrees, is phobic and racist and they need help dealing. But as with every other group suffering from social injustice, LGBTQIA+ people struggle for the right to live life the way they see fit and to fit in wherever they choose to live, vacation, and work. Some LGBTQIA+ people in fact might want help figuring out how to join in the struggle, feel like card-carrying members of the human race, with the commitment to assert that right whenever it is necessary to do so, rather than feel less than human, that they must hide. But some might indeed have to hide because they live and work in a dangerously homophobic, transphobic community. If they do not choose to join the struggle, they at least need to feel comfortable in their own bodies. That is a universal interpersonal issue. An issue of therapy. Sullivan's (1953) one-genus postulate: "Everyone is much more simply human than otherwise" (p. 32).

What's the problem with being an LGBTQIA+ person? No problem—except that people live in an extremely problematic society.

NOTES

1. Sullivan, H. S. (1972). *Personal psychopathology: Early formulations.* W. W. Norton & Co. In the era Sullivan was practicing and writing, the terms "homosexual" and "gay" referred to men and women. He worked with gay men because, he said, he didn't know enough about "gay" women. Also the term "homosexual" was consistent with that era.

2. Intimacy is defined as interpersonal closeness, not necessarily sexual.

3. As discussed in chapter six, the use of the word "love" has to do with cherishing, validation, and tender relatedness to the other's needs, not the traditional meaning of romantic love.

4. With this principle, radical for his time, Sullivan was emphasizing that "homosexuals" and people diagnosed schizophrenic must not be placed in a category of "other" and treated as such. In the current social climate, not only must his one-genus postulate be reasserted, it must particularly call attention to "recently acknowledged complexities in gender identity, development, and both the vulnerability and resilience of transgender communities; in other words, a greater understanding of the

diversity in the human condition" (Taffel, 2020, p. 17). This applies to all peoples who are oppressed and whose common humanity must be emphasized.

5. The acronyms and language are constantly in development.

6. Humans can now procreate without heterosexual physical contact through, for example, artificial insemination.

7. See, for example, Anton (2022). With the election of Donald Trump and Mike Pence in 2016, "conversion therapy" was back in the spotlight. Mike Pence's anti-LGBTQIA+ statements do indeed pose a threat to the freedom and safety of LGBTQIA+ people, particularly LGBTQIA+ people of color. As of this writing (2022), such practices are banned in several states and activists and lawmakers are concerned that hard-won protections will continue to be eroded, particularly because of the "don't say gay" legislation and the U.S. Supreme Court ruling against abortion (*Dobbs v. Jackson Women's Health Organization*).

8. See also Blechner (2009, p. 41).

9. With the caveat that some anxiety symptoms must also be medically monitored.

10. Two particularly helpful books are *Counseling Transgender and Non-Binary Youth: The Essential Guide* (Krieger, 2017), and *Sex, Sexuality and Trans Identities: Clinical Guidance for Psychotherapists and Counselors* (Jacobson et al., 2020).

11. Leslie Feinberg's *Transgender Warriors* (1997) is a comprehensive and sensitive chronicle of the historical and personal struggles of those struggling with their identity and sexuality. Along with *Stone Butch Blues* (1993), Feinberg's work has been inspirational and personally liberating for them.

12. In late 2018 the Human Rights Campaign (2018) described violence against trans people in the United States as "epidemic," with 128 trans people killed the five previous years. The overwhelming majority were trans women of color.

Chapter Seventeen

The Current Context of "Mental Disorders" and Their Treatment

In 1893, Breuer described his "talking cure" to relieve "hysterical" symptoms by the verbal expression of repressed feelings and the reexperiencing of repressed memories. Freud and others expanded upon Breuer's method and veered in different theoretical directions. Psychoanalysis was performed on "patients" by "doctors," MDs or PhDs. Further developments have taken place primarily in this medical relationship.

There have been exceptions to this. First, psychoanalysis has consequences beyond the clinical setting. Freud et al. could not avoid implications that phenomena such as repression had for issues beyond what was presented by "patients." Theories of society followed that could not be contained under the rubric of psychopathology. Ramifications occurred in medicine, psychology, philosophy, politics, sociology, and the arts.

Second, as psychoanalytic theory generalized its conclusions beyond people considered "ill," the concept of "patient" and "illness" changed. The structure and dynamics of personality, particularly the unconscious, were assumed to be ubiquitous. This threatened the status quo. As the fear-inspiring thought progression went, what if we cannot distinguish "healthy" from "sick," as in "us" and "them"?

The exploration of unconscious thoughts and feelings took hold in the 1950s, expanded in the 1960s, and leveled off in the 1970s. The release of repressed images and energies was seen as key to unlocking artistic expression. In the cultural center of New York City during the 1960s, the then-hip *Village Voice* was replete with ads for practitioners of psychoanalytic therapies, as well as newer modalities such as Gestalt and Existential.

Psychiatry has held on to the idea that its patients are "sick" based on clusters of symptoms comprising "diagnoses." The medical parallel is that determining what germ has infected the patient, based on symptoms and tests, determines their treatment. Szasz (1960, 1974) has been a compelling critic of this approach. His argument is that psychiatric labeling of people as having a disease is used by the state to control disapproved behaviors. Szasz points out that other than psychiatry, illnesses in medicine are diagnosed by provable physiological changes, not just clusters of symptoms Although his view has not gathered much support within psychiatry, it has helped spawn a movement against psychiatric treatments such as lobotomy, electroshock, involuntary hospitalization, and forced medication.[1] Aside from receiving the sympathy of humanists and others, Szasz still commands respect in mental health and the social sciences. Perusal of contemporary abnormal psychology textbooks usually finds discussion of his argument.[2] This is because his major points have not been disproved in the 60 years hence. Mental illness has not been successfully traced to physiological or genetic causes, despite the amount of research done toward that effort. Finding chemical or physiological correlates, genetic "predispositions," etc., has not proved such causes, which elude even the research supported by the pharmaceutical companies that would gain from such evidence.

Nevertheless, mainstream psychiatry has been in a frenzy of diagnosis proliferation. The first *Diagnostic and Statistical Manual of Mental Disorders* (*DSM*), published in 1952, conceptualized mental disorders primarily as dysfunctions of personality.[3] A project of the American Psychiatric Association, it listed 106 mental disorders (Grob, 1991) and relied on psychodynamic concepts and ideas from sociology and biology. *DSM-II*, published in 1968, listed 180 disorders. It largely relied on the same concepts and did not clearly distinguish between mental illness and mental health.

In the 1960s a movement toward community mental health burgeoned. Partly due to the ethic of the times and the Civil Rights Movement, psychiatric hospitalization was considered cruel and costly. That chlorpromazine had been found to hide if not decrease symptoms of "schizophrenia," and that lithium did the same for symptoms of manic-depressive psychosis, enabled decreased use of segregation. Many disorders were now manageable on an outpatient basis. Psychotropic medication became an important profit source for the pharmaceutical industry. Most psychoanalytic theorists had already thought that psychotics were not amenable to the "talking cure" and that working psychodynamically with people on massive doses of medications was daunting. The major exception was Sullivan (1962), who had worked intensively with schizophrenics in the late 1920s. Laing (1960), who worked with schizophrenics, was a major opponent of the medical approach; he was deeply influenced by existential philosophy, rejecting the medical model of mental illness.

The 1960s and 1970s also saw a surge in alternatives to psychoanalysis for long-term treatment of neuroses. Client-centered therapy (Rogers, 1951) and approaches based on existential (e.g., May et al., 1959) and Eastern philosophies amassed followings. But long-term psychotherapies were soon devastated. The conjuncture of the surge of the pharmaceutical companies into psychiatry, their expansion to the treatment of non-psychotic disorders, and the striving to contain costs by the insurance companies spurred reports that long-term psychotherapies were not cost-efficient. The concurrent rise in popularity of cognitive therapy, and later cognitive behavioral therapy (CBT) and other brief therapies, accelerated the decline of long-term therapies.

Early successes of the pharmaceutical and insurance companies were evident in *DSM-III*. Published in 1980 (American Psychiatric Association), it was almost four times as lengthy as *DSM-II*. It had a descriptive, medical approach detailing clusters of symptoms comprising 265 mental disorders (Wilson, 1993). Medical prevalence over psychodynamic approaches is exemplified by its relegation of neuroses, previously central to psychoanalytic formulations, to parenthetical additions to several disorders. A conscious aim of *DSM-III* was expanding the conditions covered by insurance companies. Major support for the contributing researchers came from the pharmaceutical companies. *DSM-IV* (American Psychiatric Association, 1994) is an elaborate classification scheme of symptoms nearly twice as long as *DSM-III*, containing 297 disorders. *DSM-V* (American Psychiatric Association, 2013) has many more.

Dozens of psychiatrists who worked on *DSM-V* had financial ties to the pharmaceutical industry. They agreed to limit their consulting relationships with companies to $10,000 a year during the *DSM-V* deliberations (Goozner, 2010). They did not agree to clear their minds of their decades-old biases—or their hopes of being rewarded by their patrons in the future for their efforts.

The prevalence of classification by symptom checklists has further trivialized psychoanalysis within psychiatry and has implications beyond. Several psychoanalytic organizations parried with the *Psychodynamic Diagnostic Manual* (PDM Task Force, 2006), another classification scheme based more on experiences of people's emotions and relationships than the *DSM* is. Any success is likely to be hampered by the collusion of pharmaceutical companies with American Psychiatric Association and insurance companies, who push to drive down costs with labor-saving inventions that pharmaceuticals offer for symptom alleviation. In the short run, the administration of medication is cheaper and sometimes may assist in psychotherapy success. Often, however, it is used as a substitute, and it provides some people some relief, albeit with side effects. Medications and their dosages are tweaked for years, sometimes until patient-doctor pairs resign themselves to controlling one or two symptoms. Sometimes the failure of the medication is attributed to the patient having been misdiagnosed now that their "true" disease has been revealed. An unfortunate outcome of this approach is that many now refer to disorders, such as bipolar, obsessive-compulsive, and attention deficit, as if they are inborn, genetically based. Conversations about those afflicted sometimes assume the same permanency of these disorders as astrological signs: e.g., "I do that because I have ADHD."

About one in four adult Americans—60 million people—suffer from a diagnosable mental disorder in a given year (Athealth, 2013). Approximately 10 million children meet the criteria for having at least one of six mental disorders (National Institute of Mental Health, 2009). Since insurance companies use *DSM* diagnoses to determine reimbursable conditions, people seeking help from any mental health professional must garner at least one diagnosis or pay out of their own pockets, a near impossibility for most. Thus, someone seeking help for emotional discomfort must be pigeonholed. Treatment of any substantial length must be justified, and insurance companies can demand (as can patients) that psychotropic medications be administered. Since the alleviation of symptoms that comprise the "disease" constitutes enough improvement for insurance companies to deny further treatment, medication and short-term behavior therapies are promoted. As of 2006, psychotropic medication accounted for more than half of all mental health care spending (Nordal, 2010). Understanding the roots of someone's psychic torment, the interpersonal relationships that have contributed to problems (and solutions), etc., take too long for today's "market-driven" solutions. The notions that improvement or cure involves bringing unconscious dynamics into awareness, fulfillment of one's potential as a human being, etc., have been eclipsed by the goal of superficial behavioral adjustment to demands of social institutions such as work, family, and school. Views of psychotherapy as adjusting social deviants to a system that needs adjustment itself are not being dismissed here. Many psychotherapies served that purpose. They do not have to. Rather, psychotherapy can facilitate people's effectiveness in changing themselves so they can expand their abilities to transform society toward a more just and equitable one.

This book's approach largely relies on ideas first expressed by Sullivan (1953), who used the term "problems of living," which Szasz would later popularize, to describe the difficulties of people who seek (or avoid) help from someone else. He called the latter "experts," astute in interpersonal relationships (Sullivan, 1954, pp. 11–13). Although Sullivan was a psychiatrist, he endeavored to take the field outside of the traditional doctor–patient relationship, with its hierarchy of power. He stressed interpersonal processes that are or can be experienced by all people regardless of classifications such as diagnoses. A core idea for Sullivan (1953) was the "one-genus postulate" that "everyone is more simply human than otherwise," and that the variety of reactions to interpersonal events result from "differences in [the] relative maturity of the persons concerned" (pp. 32–33).

Our approach to mental disorders relies heavily on Pearce and Newton (1963), who based their theory on Sullivan's. They viewed diagnoses as responses to life based on a person's sequence of development in their first few years of life (p. 239).

Their formulation is an expansion and refinement of Sullivan's "differences in relative maturity." It stresses the individual's point of fixation, the stage of growth at which development is held up. It is at this point that the integral personality forces movement in its push toward interpersonal growth. The integral personality, a dynamic organized to expand experience and satisfy needs, finds its germ in Fromm-Reichmann's (1960) drive to mental health (p. 57). The integral personality forces growth where it is most necessary—the expansion and satisfaction of the needs that were blocked in childhood (Pearce & Newton, 1963, p. 21). In this framework, people with vastly differing symptom constellations (diagnoses) may be fixated at identical points in interpersonal development. Symptoms are viewed as manifestations of security operations[4] which serve to restrict growth and maintain dissociation.

The implications of this viewpoint for treatment are enormous. Psychotropic medications may suppress some of the symptoms. The "success" of such drugs may be to save the person some embarrassment in social situations. In the best of cases, it may enable them to express their thoughts and feelings to a therapist. In the worst case, the drugs may allow the person to dissociate more of the thoughts and feelings and make them more difficult to reach by interpersonal intervention. Since the symptoms subside, the person may rely on the medication, sometimes for life, and never again attempt to grow beyond the point at which their development has been held up. Experiencing less distress, the person may terminate psychotherapy with a severely compromised version of happiness. The person has become "adjusted" or "stabilized." In the middle of these extremes, often outcomes of psychotropic medication, are that the medication has no effect or new symptoms are substituted for the ones previously manifested. The person and the physician may spend months, years, or decades trying to determine the "correct" diagnosis or tweaking the drugs or dosages involved. A good deal of time and money are often spent, with little benefit to the patient, in a search of what is supposedly the remedy for a "chemical imbalance" or hereditary defect. The cost may also include physical, cognitive, or emotional side effects that endure temporarily or permanently.

The goals of the therapy explicated here differ vastly from symptom suppression, dissociation, adjustment, and stabilization. At their center is helping the person organize the forces for growth, a dynamism oriented toward the progressive expansion of satisfaction and experience (Pearce & Newton, 1963, p. 443). Therapy attempts to alter patterns of organization that stifle growth, and to promote more satisfactory life experiences (Pearce & Newton,

1963, p. 441). Altering stifling patterns of organization is not a task that can be addressed by one or more medications or a brief series of appointments oriented primarily toward changes of behavior.

NOTES

1. See, for example, Breggin (1991).
2. Most abnormal psychology textbooks follow the *DSM*. Many college courses in abnormal psychology are attempts to teach *DSM* nosology while accepting it.
3. This discussion of the various *DSM* incarnations relies on Tsao (2009).
4. See chapter 1.

Chapter Eighteen

The Political Economy of Psychotherapy

THE CURRENT CONDITION OF PSYCHOTHERAPY

Insurance companies dictate which treatment modalities are reimbursed, how many appointments are needed, what drugs and dosages can be used, etc.[1] Few can afford to pay for psychotherapy "out of pocket." Limiting the number of sessions covered restricts effectiveness. This results from the recent rise of "managed care," which controls access to services and keeps costs down. Medication "therapy," the administration of drugs that sometimes alleviate some of the symptoms of what is assumed to be psychiatric "diseases," has become the favored modality of insurance companies. These drugs only offer symptomatic relief and do not treat the underlying causes of people's problems in living. Medication is often accompanied by dangerous side effects but costs less than psychotherapy. It takes little time to write a prescription, and side effects can be somewhat relieved by other medications.

The rationale of such "treatment" is that the "disease" is caused by a chemical imbalance. The scientific evidence for this is controversial. Correlations found between thoughts and feelings and chemical reactions in the brain do not prove causality. The implicit rationale of medication "therapy" is that people cannot change themselves or their circumstances by means of empathic understanding and analysis by psychotherapists. A result has been vast profits for pharmaceutical manufacturers.

SOME HISTORICAL BACKGROUND

As mentioned in chapter 17, the "talking cure" took hold in the 1950s, expanded in the 1960s, and leveled off in the 1970s. Brief therapies, such as cognitive Behavioral therapy (CBT) and medication "therapy," have eclipsed psychotherapy. The role of health insurance has been central.

When wages were frozen during WWII, companies facing labor shortages offered health insurance to attract workers instead. The federal government encouraged this by ruling that premiums paid by employees were tax-deductible (Rosenthal, 2017).

In 1946 a United Automobile Workers–General Motors agreement instituted company-sponsored health insurance. This broke the more progressive demand of the Congress of Industrial Organizations (CIO) for national health insurance for all workers (Leary, 2005). The Taft-Hartley Act of 1947 mandated that workers obtain health benefits only through collective bargaining with employers, not through government programs. The possibility of a state-run health system like those in European countries was outlawed.

Tying benefits to employment increased the fear of losing one's job (Navarro, 1993). The employment-insurance connection means that each time General Motors closes a plant, it saves what it paid in health insurance premiums.

The 1960s brought Medicare for the elderly and Medicaid for the poor. Stagflation (slow economic growth coupled with inflation) of the 1970s resulted in U.S. capitalists cutting health care benefits. Between 1981 and 1991, the health insurance industry's control over health policies increased, bolstered by $60 million given to congressional representatives by health companies' PACs (picture archiving and communication systems; Navarro, 1993, pp. 31–32). In the 1990s a grassroots movement arose for a government-administered single-payer system that would bypass insurance companies. President Clinton's 1992 electoral victory was buoyed by his promise of universal comprehensive health benefits, co-opting much of the single-payer movement. He appointed Hillary Rodham Clinton to head a task force that implemented the "managed-competition" approach of the Jackson Hole group, which was composed of representatives of large insurance companies, the pharmaceutical industry, other major corporations, and professional organizations. "Managed competition" is health care operated and controlled by insurance companies attempting to force providers into their networks. The theory was that insurance companies would compete for employer-paid premiums and create lower-cost plans. Instead, there have been increasing costs and cutbacks in care. Corporations, to avoid cutting into their own profits, buy into plans that have less coverage and higher deductibles while medical cost growth outpaces wage growth (O'Brien, 2021).

The corporate profits of insurance companies, including those of new entities called health care corporations, have skyrocketed. Health care is now the third largest industry in the United States, which tops the list of all but one country in per-person expenditures for health care.[2] Seventeen percent of the U.S. GDP goes to the health care industry. Per capita spending of France and Sweden is about two-thirds that of the United States. The United Kingdom spends 61 percent (World Bank, 2019). Nevertheless, the three countries cover almost their entire populations through national insurance programs (Anderson & Taylor, 2005, p. 375). In 2020, the U.S. per capita spending of $12,530 was twice the average of the countries in the Organisation for Economic Co-operation and Development, OECD(Centers for Medicare & Medicaid Services, 2021).

Part of the triumph of the insurance companies is due to HMOs (health maintenance organizations), which were created beginning in the 1950s to keep costs down. Since then, they have grown enormously, from 26 million subscribers in 1986 to 55 million in 1996 (Anderson & Taylor, 2005, p. 375). Insurance companies often sponsor HMOs, and people are forced or enticed into HMOs by lower premiums than plans offering freer choice of providers.[3] HMOs control all aspects of health care, including the selection of providers, authorization of treatment plans, and monitoring of treatment. They limit the ability of practitioners to determine treatments and patients' ability to choose providers. They favor the least expensive treatments. In the mental health field, this means medication rather than psychotherapy, and very short-term rather than long-term psychotherapy.

The profits of pharmaceutical corporations skyrocketed. The drug industry had already been the most profitable in the country since the early 1980s . The ascendancy was documented by Angell (2004), who reports that in 2002, the combined profits of the 10 drug companies in the Fortune 500 exceeded the profits of all 490 other firms combined. She details how industry-friendly legislation, beginning in 1980 with the Bayh-Dole Act, facilitated their success. It allowed universities and small businesses to patent discoveries emanating from research sponsored by the National Institutes of Health (NIH), the major distributor of dollars for medical research. Before that, taxpayer-financed discoveries were in the public domain. After that, universities could patent their discoveries and grant-exclusive licenses to pharmaceuticals for royalties. Other legislation allowed NIH to make deals with pharmaceuticals to transfer NIH discoveries to industry. Medical schools and teaching hospitals were transformed into "partners of industry." The Joint Economic Committee of Congress found that *publicly* funded research led to 15 of the 21 drugs introduced between 1965 and 1992 considered to have the highest therapeutic value (Goozner, 2000). Pharmaceuticals reaped the profits.

In 1995, an internal NIH memo lifted the limits on outside income of its personnel, reversed prohibitions against taking stock or options, and freed its leaders to make personal deals with companies (Willman, 2003). Between 2000 and 2004, at least 530 NIH scientists—upon whose recommendations doctors rely—took fees, stocks, or options from biomedical companies (Willman, 2004).[4] A 2002 survey of medical experts who write practice guidelines found that nine of 10 had financial relationships with drug manufacturers, and six of 10 were tied to companies whose drugs were considered or recommended in the guidelines they wrote (Stolberg, 2002). The financial ties were rarely disclosed.

Angell (2004) also states that, starting with the Hatch-Waxman Act of 1984, laws extended the monopoly rights of brand-name drugs, another boon to pharmaceutical mega-profits. With these came the increasing ability of drug companies to control Food and Drug Administration (FDA) decisions made regarding the safety of medications. Pharmaceutical lobbyists made the FDA a de facto partner in industry and successfully pushed FDA fast-track approval of new drugs (Willman, 2004). This was facilitated by the 1992 Prescription Drug User Fee Act. Pharmaceuticals agreed to pay the FDA $300,000 for each new medication, and in return, the FDA promised speedier approval of new medicines (Abramson, 2004).

Exemplifying this partnership, Angell points to FDA committees that review new drug applications. At least one member at 92 percent of the meetings had a conflict of interest, and half or more at 55 percent of the meetings had conflicts (Cauchon, 2004, p. 1A, as cited by Angell [2004]). Ten of 32 panelists advising FDA about removing pain control pills associated with heart attacks from the market were consultants for pharmaceuticals. Without their votes, Vioxx and Bextra would have been pulled. They were not, and the stocks of the drugs' makers soared after the vote (Harris & Berenson, 2005).

The most powerful in Washington, the drug lobby spent $245,812,399 in 2016, more than any other industry. In 2014 it contributed over $50.7 million to candidates (Center for Responsive Politics: Lobbying, 2017). The president and CEO of Pharmaceutical Research and Manufacturers of America (PhRMA) from 2005 to 2010 was former Louisiana congressperson W. J. Tauzin, appointed as a reward for making sure that the new Medicare prescription drug law precluded discounts for Medicaid and Medicare, and barred the importation of cheaper drugs from Canada (Martin, 2004). PhRMA's power precludes the possibility of regulating drug prices. All other developed nations have some form of such regulation.

The rampant march of the profit-making insurance and drug corporations has been merciless in its effects upon mental health research. George Albee, a past president of the American Psychological Association, summarizes the situation:

> Unfortunately, in psychiatry, much that passes as research is financed by the pharmaceutical corporate giants. They pay for the research. They pay the referees who judge the research. They underwrite the cost of the conferences where results are announced and the cost of publishing the psychiatric journals where they are published. The usual freedoms of scientific inquiry are missing. (Albee, 2002)

The Results: Drug Company Dominance of the Mental Health Field

The power of pharmaceuticals acutely impacts the mental health field. Breggin (1991) documents its influence upon the American Psychiatric Association, whose journals, conferences, and projects are funded by pharmaceuticals. This started primarily because of the association's loss in income in the early 1970s, as it was losing the competition for psychotherapy patients to lower-cost providers like psychologists and social workers. In 1980 APA decided to encourage pharmaceuticals to support scientific activities. This unholy alliance has promoted the self-serving view that has been pushed within psychiatry for most of its existence: that mental illnesses have biochemical etiologies, and thus biochemical treatments.

The American Psychiatric Association also aligned itself with the National Alliance for the Mentally Ill (NAMI), which consists of parents of "mentally ill" offspring who deny any parental role contributing to interpersonal or emotional problems of their grown children. NAMI promotes genetic and biological explanations of interpersonal behavior, and drug treatment and electroshock to control it. Major drug corporations contribute to NAMI (Breggin, 1991). Albee (1990) warned the mental health field against the alliance of NAMI and biological psychiatry in dismissing family dynamics as causes of severe mental problems. NAMI's counterpart in the realm of children's problems is Children with Attention Deficit Disorders (CH.A.D.D.). Because CH.A.D.D. advocates the neurological etiology of attention deficits, it deflects blame from parents. Socio-economic factors, problems with parenting and/or schools, etc. are downplayed. CH.A.D.D. receives funding from pharmaceuticals, such as CIBA-Geigy, the manufacturer of Ritalin.

Psychiatrists reap their share of the NIH/pharmaceutical bonanza. For example, P. Trey Sunderland III, a senior researcher at NIH, endorsed a Pfizer-marketed Alzheimer's drug in a 2003 NIH national television broadcast. He omitted that his research was done in collaboration with Pfizer and had received $508,050 in reimbursement from the company (Willman, 2004). Psychologists, through their own professional organization, have pushed for parity in benefit reimbursement so that mental health services can be covered as much as medical ones. However, whereas many psychologists had opposed the medicalization of mental health, now they primarily have taken a "if you can't beat 'em, join 'em" stance, pushing for their own right to prescribe.[5]

Over six billion prescriptions were dispensed in the United States in 2020 (IQVIA Institute, 2021) for everything from lowering cholesterol to raising penises. The success of the drug industry also typifies a sleight of hand that the drug companies have become quite adept at: inventing new diagnoses to accommodate their marketing ambitions. In Angell's words, "Once upon a time, drug companies promoted drugs to treat diseases. Now . . . they promote diseases to fit their drugs" (Angell, 2004, p. 86). "Erectile dysfunction" removes the problem of "impotence" from the mental and emotional field completely, over-biologizing and chemicalizing interpersonal interactions.

The same dangerous inventiveness fills the *DSM*, the official authority of psychiatry. Recent additions include adolescent rebelliousness, arithmetic learning problems, childhood hyperactivity, and attention deficit disorders (Albee, 2002). Angell documents how GlaxoSmithKline pushed Paxil to treat their invented "social anxiety disorder." The original *DSM* listed about 60 disorders, while the latest (American Psychiatric Association, 2013) has about five times as many.[6] Recent marketing of treatments for invented diseases, including "restless leg syndrome," "female sexual dysfunction," and "low testosterone," is reviewed in Walsh (2018).

New "diseases" spread like the plague, while old ones—depression, schizophrenia, etc.—became framed in chemical terms in television commercials and drug company publicity adopted by psychiatry. A brochure distributed in a major psychiatric facility in New York is published by Pfizer and typifies the backwardness of the "science" behind it by stating, "The importance of dopamine [a chemical that carries messages within the brain] in psychotic symptoms is clear from the fact that medications that are used to treat psychotic symptoms affect dopamine to some degree" (Pfizer, 2001). This is akin to saying that histamines are important to understanding insomnia because some antihistamines cause drowsiness.

Marketing of psychiatric drugs has extended toward younger and younger children. Spending on drugs to treat children and adolescents for behavior-related "disorders" rose 77 percent between 2000 and 2003, mostly for depression and attention deficit disorder (Freudenheim, 2004). Sixty-five percent of children and adolescents taking behavioral medicines were on antidepressants in 2004, despite FDA warnings of side effects such as suicide. Attention disorder drug use by children *under age five* rose 49 percent in that period. Twenty-nine million prescriptions were written in 2004 for Ritalin and similar stimulants—23 million of them for children. A study of 12 children who took Ritalin for three months found chromosome damage in each child, suggesting increased cancer risk. Ritalin "expert" Lawrence Greenhill, who consults for the companies that make stimulants, questioned why the government became so concerned about chromosome damage and the risk of cancer (Harris, 2005b). By 2017 more than seven million children were on psychiatric medication (Citizens Commission on Human Rights, 2017). Pharmaceuticals also buy influence from state mental health officials, resulting in the overmedication of children with anti-psychotic drugs (Waters, 2005).

The Economic Context of These Developments

The industrialization of health care and, within it, "mental health" care must be viewed within the context of the advance of the capitalist mode of production. The tide that has swept away many crafts and the family farm, and transformed the family itself, has tumultuously changed health care and medical research. Capitalism succeeded in commodifying much that was heretofore unthinkable—water, even air, in the form of pollution credits. Why not health?

Technological Innovation and Scientific Research

Technological innovation and scientific discovery have been crucial to the advancement of capitalism. Marx astutely analyzed this during early capitalism: "[M]odern industry . . . makes science a productive force distinct from labor and presses it into the service of capital" (Marx, 1967 [1867], p. 361). "Invention then becomes a business, and the application of science to direct production itself becomes a prospect which determines and solicits it" (Marx, 1973, p. 704). Marx saw the force behind this development in capitalists who, in order to cut costs, strive to increase productivity via technical innovation, particularly mechanization, to undersell other capitalists or firms. They then could expand their market share and profits relative to others, allowing their survival. Their competitors would then be forced to adopt the new innovations.

Mandel (1978) describes how as capitalism matured, research and development became organized as autonomous investment, first as a branch of each company, then as independent enterprises themselves. Noble (1977) built upon Braverman's (1998) analysis of how industry monopolized science, controlling the products of technology by controlling patents and directing the process of scientific production by means of organized and regulated industrial research. By the middle of the 20th century, technology and science had submitted to corporate concerns. This is attested to not only by left-wing analysts such as Mandel, Noble, and Braverman but also by economic historian Nathan Rosenberg (1982). He writes:

> Industrial societies have created a vast technological realm that is very closely shaped by economic needs and incentives. This technological realm, in turn, provides numerous ways in which daily economic life has become closely linked with science. That realm defines the directions that promise large financial rewards and provides many problems and empirical observations that stimulate creative scientific research. These statements are supported by the increasing institutionalization of research in private industrial laboratories. . . . [D]ecisions in the pursuit of science are subjected, in these profit-making firms, to a calculus of private costs and benefits. (p. 159)

Note that the "economic needs" referred to by Rosenberg have no necessary correspondence to any interpersonal, biological, or other kinds of "needs." They may overlap with them, for example, when food produced by corporate agriculture has some nutritional value. But "economic needs" may be constructed by the same agents that provide their fulfillment. There are countless technological inventions being created for which the "need" (aka "demand") is manufactured and marketed with it. Commercials pound away about our "need" for cellular phones with cameras that download music, and the "need" for sufferers of the newly invented "social anxiety disorder" to take Paxil. For pharmaceuticals, like all capitalist firms, "need" is profit, and dictates the direction of research: "[T]he pharmaceutical industry is supremely uninterested in finding drugs to treat tropical diseases . . . since those who suffer from them are in countries too poor to buy drugs," states Angell (2004).

In contrast, the profitability of drugs that treat penile flaccidity has led to the investment of extraordinary sums in research, development, and marketing and inspired (so far unsuccessfully) attempts to bridge the "gender gap" in the "sexual dysfunction" market to fulfill economic "need."[7]

The subjugation of science to capitalists' profit demands, foretold by Marx and elaborated by Rosenberg and others, merits a revised description of what is called "scientific research." First, incentives to fudge are eclipsing ethical concerns. More than 15 percent of thousands of NIH scientists responding to a survey *admitted* they had changed studies' designs or results to satisfy sponsors (Weiss, 2005, p. A03). Determining how many actually fudge would require more sophisticated techniques. Secondly, 13.5 percent of scientists in the same survey admitted they knew their research designs would not yield accurate results. Again, these are just the admitted transgressions. Even so, how "scientific" can such knowledge be? Martinson, one of the surveys' investigators, concludes, "Science has changed a lot in terms of its competitiveness, the level of funding and the commercial pressures on scientists. We've turned science into a big business but failed to note that some of the rules of science don't fit well with that model" (Weiss 2005, p. A03).

Thus, the health care industry, spurred by profit-seeking insurance and drug corporations, has followed the path of other industries within the capitalist economy. Profits determine the direction of innovation and research. Each firm tries to expand its market share to survive against competitors. New products are then built upon or changed slightly by competitors. Since patents are central to their profitability through monopoly pricing, pharmaceuticals patent minor changes to existing drugs and claim that their "new" one works better. Since they control the research, even to the extent of falsifying evidence, pursuit of science is subjected to calculations of profit, and profits allow them to buy further influence in government.

THE COMMODIFICATION OF CARE

In capitalist societies not only physical goods become commodified; so do services. Marx 1967 [1867]) wrote, "A service is nothing more than the useful effect of a use-value, be it of a commodity, or be it of labor" (pp. 299–300). Braverman (1998) states that when the useful effect of labor is not an object but is sold directly to the consumer, the effect of the labor becomes the commodity, and "[w]hen the worker does not offer this labor directly to the user of its effects, but instead sells it to a capitalist, who re-sells it on the commodity market, then we have the capitalist form of production in the field of services" (p. 248).

Services become commodities produced and sold for profit, increasingly true for health care, which produces not only medicines, hospitals, and dialysis machines, but also *care*. Care includes surgery, advice, TLC, counseling, laboratory testing, etc. Some is aided by computers and other devices, but all involves human labor. The labor is increasingly paid for in wages and fees by firms that reap profits from the labor that they buy. The providers of that labor, who own no part of these companies, become proletarianized—they become workers whose only way to earn income is to sell their labor power. Whether they are being compensated well, as are most physicians, or poorly, as are many other health workers, they are workers. In the mental health field, the product that is commodified and profited from consists of the relief of symptoms, control of behavior, etc., and is marketed wherever demand exists or can be created.

As in other profit-making industries, health care firms depend upon their workers being paid less than the value they create by their productive activity. Much of that surplus value becomes profit. The commodification of health care and the proletarianization of its workers are the result of the conversion of "the helping professions" into a capitalist industry.

TURNING THE TIDE

The moral outrage expressed by Szasz (1960) concerning the abuses of psychiatry resonated with compassionate observers in the mental health field, as well as with social observers. Psychiatry's abuses have since become less visually appalling, as medicines have replaced straightjackets as tools of control. Medicalized control is not only more convenient; it is more insidious and widespread. More recent expressions of outrage, such as Breggin (1991), are as justifiable as were those of the Luddites, who destroyed machines in the early 1800s. Those machines formed the material mode of existence for the rising capitalist mode of production. "It took both time and experience before the workers learnt to distinguish between machinery and its employment by capital, and therefore to transfer their attacks from the material instruments of production to the form of society which utilizes those instruments" (Marx, 1967 [1867], pp. 554–555).

Breggin's well-intentioned pleas for therapy, empathy, and love to replace drugs, electroshock, and biochemical theories similarly blur the distinction between the instruments of production and the form of society using them. In the mental health field, the pushback against these abuses needs to be focused on the profit system from which they stem.

The treatment of mental disorders is part of profit maximization. The system of agencies, political institutions, and laws serves the accumulation of profits. The capitalist class is like an addict who requires ever bigger doses to satisfy the urge. Capitalists can be influenced by persuasion as easily as a vampire can be convinced to relinquish blood-sucking. A stake through its heart—or, in the case of the capitalist system, a radical transformation—is the treatment required.

The implementation of such treatment demands organizing the associations of providers and the people they work with—the producers and consumers of care—in mental health and health care in general. Some steps in organizing the providers have already been taken, despite the "professionalism" that has kept health workers from uniting to fight for better pay and benefits. This elitist ideology, promulgated by employers, warns doctors, nurses, etc., not to sully themselves by joining unions. In the name of being professionals, when they did not challenge employers' offers, many remained underpaid.

However, about 40 years ago, nurses began to organize. According to the U.S. Bureau of Labor Statistics, 20.4 percent of RNs and 10 percent of LPNs/LVNs currently identify as union members (Nursing.org, 2022). Unionized nurses can earn an average of $220-$400 more per week than non-unionized nurses (Soliant.com, 2020). There have even been inroads in the unionization of physicians (Sherer, 1999).

SUMMARY

The ascendant power of capital makes it a formidable opponent to human needs. The number of victims of commodification and proletarianization of everything and everyone in its path continues to rise. A renewal of truly helpful mental and physical care is tied to the success of these victims in eliminating capitalist exploitation.

NOTES

1. Updated and reprinted from Singer (2007).
2. The island country of Tuvalu spends 24 percent (World Bank, 2019).
3. See, for example, Freudenheim (1995, p. C2).
4. In 2005, the NIH director banned agency scientists from consulting for drug companies while assuring that he would "re-examine the new rules . . . to make sure they have not had negative effects on the agency's ability to recruit top scientists" (see Harris, 2005c). He also softened a proposed rule requiring 6,000 NIH scientists to sell their shares in drug and biotechnology companies. Instead, only the top 200 officials must keep their holdings in any one drug firm below $15,000 (Harris, 2005a).
5. See, for example, American Psychiatric Association (2013).
6. But the American Psychiatric Association "cured" millions of "sick" Americans by dropping "homosexuality" from the *DSM* in 1973.
7. See, for example, Harris (2004, p. C1) and Pollack (2004, p. C1).

Chapter Nineteen

A Comparison of Revolutionary and Interpersonal Theories

People, raised by people, create interpersonal relationships that produce social change. This change affects how human needs are satisfied or blocked. Need satisfaction ranges from basic survival, like food, water, clean air, and good health, to increasingly complex social interactions with ever-widening circles of people.

Social change, satisfying needs of more and more people, becomes revolutionary when it breaks the bonds of restrictive social structures. In the same manner, if personal satisfaction grows beyond restrictions set in early relationships, it is revolutionary. The struggle to get needs met against the forces that deny those needs is a continuous process; it never stops.

Interpersonal theory is in the tradition of revolutionary theory, discussed by Marx and Engels in the late 19th century, and since then by many revolutionary thinkers in liberation struggles around the world. It shares some assumptions with the Soviet psychologist Lev Vygotsky and some of his more recent followers.[1]

One assumption is that people and society are constantly changing. This change is dialectic, determined by cause and effect, action and reaction, always creating something new, and that change is developmental, based on the force of human needs versus the restrictions against their satisfaction. It studies how people interact with the surrounding world, how they struggle against the barriers to satisfaction, break down those barriers or fail, only to rise up and try again.

In interpersonal theory, development is individual evolution in an interpersonal context based on the interaction between a person's needs and restrictions placed on the satisfaction of those needs by others in that context.

An interpersonal example:

A baby, given the opportunity to play and explore, begins to move from crawling after things to trying to stand, experimenting with walking and falling and getting up again, to moving more efficiently in space, all facilitated with the encouragement of its caretaker(s) in a social context. To the degree that the caretaker(s) encourage the process and provide the opportunity, the baby will become mobile, learning to walk, run, and explore. Given the opportunity, the process is continually expanding. If validation and opportunity are limited, the outcome will be affected to the degree of the limitation, until the next opportunity arises.

In interpersonal theory, human beings are always changing, growing, or deteriorating.[2] In Marxist theory, constant pressure for change from below pushes for expansion while pressure from restrictive forces pushes for reactionary constriction. Validation for expansion in society comes from recognition by growing numbers of people that it is not only desirable for more people to meet their needs, but that it is possible and necessary. That recognition is called social consciousness.

When change occurs on a mass basis, it may become a movement or a trend. If it continues to grow, it can become an uprising or a revolution. It may make some gains, or it may fail, but the outcome is also based on the context in which it occurs.

A political example:

In his historic work, *Black Reconstruction in America*, W.E.B. Du Bois (1998) referred to the mass escape from slavery as a general strike for freedom. The intervention of Black soldiers in the Civil War, including the great Harriet Tubman as a Union spy, was decisive in terms of the military defeat of the slavocracy. The Civil War in class terms was the inevitable war not just against North vs. South geographically, but a clash between two social systems vying to see which one would come out on top in controlling the means of producing everything in society. The short-lived Reconstruction Period was probably the most revolutionary period in the United States, when Black people were making strides to win their bourgeois democratic rights. Black people built their own schools and were gaining political power through the elections to state legislatures in the South. In some areas, Black people were being armed by the Union Army to protect themselves against attacks from the remnants of the slavocracy that were regrouping in order to regain state power.

Once the new federal government, led by President Andrew Johnson, a Confederate sympathizer, withdrew the Union Army, this retrenchment tragically gave new life to the former slavocracy to usher in a reign of white supremacist terror on the Black population. This resulted in the overturn of virtually all the progressive gains, replaced by semi-slavery conditions in the South which gave rise to the KKK, lynchings, sharecropping, low wages—racist Jim Crow became legalized by the U.S. Supreme Court in 1898, forcing millions of Black

> folks to migrate from the South to the North. The overthrow of Reconstruction was nothing less than a counter-revolution. (Dowell, 2018)[3]

The needs do not go away; no matter how strong the personal or societal repudiation of needs, the push for greater satisfaction of needs continues. There is also the awareness of the conflict, now awakened, including awareness there has been some progress, however brief.

The change can be gradual, but when it is a question of changing basic structure, be it personal or societal, change is likely to be a more massive struggle, destroying old repressive patterns and reorganizing the individual or the society to meet more needs. Even then, it is usually only partial, leaving more struggle ahead.

In interpersonal theory, growth is determined by validation of needs and functions to meet those needs. Validation of a function is a process of communication between people. It goes smoothly or in a skewed or limited form, depending upon how the expansion of that function was originally experienced by the validator and, consequently, the person being validated. Conscious experience is validated experience. It is limited by what is conceivable to a person,which is determined by validation from primary relationships in the process of development.

In the same way, social consciousness, the awareness of great numbers of people about what is possible for them, comes from validation and demonstration of that possibility. The validators that push the boundaries of social consciousness are the revolutionaries, in the form of activists, artists, anyone communicating something new that strikes a chord. Here is an example from an activist of how a great artist dramatically expanded her social consciousness:

> I was a white kid in Oak Park, just across the 8 Mile Road line dividing Detroit and its suburbs. I was 10 years old in 1964 when I first found Aretha Franklin's music, 13 at the time of "Respect" and the Black rebellion. Those two related things—the Black uprising and Aretha's defiant, soul-stirring music—played a big part in raising my consciousness, giving rise to my anti-racist solidarity and starting me along the revolutionary road. (Ettinger, 2018, p. 3)

If the society at large is ready to hear the news, it will spread. For that reason, Lenin called the newspaper of the Bolshevik Party *Iskra*, *The Spark*, and Mao, judging the readiness of the Chinese masses to welcome the ideas of socialist revolution, invoked the phrase "A single spark can start a prairie fire." If the society as a whole is not ready, the new message of hope will not have a broad response in the moment, but the message, if preserved, will not only add to the force of later messages but also inspire them.

On an individual level, needs that have not been validated exist outside of awareness. To the degree they are not acceptable to the primary validator(s), they are also unavailable to awareness in their offspring. However, the needs don't go away. They are still pressing for satisfaction because their satisfaction is required for increased functioning, i.e., further development. The needs may not be consciously experienced, except via fantasies, dreams, and fugue states,[4] or if there is unavoidable contact with an experience that requires functioning that has been heretofore forbidden.

> Ann grew up in a reclusive family. She learned early not to trust her neighbors and to see herself as a loner, careful about whom she played with. She made friends one at a time, usually avoiding groups of people, and was uncomfortable with strangers. She sometimes fantasized about being part of a guerrilla movement or a band of outlaws, but she never actually belonged to any group. Things changed when she was sent to sleep-away camp at age 14, against her objections. At camp, she was inundated with strangers and forced to participate in group activities. She suddenly spiked a high fever and was confined to the infirmary for the first week. She slept almost constantly, enduring terrifying nightmares. When she rejoined the group, she plunged into activities as she had never done before. She learned how to deep-water swim and play baseball.
>
> Fortunately, the camp was staffed by people who were sensitive to the needs of the campers and had available counselors who were good at group dynamics, providing activities that were fun. They were also good at listening to campers that needed to talk.
>
> Ann confided to a counselor that she was very cautious about making friends, first assessing how they reacted to her before she tried committing to a friendship. The counselor said that was nonsense, that she had to go full force and not be afraid to be interested in people. Ann took the advice to heart. The following fall, with new experiences of camp friendships under her belt, she continued practicing being friendly to strangers at her new school. She noticed that being open and friendly felt freeing and that, for the most part, she got good responses back. She integrated this new social function, the ability to be comfortable with strangers, and also the ability to participate in group activities.

Needs are constantly pushing for a place in the sun depending on which functions are most urgently emerging at the time. The emergence of previously dissociated needs is a stormy process. They were originally dissociated because they made the caretaker(s) anxious. As the needs were pushed out of awareness, the forbidding gestures[5] and the despairing assumptions connected to those needs were also relegated to the margins of awareness or were completely dissociated.

When the reemergence of the need to function in a particular way becomes clearly felt in focal awareness, despairing thoughts and feelings associated with that previously forbidden need emerge as well. In addition, the organization of consciousness becomes disrupted in the process of the shifting pattern of what one considers oneself. "Who I am" (the self-system[6]) is expanding.

One strenuously begins to question many of the basic assumptions they have upheld about living. They simultaneously experience great disorganization and powerful negative feelings. Sullivan (1953) has called them "uncanny emotions": awe, horror, loathing, and dread (pp. 163–165). The form these feelings take is determined by the specific experiences a person had in the process of originally dissociating the needs. The despairing feelings are part of the security apparatus, the basis for all operations a person goes through to stave off recognition of any forbidden need.

The despairing assumptions and the security operations that flow from them are like the security forces of the state, the police, the prison system, ICE, FBI, CIA, as well as extra-legal forces like the KKK, that guard against the recognition and satisfaction of needs of the more disenfranchised in society.

Pearce and Newton (1963) call despair the "central paranoia" and describe it as the "fear of death," "fear of disorganization," and "dissociation of the need for tenderness" (p. 170). These abhorrent feelings, learned in early infancy when the human being is most vulnerable, form the underpinning of the defensive structure. They are aroused at the point that the new, previously dissociated feelings spring into awareness. Usually these feelings are to be avoided at all costs, but when the press of needs is greater than the desire to avoid noticing them, there is a struggle between the integral personality,[7] which is pressing for need recognition, and the defensive structure. The person experiences their own despair full force but is also pulled to express the need and learn to satisfy it, despite their despair. It is truly a revolution of the psyche.

The outcome of that personal revolution depends on what social support, i.e., later validation, is available for reintegration of the new needs and functions. If the "revolutionary" transition is not perceived as such by any other people, it's very possible that the person's security system will be strengthened. They will regard brief emergence into awareness of new needs and functionality with some derision, perhaps an example of their "perverse nature," a "dangerous weakness," or "moral failure." It will require more strenuous circumstances to allow the new aspects of oneself back into awareness. Since the need still exists, it will take greater vigilance and more stringent measures to keep it out of awareness. However, if there is any validation for that emerging need, some aspect of it will remain available to consciousness.

Such eruption of needs into awareness occurs most frequently in adolescence, when there is great physiological change and, for most, sexual urges become intense, almost impossible to ignore. They need to be integrated into the rest of the adolescent's repertoire of relatedness. In early and late adolescence it is urgent to establish relationships outside the family, to play a wider role in society, requiring an expansion of functions to relate to the world beyond. Such eruptions of need are felt earlier, at the point a child begins nursery school or begins to be confronted with the need to relate to one's peers. They also occur during any radical adult change in a person's life, such as having children or drastically changing one's lifestyle. Depending on the intensity of exposure to new circumstances and the availability of new validation, the experience of the need for reorganization of one's personality can occur at any time in life.

The revolutionary upheaval accompanying change on an individual level parallels what occurs in societal push for change. On a societal level, it can and usually does mean revolutionary war, with all its attendant violence and upheaval. It also can mean ideological struggle between those trying to express their needs and the repressive forces trying to keep them down. The outcome, as mentioned before, depends on the balance of forces.

However not all wars are revolutionary wars. There are wars of conquest and competitive wars between rivals over who should dominate. Sometimes such wars are advertised as "revolutionary" to the masses of people who are expected to provide the raw material to fight them. People wage legitimate revolutionary wars (as in, for example, China, Cuba, DPRK [North Korea], USSR [Soviet Union], and Vietnam) to improve the well-being and expand the independence and autonomy of more and more people in a material way that can be measured.

SULLIVAN'S ONE-GENUS POSTULATE: "EVERYONE IS MUCH MORE SIMPLY HUMAN THAN OTHERWISE"

A major principle of interpersonal theory is that all people have the same needs and ways of growing and deteriorating despite superficially different appearances and external behavior (Sullivan, 1953, pp. 32–33).[8] The assumption makes it possible to understand any human behavior, no matter how ostensibly bizarre, based on a knowledge of the individual's history. It also makes it possible to help anyone get their needs met given the right circumstances.

Revolutionary theory also assumes that all human beings have an equal right to health, education, shelter, and opportunity "from each according to their ability, to each according to their needs,"[9] despite differences in race, gender identity, sexuality, ability, and country of origin. No one is left out. To be effective in making lasting social change, solidarity is necessary among all those who are oppressed, regardless of superficial differences. In unity, there is strength. It's not a coincidence that imperialist forces who take over other countries encourage ethnic and religious hatred that divides the population to weaken it (for example, in Iraq, Ireland, Yugoslavia, and throughout the African continent).

Social consciousness plays a large part in relation to concepts of unity. When Marx first wrote, he was referring to European workers as the Proletariat. He expanded his position with the statement, "Labor in the white skin can never free itself as long as labor in the black skin is branded" (Marx, 1967 [1867], p. 169). At the time he wrote, the concept of enslavement was commonly accepted. It took half a century to expand the slogan "Workers of the World Unite!" to "Workers and Oppressed of the World Unite! You have nothing to lose but your chains!" It took another century for the slogan "Black Lives Matter" to be commonly used, and that struggle continues today in the consciousness of many.

At the beginning of the 20th century, only a married, heterosexual orientation was legal in industrialized countries. All other forms of sexual relatedness were relegated to "unacceptable" or even "bestial," often declared illegal, and certainly frowned upon. Awareness and acceptance of LGBTQIA+ sexual and gender expression have slowly increased over the past century, particularly since the Stonewall Rebellion and the Gay Liberation Movement of the 1970s. What was considered a serious crisis for an adolescent 50 or 60 years ago is now commonplace in many homes (depending upon where they are) as young people increasingly explore openly with gender identity and sexuality. However, statistics show that, as with people of color, it is still dangerous to be a trans person in the United States (Human Rights Campaign, 2018). The struggle for freedom of gender and sexual expression is far from over.

Awareness of the humanness of more and more people increases slowly, but as it does, it creates more identification between groups of people and potential strength and unity of purpose in social movements. It follows that the more people one identifies with, the greater the possibility for inspiration and change. The West Virginia teachers' strike inspired the Oklahoma teachers' walk-out, and suddenly people who may have never thought about Puerto Ricans before recognized the importance of the Puerto Rican teachers' struggles and identified with them. The awakening is indeed like a spark that starts a prairie fire, from Puerto Rico and West Virginia to Jersey City, Arizona, and Oklahoma. Who knows where it will end?

What is disparagingly labeled as "identity politics" by the corporate press is the increased recognition of the ways people are oppressed by category and of the need to unite and uplift all identities. The universality of cause only makes the masses of oppressed people stronger.

DEVELOPMENT IN AN ORDERLY SEQUENCE

As explicated throughout *Evolving Self*, biological functions must be validated in infancy, but other functions, such as curiosity and playfulness, are also needed to thrive and grow (Pearce & Newton, 1963, pp. 77–90; Trevarthen, 2009). Without curiosity and a sense of play, a baby cannot relate to the world with perceptual-motor coordination while exploring the object world. Relating comfortably to objects is necessary before one can begin to feel competent and interact successfully with other children and authorities. Successful interactions with other children allow the possibility for feeling like a member of the human race. Feeling like a peer is the basis for feeling like a full member of a specific group of people. In turn, feeling like a member of a group is a prerequisite for being able to compromise, compete, and cooperate, i.e., to interact successfully within that group in working toward goals. Feeling comfortable as a group member allows one to form more intimate friendships within that group, identifying with others empathically. Being able to make intimate friends allows one to form a "chumship" with a person one admires and identifies with. The increased self-confidence and self-esteem that comes from the chumship experience allows a person to expand that relatedness to other individuals and groups of people indefinitely. "There are functions just beyond a person's learned ability that would be the next step in interpersonal development" (Pearce & Newton, 1963, p. 58). That is, there is an ongoing push in people to expand their functions to the limit of what they can conceive is possible.

The transition to the next level of functioning, beyond what is conceivable at the moment, may be easy or difficult depending on the strength of the self-system's security operations. Simultaneously, the integral personality, based on the press of the individual's emerging needs, is focused on this zone of experience, pushing the person to find a way to satisfy those needs. If the limit is pushed further along, consciousness expands. "Human society also develops based on a dynamic process of cause and effect" (Engels, 1902). "Marx and Engels not only discovered the laws governing capitalist society in particular, but also the driving forces of social development of humanity since its rudimentary beginnings on earth" (Ballan, 1971, p. 5).

> [Engels] found that the family, like any other historical phenomenon, was by no means a frozen, ossified, permanent, changeless institution based on moralistic or religious conception. Quite the contrary. . . . Its development and transformation flowed from the material conditions of life and was most vitally affected by profound changes in the development of production. (Ballan, 1971, p. 6)

> The increase of production in all branches—stock raising, agriculture, domestic handicrafts—enabled human labor power to produce more than was necessary for its maintenance. . . . The addition of more labor power became desirable. It was furnished by war; the captured enemies were transformed into slaves. Under the given historical conditions, the first great division of social labor, by increasing the productivity of labor, adding to the wealth, and enlarging the field of productive activity, necessarily carried slavery in its wake. Out of the first great division of social labor arose the first great division of society into two classes: masters and servants, exploiters and exploited. (Engels, 1902, p. 167)

Engels (1902) describes the development of the stages of servitude: "Slavery is the first form of exploitation, characteristic of the antique world. Then followed feudalism in the Middle Ages, and wage labor in recent times. These are the 3 great forms of servitude, characteristic of the 3 great epochs of civilization. Their invariable mark is either open or, in modern times, disguised slavery" (p. 182). Engels goes on to describe how these divisions affected social consciousness in the family:

> The herds and the other new objects of wealth brought about a revolution in the family. Procuring the means of existence had always been the man's business. The tools of production were manufactured and owned by him. The herds were the new tools of production, and their taming and tending was his work. Hence, he owned the cattle and the commodities and slaves obtained in exchange for them. All the surplus now resulting from production fell to the share of the man. The woman shared in its fruition but she could not claim its ownership. The "savage" warrior and hunter had been content to occupy the second place in the house, to give precedence to the woman. The "gentler" shepherd, standing on his wealth, assumed the first place and forced the woman back into the second place. . . . The former domestic relation was now reversed, simply because the division of labor outside of the family had been altered. The same cause that once had secured the supremacy in the house for women, viz., the confining of women's activity to domestic labor, now assured the supremacy of the men in the households. The domestic labor of women was considered insignificant in comparison to men's work for a living. . . . At this early stage, we can already see that the emancipation of women and their equality with men are impossible and remain so, as long as women are excluded from social production and restricted to domestic labor. The emancipation of women becomes feasible only when women are enabled to take part extensively in social production, and when domestic duties require their attention in a minor degree. This state of things was brought about by the modern great industries, which not only admit of women's liberal participation in production, but actually call for it and, besides, endeavor to transform domestic work also into a public industry. (p. 167)

Ballan (1971) relates Engels's thinking to the changing structure of the family under capitalism:

> The family has of course undergone changes, and these changes are concomitant with the stages of development of class society. Just as class society has been transformed from slave society to feudal society, and then to capitalist society, each stage demarcated by a qualitative advance in the development of the means of production, so it is that the family, as an economic unit of private property, has also changed. (p. 21)

In the first stages of the capitalist era there was the need for education of the workers to produce profit. There was vast improvement of technology and, consequently, increased awareness of vast numbers of people, that is, awareness of each other, historically as well as currently. The opening up of new markets included more and more people open to exploitation. The drive to profit also created greater boom and bust cycles as the market's ability to absorb any more surplus dried up. In the ensuing era of capitalist decay, labor has become so productive that fewer skilled workers are required to produce profit for highly technical work to maintain capitalist society. For that reason, the trend is for the ruling class to cut back on the needs of the workers and the oppressed, who have become "superfluous." Universal human needs, such as health care, housing, and education, have increasingly become more and more for profit and out of reach for most people. In addition, the exploitation of greater areas of the world has created increasing environmental disaster everywhere. All this lays the groundwork for the potential of a new revolution to create a society based on human needs rather than profit.

Human behavior, motivated by material needs and society, is more efficient at satisfying needs for the greatest number when it is organized collectively and cooperatively.

Interpersonally speaking, human beings are constantly changing in a causal sequence (development). A person or a society is either growing or deteriorating.

THE INTEGRAL PERSONALITY—GUERRILLA FIGHTER FOR PERSONAL GROWTH

The integral personality (Pearce & Newton, 1963, p. 21–22) is the total of all aspects of experience, dissociated and in awareness. All experience a person has is contained in the integral personality. It is called integral because it integrates everything: the self-system, the central paranoia, and the dissociated, which all relate to the integral personality in a particular way. It is seen as integrating all experience, both conscious and unconscious. The integral personality is motivated by the press of need and moves a person to find ways to begin to satisfy that need. It incorporates all experience, hopeful as well as despairing. Because needs press for satisfaction, the integral personality focuses on one's most pressing needs and how they are being blocked in order to organize ways to break through the security system. In the individual, it is the integral personality that pushes a person to move, sometimes unwittingly, in the direction of potential satisfaction of need, even when that need is dissociated. The integral personality also exposes the individual's restrictive, despairing assumptions and the myriad ways the person limits their own functioning. The exposure can be through dreams, rumination, or the unconscious push to be in situations that make one's limitations obvious. A person finding themself placed in the uncomfortable position of having their limitations exposed can choose to use the opportunity or run from it. For example,

> Carol moved into a dorm at a university where she would be sleeping away from home for the first time since she was 12. She came from a small town where she had rarely come into contact with strangers.
>
> The first few weeks of college, she began to engage with her roommates, teachers, and classmates. She enjoyed herself, intrigued by the new people she met and challenged by the new ways people interacted. Simultaneously, she was increasingly anxious, dizzy, disoriented, and feeling increasingly disloyal to her parents, whom, she felt, would not approve of some of the people she met or how they behaved. One night, she had a nightmare that she was murdering her parents. She awoke suddenly, the image of the nightmare vivid before her eyes. She couldn't shake the mood of the nightmare and for the next few days she felt increasingly guilty and frightened. The fun she had started to feel was slipping away, replaced by dread. She suddenly had the thought, "I can't stay here! I have to go home."
>
> This situation could progress in varying ways. She could confide in someone at the college, a roommate, a counselor, or even a friend back home, who might be able to label her anxiety as temporary homesickness. A counselor might even link her nightmare to her own despair that moving into a wider world would "kill" her parents. Her parents themselves might be a source of validation, telling her they were excited for her to go to the university and meet all those new people, assuring Carol she wasn't "killing" them and urging her to stick it out. Or, less hopefully, the people she chose to confide in might buy her nightmare, suggesting she go home, not bite off more than she can chew.
>
> Depending on how much she has integrated the ability to relate to peers, she could continue to be enthusiastic, using her newfound contacts to get her past her anxiety. Or she could isolate herself socially and in class but stick it out, later remembering her time at the university as lonely and depressing. She could stay at the university and get drunk a lot, keeping her experience foggy and distant, placing herself in jeopardy, and avoiding meaningful interaction. She could

drop out and go home. Much would depend on prior and current validation for enjoying new friends, as well as the opportunity for meeting people who could give her support.

Psychotherapy, in interpersonal theory, is a method for reorganization of a person's life to include more satisfaction, an increasingly deeper capacity for intimacy with a wider range of people, to help a person make revolutionary change in living, breaking with whatever prohibitions were in one's childhood and committing to ever-expanding growth (Pearce & Newton, 1963, p. 438): "Successful analysis involves becoming accustomed to revolution" (Pearce & Newton, 1963, p. 440). Therapy is not the only way in which such personal revolution can be accomplished. Any situation in which a person can be exposed to interpersonal validation, learn to tolerate the disorganization and anxiety involved in making meaningful interpersonal changes, can be effective in producing more hopeful, even revolutionary living.

The political analogy to the integral personality is the collective experience of the masses of people, expressed in their oral and written history, their mythology, and their tradition. A validator in society can be a revolutionary leader or group of people, past or present, who awakens people to new needs and inspires them to try new ideas, identify with the oppressed, and resonate with them. They can be a visual or theatrical artist, a writer, an activist, or a philosopher. It can be an organized group of revolutionaries, an organization, a political party, or a tendency that resists repression and has the vision and the dedication to reorganizing society to meet the needs of all the people. The revolutionaries make the uncomfortable statements, the "impossible" demands, and move a society to expand, to change. "Be realistic, demand the impossible!" (Che Guevara).

As social consciousness begins to change and become inclusive of more and more people, it uncovers issues that had not previously been obvious before, new needs. The revolutionary group points out the ways those issues are hidden, the misperceptions, and the limited assumptions that form the restrictive aspects of society.

SUMMARY

Revolutionary socialist and interpersonal theories describe interactions between people, the development of individuals and society based on cause and effect. Both theories include the concept of constant change for expansion or constriction in human functioning based on the conflict of human needs versus repression of those needs. Both theories address the crucial role of changing consciousness in the individual and the society as part of the process of change and the role of validation in the process of changing consciousness. Revolutionary socialist and interpersonal theories stress the importance of the universality of human needs and the need for unity among all people(s).

NOTES

1. See, for example, *Beyond the brain: An agentive activity perspective on mind, development, and learning* (Arievitch, 2017); "Vygotsky and Lenin on Learning: The Parallel Structures of Individual and Social Development" (Au, 2007); "Marxist psychology and dialectical method" (Elhammoumi, 2015); and "Quasi-appropriation of dialectical materialism: A critical reading of Marxism" (Rodrigues et al., 2014).

2. If a person allows the new experience to come into awareness, the person can expand the ability to function, to relate to people; on the other hand, a person may effectively put a damper on the new experience, reasserting and strengthening the old restrictions. There is either growth or deterioration.

3. Extracted from a seminar on *Black Reconstruction in America* by W.E.B. Du Bois conducted by LeiLani Dowell in New York City (2018).

4. A fugue state is a period in which experience of dissociated material is in awareness. It may be accompanied by powerful feelings of paranoia and terror or blankness or depression. It may or may not be remembered. It is like being in a waking nightmare or dream (Pearce & Newton, 1963, p. 347).

5. A forbidding gesture is a non-verbal mode of communication that expresses dissatisfaction or disgust with what another is doing or saying. For example, a significant parenting one signals dissatisfaction by stiffening when their toddler tries to climb on their lap, or the adult walks away when the child tries to show them something they drew. Often the gestures are spontaneous, and although keenly felt by the child, they are not in the adult's awareness. A person cannot remember the actual gestured message from infancy, but now, as an adult, they might be able to get in touch with the mood-memory and be able to connect that mood-memory to stories about their infancy.

6. The self-system is one's sense of self at any particular moment. It has productive and restrictive characteristics. It is available to grow from experience or to ward off growth from experience by omission or distortion. The self-system is the part of personality that organizes awareness. If the self-system could be frozen in time, it would consist of what a person has available to consciousness, that is, awareness of what one can do and who one believes oneself to be in relation to self, other people, and the world.

7. The integral personality is motivated by the press of need and moves a person to find ways to begin to satisfy that need (see below).

8. Sullivan's most basic postulate in his theoretical approach is, "Everyone is much more simply human than otherwise." With this principle, radical for his time, Sullivan was emphasizing that "homosexuals" and people diagnosed schizophrenic must

be not be placed in a category of "other" and treated as such. In the current social climate, not only must his one-genus postulate be reasserted, it must particularly call attention to "recently acknowledged complexities in gender identity, development, and both the vulnerability and resilience of transgender communities; in other words, a greater understanding of the diversity in the human condition" (Taffel, 2020, p. 17). This applies to all peoples who are oppressed and whose common humanity must be emphasized.

9. "From each according to his ability, to each according to his needs" is a slogan popularized by Karl Marx (1970) in his 1875 *Critique of the Gotha Programme*.

Bibliography

Abramson, J. (2004). *Overdosed America: The broken promise of American medicine*. HarperCollins.

Albee, G. (1990). The futility of psychotherapy. *Journal of Mind and Behaviour, 11*, 369–384.

Albee, G. W. (2002). *Another surprise from American psychiatry*. Austin Community College. https://www.austincc.edu/ddydek/dsmcritique.htm

American Psychiatric Association. (1980). *Diagnostic and statistical manual of mental disorders (DSM-III)*. American Psychiatric Publishing.

American Psychiatric Association. (1987). *Diagnostic and statistical manual of mentaldisorders (DSM-IV-R)*. American Psychiatric Association.

American Psychiatric Association. (1994). *Diagnostic and statistical manual of mental disorders (DSM-IV)*. American Psychiatric Association.

American Psychiatric Association. (2013). *Diagnostic and statistical manual of mental disorders (DSM-V)*. American Psychiatric Association Publishing.

American Psychological Association. (December). Criteria for evaluating treatment guidelines. *American Psychologist, 57(12)*, 1052–1059.

Anderson, M. L., & Taylor, H. F. (2005). *Sociology: The essentials* (3rd ed.). Thomson-Wadsworth.

Angell, M. (2004). *The truth about the drug companies: How they deceive us and what to do about It*. Random House.

Annie E. Casey Foundation. (2019). *2019 KIDS COUNT data book*. https://www.aecf.org/resources/2019-kids-count-data-book/

Anton, B. S. (2022). Proceedings of the American Psychological Association for the legislative year 2009: Minutes of the annual meeting of the Council of Representatives and minutes of the meetings of the Board of Directors. *American Psychologist, 65(5)*, 385–475. https://doi.org/10.1037/a0019553

Arievitch, I. M. (2017). *Beyond the brain: An agentive activity perspective on mind, development, and learning*. Sense Publishers.

Athealth. 2013. *The numbers count: Mental health disorders in America*. https://athealth.com/topics/the-numbers-count-mental-health-disorders-in-america/

Au, W. (2007). Vygotsky and Lenin on learning: The parallel structures of individual and social development. *Science and Society, 71*(3), 273–298.

Ballan, D. (1971). *Feminism and Marxism.* World View Publishers.
Beebe, B. (1973). *Ontogeny of positive affect in the third and fourth months of the life of one infant.*[Doctoral dissertation, Columbia University].
Beebe, B., & Gerstman, L. (1980). The "packaging" of maternal stimulation in relation to infant facial-visual engagement: A case study at four months. *Merrill-Palmer Quarterly, 26*, 321–329.
Beebe, B., Knoblauch, S., Rustin, J., & Sorter, D. (1965). *Forms of intersubjectivity in infant research and adult treatment.* Other Press.
Beebe, B., & Sloate, P. (1982). Assessment and treatment of difficulties in mother-infant attunement in the first three years of life: A case history. *Psychoanalytic Inquiry, 1*(4), 601–23.
Beebe, B., Sorter, D., Rustin, J., & Knoblauch, S. (2003). A comparison of Meltzoff, Trevarthen, and Stern. *Psychoanalytic Dialogues, 13*(6), 777–804. https://doi.org/10.1080/10481881309348768
Bérubé, A. (1990). *Coming out under fire: The history of gay men and women in World War II.* The Free Press.
Blakeslee, S. (2006, January 10). Cells that read minds. *The New York Times.*
Blechner, M. J. (2009). *Sex changes: Transformations in society and psychoanalysis.* Routledge.
Blechner, M. J. (2013). New ways of conceptiulaizing and working with dreams. *Contemporaty Psychoanalysis, 29*(2), 259–275.
Boswell, J. E. (1980). *Christianity, social tolerance, and homosexuality: Gay people in Western Europe from the beginning of the Christian era to the fourteenth century.* University of Chicago Press.
Bowlby, J. (1982). *Attachment and loss* (2 end., Vol. 1: Attachment). Basic Books.
Braverman, H. (1998). *Labor and monopoly capital: The segradation of work in the twentieth century..* Monthly Review Press.
Brazelton, T. B. (1982). Joint regulation of neonate-parent behavior. In E. Z. Tronick (Ed.), *Social interchange in infancy: Affect, cognition and communication (pp. 7–22).* University Park Press.
Brazelton, T. B., Koslowski, B., & Main, M. (1974). The origins of reciprocity: The early mother-infant interaction. In M. Lewis & L. A. Rosenblum (Eds.), *The effects of the infant on its caregiver (pp. 49–76).* Wiley.
Breggin, P. (1991). *Toxic psychiatry: Why therapy, empathy and love must replace the drugs, electroshock and biochemical theories of the 'New Psychiatry.'* St. Martin's Press.
Buck, R. (1984). *The communication of emotion.* Guilford.
Buechler, S. (2008). *Making a difference in patients' lives.* Routledge.
Butterwoth, G., & Castello, M. (1976). Coordination of auditory and visual speace in newborn human infants. *Perception, 5*, 155–160.
Cauchon, D. (2004, September 25). FDA advisors tied to industry. *USA Today*, p. 1A.
Center for Responsive Politics. (2017). *Lobbying*. https://www.opensecrets.org/lobby/top.php?showYear=2016
Center for Responsive Politics. (n.d.). *Pharmaceuticals / Health products*. https://www.opensecrets.org/industries/indus.php?ind=H04.

Centers for Medicare & Medicaid Services. (2021) National Health Expenditure Data: *Historical.* https://www.cms.gov/Research-Statistics-Data-and-Systems/Statistics-Trends-and-Reports/NationalHealthExpendData/NationalHealthAccountsHistorical

Chen, E. Miller, G. E., Kobor, M. S., & Cole, S. W. (2011). Maternal warmth buffers the effects of low early-life socioeconomic status on pro-inflammatory signaling in adulthood. *Molecular Psychiatry, 16*(7), 729–737.

Chung, H. Y., Cesari, M., Anton, S., Marzett, E., Giovannini, S., Seo, A., et al. (2009). Molecular inflammation: Underpinnings of aging and age-related diseases. *Ageing Research Reviews, 8*(1), 18–30.

Citizens Commission on Human Rights. (2017). *Number of children and adolescents taking psychiatric drugs in the U.S.* https://www.cchrint.org/psychiatric-drugs/children-on-psychiatric-drugs/.

Cohen, L. B., & Cashon, C. H. (2003). Infant perception and cognition. In I. Weiner (Ed.), *Handbook of psychology.* John Wiley & Sons. https://doi.org/10.1002/0471264385.wei0603

Conci, M. (2013). *Sullivan revisited. Life and work. Harry Stack Sullivan's relevance for contemporary psychiatry, psychotherapy and psychoanalysis.* (L. Cohen, D. Lee, & M. Bacciagalucci, Trans.) Tangram Edizioni Scientifiche Trento.

Cytryn, L., & McKnew, D. (1996). *Growing up sad: Childhood depression and its treatment* (1st ed.). W. W. Norton & Co.

Damasio, A. (2018). *The strange order of things: Life, feeling, and the making of cultures.* Pantheon Books.

DeCasper, A. J., & Fifer, W. P. (1980). Of human bonding: Newborns prefer their mother's voices. *Science, 208*, 1174–1176.

Delafield-Butt, J., Trevarthen, C., Rowe, P., & Gillberg, C. (2019). Being misunderstood in autism: The role of motor disruption in expressive communication, implications for satisfying social relations. *Behavioral and Brain Sciences, 42,* E86. https://doi.org/10.1017/S0140525X1800242X

Dowell, L. (2018). Extracted from a Seminar on Black Reconstruction in America by W.E.B. Du Bois. Conducted at The Solidarity Center, New York City.

Du Bois, W. (1998). *Black reconstruction in America 1860–1880.* The Free Press.

Duncan, S., & Fiske, D. W. (1977). *Face-to-face interaction: Research, methods, and theory.* Lawrence Erlbaum Associates.

Eibl-Eibesfeldt, I. (1989). *Human ethology.* Aldine de Gruyier.

Elhammoumi, M. (2015). Marxist psychology and dialectical method. In I. Parker (Ed.), *Handbook of critical psychology* (pp. 271–279). Routledge.

Emde, R., Polack, P., & Spitz, R. (1965). Anaclitic depression in an infant raised in an institution. *American Academy of Child Psychiatry, 4*, 545–553.

Engels, F. (1902). *The origin of the family, private property and the state.* (E. Untermann, Trans.) Charles H. Kerr & Co.

Ettinger, S. (2018). *WW pays tribute to the activism of Queen of Soul, Aretha Franklin. Workers World Party Newspaper, 60*(34), 3. https://www.workers.org/2018/08/23/ww-pays-tribute-to-the-activism-of-queen-of-soul-aretha-franklin/

Evans, B. (1996). *Harry Stack Sullivan.* Routledge.

Faderman, L. (2015). *The gay revolution: The story of the struggle.* Simon & Schuster.

Faraone, S., Tsuang, M., & Tsuang, D. (1999). *Genetics of mental disorders: A guide to students, clinicians, and researchers.* The Guilford Press.

Feinberg, L. (1992). *Transgender liberation: A movement whose time has come.* World View Forum.

Feinberg, L. (1993). *Stone butch blues.* Firebrand Books.

Feinberg, L. (1997). *Transgender warriors: Making history from Joan of Arc to Dennis Rodman.* Beacon Press.

Feinberg, L. (1999). *Trans liberation: beyond pink or blue.* Beacon Press.

Feinberg, L. (2003). What price for truth? *Workers World, 45*(15), 2.

Feinberg, L. (2004–2008). Lavender & red. *Workers World.* https://www.workers.org/books2016/Lavender_and_Red.pdf

Feist, G., & Rosenberg, E. (2014). *Psychology: Perspectives and connections (3rd ed.).* McGraw Hill.

Feist, G., & Rosenberg, E. (2021). *Psychology: Perspectives and connections (*5th ed.). McGraw Hill.

Fields, D. R. (2009). *The other brain.* Simon & Schuster.

Fox, N., & Hane, A. A. (2008). Studying the biology of human attachment. In J. Cassidy, & P. R. Shaver (Eds.), *Handbook of attachment: Theory, research and clinical applications* (pp. 811–829). Guilford Press.

Freud, S. (1913). *Interpretation of dreams.* (A. Brill, Trans.) Macmillan.

Freud, S. (1951). Historical notes: A letter from Freud. *The American Journal of Psychiatry 107*(10), 786–787.

Freudenheim, M. (1995). Efforts grow to steer elderly retirees to HMOs. *The New York Times*. http://www.nytimes.com/1995/06/13/business/efforts-grow-to-steer-elderly-retirees-to-hmo-s.html

Freudenheim, M. (2004). Behavior drugs lead in sales for children. *The New York Times*. http://www.nytimes.com/2004/05/17/business/behavior-drugs-lead-in-sales-for-children.html

Fromm-Reichmann, F. (1960). *Principles of intensive psychotherapy.* University of Chicago Press.

Gallese, V. (2005). "Being like me": Self-other identity, mirror neurons, and empathy. In S. Hurley & N. Chater (Eds.), *Perspectives on imitation: From neuroscience to social science* (Vol. 1, pp. 101–118). MIT Press.

Goldman, A. I. (2006). *Simulating minds: The philosophy,psychology, and neuroscience of mindreading.* Oxford University Press.

Goldstein, F. (2012). *Capitalism at a dead end.* Word View Forum.

Goodrich, B. G. (2010). We do, therefore we think: Time, motility, and consciousness. *Reviews in the Neurosciences, 21*(5), 331–361. https://doi.org/10.1515/REVNEURO.2010.21.5.331

Goozner, M. (2000). *The price isn't right.* The American Prospect. http://prospect.org/article/price-isnt-right

Green, H. (1964). *I never promised you a rose garden.* New American Library/Signet.

Grob, G. N. (1991). Origins of *DSM-I*: A study in appearance and reality. *American Journal of Psychiatry, 148*(4), 421–31.

Harris, G. (2004). Pfizer gives up testing Viagra on women. *The New York Times,* p. C1. https://www.nytimes.com/2004/02/28/business/pfizer-gives-up-testing-viagra-on-women.html

Harris, G. (2005a). Health agency tightens rules governing federal scientists. *The New York Times.*

Harris, G. (2005b). Report of Ritalin risks prompts a federal study. *The New York Times.* https://www.nytimes.com/2005/07/01/health/report-of-ritalin-risks-prompts-a-federal-study.html

Harris, G. (2005c). A businessman-scientist shakes up the health institutes. *The New York Times.* https://www.nytimes.com/2005/08/30/health/policy/a-businessmanscientist-shakes-up-the-health-institutes.html

Harris, G., & Berenson, A. (2005). *10 voters on panel backing pain pills had industry ties. The New York Times, Late Edition,* pp. A1. http://www.nytimes.com/2005/02/25/politics/10-voters-on-panel-backing-pain-pills-had-industry-ties.html

Harris, S. (1980). A theoretical approach to the halfway house. In E. Jansen, *The theoretical approach to the halfway house* (pp. 121–131). Croom Helm, Ltd.

Harvey, J. (2009). *Seminar on dreams* [Unpublished transcript], New York City.

Havens, L. (1976). *Participant observation.* Aronson.

Havens, L. (1977). Harry Stack Sullivan's contribution to clinical methods. *Contemp. Psycholan., 13*, 360–364.

Hobson, J. A. (1977). The brain as a dream-state generator: An activation-synthesis hypothesis of the dream process. *Am J Psychiatry, 134*(12), 1335–1348.

Hubel, D. H., & Wiesel, T. N. (1964). Effects of monocular deprivation in kittens. *Neurophysiology Laboratory 248*, 492–497.

Human Rights Campaign. (n.d.). *Sexual orientation and gender identity definitions.* https://www.hrc.org/resources/sexual-orientation-and-gender-identity-terminology-and-definitions

Human Rights Campaign. (2018). *Violence against the transgender community in 2017.* https://www.hrc.org/resources/violence-against-the-transgender-community-in-2017

Hyman, S. (2000). The genetics of mental illness: Implications for practice. *Bull World Health Organ., 78*(4), 455–463.

Insel, T. R., & Wang, P. S. (2010). Rethinking mental illness. *JAMA, 303*(19), 1970–1971. https://doi.org/10.1001/jama.2010.555

Interpersonal Psychotherapy Institute. (2016). *About IPT.* https://iptinstitute.com/about-ipt/

IQVIA Institute (2021). The Use of Medicines in the U.S., https://www.iqvia.com/insights/the-iqvia-institute/reports/the-use-of-medicines-in-the-us, May 27, 2021.

Jacobson, G. J., Niemira, J. C., & Violeta, K. J. (Eds.). (2020). *Sex, sexuality and trans Identities: Clinical guidance for psychotherapists and counselors.* Jessica Kingsley Publishers.

Jaswal, V., & Akhtar, N. (2019). Being versus appearing socially uninterested: Challenging assumptions about social motivation in autism. *Behavioral and Brain Sciences, 42,* E82. https://doi.org/10.1017/S0140525X18001826

Johnson, C., & Stevens, M. (2003). *Script partners: What makes film and TV writing teams work.* Michael Wiese Productions.

Keene, C. (1959). *The secret of the old clock.* Grosset & Dunlap.

Keller, H. (1903). *The story of my life.* Doubleday.

Kendon, A. (1980). Gesticulation and speech: Two aspects of the process of utterance. In M. Key (Ed.), *Relationship of verbal and non-verbal communication* (pp. 207–228). De Gruyter Mouton.

Krieger, I. (2017). *Counseling transgender and non-binary youth.* Jessica Kingsley Publishers.

Kvarnes, R., & Parloff, G. (1976). *A Harry Stack Sullivan case seminar.* Norton.

Leach, P. (2010). *Your baby and child: From birth to age five.* Alfred A. Knopf.

Leary, E. (2005). Crisis in the U.S. labor movement: The roads not taken. *Monthly Review, 57*(2), 28–37.

Levenson, E. (1991, updated 2016). *The purloined self: Interpersonal perspectives in psychoanalysis.* Routledge.

Lionells, M., Fiscalini, J., & Stern, D. (2015). *Handbook of interpersonal psychoanalysis (2nd ed.).* Routledge.

Lippman, P. (1996). On dreams and interpersonal psychoanalysis. *The International Journal of Relational Perspectives, 6*(6), 831–846. https://doi.org:10.1080/10481889609539155

Malloch, S., & Trevarthen, C. (2018). The human nature of music. *Frontiers in Psychology, 9*, 1680. https://doi.org/10.3389/fpsyg.2018.01680

Malloy, S. (2016). *A convenient myopia: SEEK, Shaughnessy, and the rise of high-stakes testing at CUNY.* CUNY Academic Works. http://academicworks.cuny.edu/gc_etds/1513

Mandel, E. (1978). *Late capitalism.* Verso.

Martin, P. (2004). *Top house republican becomes chief US drug company lobbyist. World Socialist.* http://www.wsws.org/en/articles/2004/12/tauz-d18.html

Marx, K. (1967 [1867]). *Capital.* International Publishers.

Marx, K. (1970). *Critique of the Gotha Programme. Marx/Engels archive, 3*. Progress Publishers. https://www.marxists.org/archive/marx/works/1875/gotha/ch01.htm

Marx, K. (1973). *Grundrisse.* Random House.

Maturana, H., & Varela, F. (1980). *Autopoesis and cognition.* D. Reidel.

May, R., Angel, E., & Ellenberger, H. F. (1959). *Existence: A new dimension in psychiatry and psychology.* Basic Books.

McCubbin, B. (1979). *The gay question: A Marxist appraisal* (2nd ed.). World View Publishers.

McGuffin, P., & Murray, R. (Eds.). (2013). *The new genetics of mental illness.* Butterworth-Heinemann.

Meltzoff, M., & Moore, M. K. (1983). The origins of imitation in infancy: Paradigm, phenomena and theories. In L. P. Lipsitt (Ed.), *Advances in infancy research (Vol. 2, pp. 265–301).* Ablex.

Mercer, M. A. (2017). *Preventing infant deaths: What can we learn from Cuba? Huffington Post.* http://www.huffingtonpost.com/mary-anne-mercer/preventing-infant-deaths-_b_6812102.html

Merriam-Webster Dictionary. (n.d.). Interpersonal. https://www.merriam-webster.com/dictionary/interpersonal

Mullahy, P. (1948). *Oedipus, myth and complex: A review of psychoanalytic theory.* Grove Press.

Mullahy, P. (Ed.). (1952). *The contributions of Harry Stack Sullivan: A symposium on interpersonal theory in psychiatry and social science.* Hermitage House.

Mullahy, P. (Ed.). (1957). *A study of interpersonal relations: New contributions to psychiatry.* Grove Press.

Mullahy, P. (1963). Book reviews. *Psychiatry, 26*(4), 394–404. https://doi.org/10.1080/00332747.1963.11023368

Mullahy, P. (1980). *Psychoanalysis and interpersonal psychiatry: The contributions of Harry Stack Sullivan.* Jason Aronson, Inc.

Murray, L., & Andrews, L. (2005). *The social baby: Understanding babies' communication from birth.* CP Publishing.

Nagy, E. (2011). The newborn infant: A missing stage in developmental psychology. *Infant and Child Development, 20*, 3–19.

Nagy, E., & Molnár, P. (2004). Homo imitans or homo provocans? Human imprinting model of neonatal imitation. *Infant Behavior and Development, 27*, 54–63.

National Institute of Mental Health. (2009). *National survey tracks rates of common mental disorders among American youth.* https://www.nih.gov/news-events/news-releases/national-survey-tracks-rates-common-mental-disorders-among-american-youth

Navarro, V. (1993). *Dangerous to your health: Capitalism in health care.* Monthly Review Press.

Noble, D. (1977). *America by design: Science, technology, and the rise of corporate capitalism.* Alfred A. Knopf, Inc.

Noe, R. A., Dachner, A. M., Saxton, B., & Keeton, K. E. (2011). *Team training for long-duration missions in isolated and confined environments: A literature review, an operational assessment, and recommendations for practice and research.* National Aeronautics and Space Administration. https://www.researchgate.net/publication/272179167_Team_Training_for_Long-duration_Missions_in_Isolated_and_Confined_Environments_A_Literature_Review_an_Operational_Assessment_and_Recommendations_for_Practice_and_Research

Nordal, K. C. (2010). Where has all the psychotherapy gone? *Monitor on Psychology, 41*(10), 17.

Nugent, K., & Morell, A. (2011). *Your baby is speaking to you: A visual guide to the amazing behaviors of your newborn and growing baby.* Houghton Mifflin.

Nursing.org. 2022. *Should I join a Nurses Union? Pros and Cons.* https://nurse.org/articles/pros-and-cons-nursing-unions/

O'Brien, S. 2021. *Average family premiums for employer-based health insurance have jumped 47% in the last decade, outpacing wage growth and inflation.* CNBC.

https://www.cnbc.com/2021/11/11/premiums-for-employer-health-insurance-have-jumped-47percent-in-10-years.html

Ontario Human Rights Commission. (n.d.). *Gender identity and gender expression.* https://www.ohrc.on.ca/en/policy-preventing-discrimination-because-gender-identity-and-gender-expression/3-gender-identity-and-gender-expression

Ouellette, D. (2017). *Ron Carter: Finding the right notes.* Retrac Productions, Inc.

PDM Task Force. (2006). *Psychodynamic diagnostic manual.* Alliance of Psychoanalytic Organizations.

Pearce, J., & Newton, S. (1963). *The conditions of human growth.* Citadel Press.

Pfizer. (2001). Understanding schizophrenia. *Trust (Treatment Resources for Understanding Schizophrenia Therapy) Brochures.*

Piaget, J., & Inhelder, B. (1969). *The psychology of the child* (2nd ed.). Basic Books.

Pollack, A. (2004). *Panel to review drug for low female sex drive. The New York Times*, p. C1. https://www.nytimes.com/2004/12/02/health/02patch.html

Reik, T. (1949). *Listening with the third ear: The inner experience of a psychoanalyst.* Farrar, Straus and Giroux.

Ribble, M. A. (1938). Clinical studies of instinctive reactions in new born babies. *American Journal of Psychiatry, 95*, 149–158.

Ribble, M. A. (1965). *The rights of infants: Early psychological needs and their satisfaction* (2nd ed.). Columbia University Press.

Rifkin, J. (2010). *The empathic civilization: The race to global consciousness in a world in crisis.* Polity Press.

Rodrigues, A., Camillo, J., & Mattos, C. (2014). Quasi-appropriation of dialectical materialism: A critical reading of Marxism in Vygotskian approaches to cultural studies in science education. *Cultural Studies of Science Education, 9*, 583–589. https://doi.org/10.1007/s11422-014-9570-7

Rosenberg, N. (1982). *Inside the black box: Technology and economics.* Cambridge University Press.

Rosenthal, E. 2017. *An American sickness: How healthcare became big business and how you can take it back.* Penguin Press.

Rogers, C. (1951). *Client-centered therapy: Its current practice, implications and theory.* Constable.

Schrefer, E. (2022). *Queer ducks (and other animals): The natural world of animal sexuality.* HarperCollins Publishers.

Sherer, R. A. (1999). Physicians' unions: A growing power. *Psychiatric Times*. http://www.psychiatrictimes.com/articles/physicians-unions-growing-power

Singer, D. (2007). The political economy of psychotherapy. *New Politics, XI(2)*. http://newpol.org/content/political-economy-psychotherapy

Soliant.com. 2020. *The Pros and Cons of Nursing Unions, https://www.soliant.com/blog/the-pros-and-cons-of-nursing-unions/.* https://www.soliant.com/blog/the-pros-and-cons-of-nursing-unions/

Solms, M. (2021). *REM sleep and dreaming.* https://www.youtube.com/watch?v=pcgwAfo4ZDU

Spitz, R. A. (1945). Hospitalism: An inquiry into the genesis of psychiatric conditions in early childhood. *Psychoanalytic Study of the Child, 1*, 53–74.

Spitz, R. A. (1946a). Anaclitic depression. *Psychoanalytic Study of the Child, 2*, 313–342.
Spitz, R. A. (1946b). Hospitalism: A follow-up report. *Psychoanalytic Study of the Child, 2*, 113–118.
Stern, D. B. (2015). *Relational freedom: Emergent properties of the interpersonal field.* Routledge.
Stern, D. B., & Hirsch, I. (Eds.). (2017). *The interpersonal perspective in psychoanalysis, 1960s–1990s.* Routledge.
Stern, D. N. (1971). A micro-analysis of mother-infant interaction: Behaviors regulating social contact between a mother and her three-and-a-half-month-old twins. *Journal of American Academy of Child Psychiatry, 13*, 402–421.
Stern, D. N. (1974). Mother and infant at play: The dyadic interaction involving facial, vocal and gaze behaviors. In M. Lewis & L. A. Rosenblum (Eds.), *The effect of the infant on its caregiver.* Wiley.
Stern, D. N. (1977). *The first relationship: Infant and mother.* Harvard University Press.
Stern, D. N. (1994). One way to build a clinically relevant baby. *Infant Mental Health Journal, 15*(1), 9–25.
Stern, D. N. (2000). *The interpersonal world of the infant: A view from psychoanalysis and developmental psychology.* Basic Books.
Stern, D. N. (2004). *The present moment: In psychotherapy and everyday life.* Norton.
Stern, D. N. (2018). *The interpersonal world of the infant.* Routledge.
Stickgold, R. (2021). Why do we dream? [Video] YouTube. https://www.youtube.com/watch?v=1-gFlSUDxPo
Stolberg, S. G. (2002). Study says clinical guides often hide ties of doctors. *The New York Times.* https://www.nytimes.com/2002/02/06/us/study-says-clinical-guides-often-hide-ties-of-doctors.html
Sullivan, H. S. (1953). The *interpersonal theory of psychiatry.* W. W. Norton.
Sullivan, H. S. (1954). *The psychiatric interview.* W. W. Norton.
Sullivan, H. S. (1962). *Schizophrenia as a human process.* W. W. Norton & Company.
Sullivan, H. S. (1966). *Conceptions of modern psychiatry.* W. W. Norton & Company.
Sullivan, H. S. (1972). *Personal psychopathology: Early formulations.* W. W. Norton & Company.
Supreme Court Opinion on Same Sex Marriage. (2015). *Washington Post.* http://apps.washingtonpost.com/g/documents/preview/1605/desktop/?das
Szasz, T. (1974). *The myth of mental illness.* HarperCollins Publishers.
Szasz, T. S. (1960). The myth of mental illness: Foundations of a theory of personal conduct. *American Psychologist, 15*(2), 113–118.
Taffel, R. (2020). Preface. In G. J. Jacobson, J. C. Niemira, & K. J. Violeta (Eds.), *Sex, sexuality and trans identities: Clinical guidance for psychotherapists and counselors* (pp. 15–18). Jessica Kingsley Publishers.
Taras, H. L., Frankowski, B. L., McGrath, J. W., Mears, C. J., Murray, R. D., & Young, T. L. (2003). Out-of-school suspension and expulsion. *Pediatrics, 112*(5), 1206–1209. https://doi.org/10.1542/peds.112.5.1206

Tasman, A., Kay, J., Lieberman, J., First, M., & Riba, M. (Eds.) (2015). *Psychiatry (4th ed.).* John Wiley & Sons.

Teyber, E., & Teyber, F. H. (2016). *Interpersonal process in therapy: An integrative model* (7th ed.). Cengage Learning.

Trevarthen, C. (1977). Descriptive analyses of infant communicative behavior. In H. R. Schaffer (Ed.), *Studies in mother-infant interaction (pp. 227–270).* Academic Press.

Trevarthen, C. (1979). Communication and cooperation in early infancy: A description of primary inter-subjectivity. In M. Bullowa (Ed.), *Before speech: The beginning of interpersonal communication* (pp. 321–348). Cambridge University Press.

Trevarthen, C. (1980). The foundations of intersubjectivity: Development of interpersonal and cooperative understanding in infants. In J. M. Anglin, J. S. Bruner, & D. R. Olson (Eds.), *The social foundation of language and thought: Essays in honor of Jerome Bruner (pp. 316–342).* Norton.

Trevarthen, C. (1989). Development of early social interactions and the affective regulation of brain growth. In C. von Euler, H. Forssberg, & H. Lagercrantz (Eds.), *Neurobiology of early infant behaviour (Wenner Gren Center International Symposium Series)* (Vol. 55, pp. 191–216). Macmillan/Stockton Press.

Trevarthen, C. (1993a). The function of emotions in early infant communication and development. In J. Nadel & L. Camaioni (Eds.), *New perspectives in early communicative development* (pp. 48–81). Routledge.

Trevarthen, C. (1993b). *Neurobiology of early infant behavior* (Vol. 55). (C. Von Euler, H. Forssberg, & H. Langercrantz, Eds.) Stockton.

Trevarthen, C. (2006). The self born in intersubjectivity: The psychology of an infant communicating. In U. Neisser (Ed.), *The perceived self: Ecological and interpersonal sources of self knowledge* (pp. 121–173). Cambridge University Press.

Trevarthen, C. (2007). Moving experiences: Perceiving as action with a sense of purpose. In G. Pepping & M. Grealy (Eds.), *Closing the gap: The scientific writings of David N. Lee* (pp. 1–20). Erlbaum.

Trevarthen, C. (2009). *Why attachment matters in sharing meaning*. Institute for Research and Innovation in Social Services. https://www.iriss.org.uk/resources/irissfm/why-attachment-matters-sharing-meaning-colwyn-trevarthen

Trevarthen, C. (2011a). The generation of human meaning: How shared experience grows in infancy. In A. Seemann (Ed.), *Joint attention: New developments in philosophy, psychology, and neuroscience* (pp. 73–113). MIT Press.

Trevarthen, C. (2011b). What is it like to be a person who knows nothing? Defining the active intersubjective mind of a newborn human being. *Infant and Child Development, 20*, 119–135. https://doi.org/10.1002/icd.689

Trevarthen, C. (2017). The affectionate intersubjective intelligence of the infant, and its innate motives for relational mental health. *International Journal of Cognitive Analytic Therapy and Relational Mental Health, 1*(1), 11–53.

Trevarthen, C. (2019a). Sander's life work, on mother-infant vitality and the emerging person. *Psychoanalytic Inquiry, 39*(1), 22–35.

Trevarthen, C. (2019b). The psychobiology of the human spirit. In G. Apter, E. Devouche, & M. Gratier (Eds.), *Early Interaction and Developmental Psychopathology* (Vol. 1, pp. 1–18). Springer.

Trevarthen, C., Gratier, M., & Osborne, N. (2014). The human nature of culture and education. *Wiley Interdisciplinary Reviews: Cognitive Science, 5*, 173–192.

The Trevor Project. (2021). *Understanding asexuality*. https://www.thetrevorproject.org/resources/article/understanding-asexuality/

Tsao, E. (2009). Inside the *DSM*: The drug barons' campaign to make us all crazy. *Counterpunch*. https://www.counterpunch.org/2009/08/20/the-drug-barons-campaign-to-make-us-all-crazy/

U.S. Department of Health and Human Services, Administration for Children and Families, Administration on Children, Youth and Families, Children's Bureau. (2013). *Child mistreatment 2012*. http://www.acf.hhs.gov/sites/default/files/cb/cm2012.pdf

Vygotsky, L. S. (1997). *The collected works of L.S. Vygotsky: Problems of the theory and history of psychology* (Vol. III). (R. Rieber, Ed.) Plenum.

Wald, J., & Losen, D. J. (2003). Defining and re-directing a school-to-prison pipeline. *New Directions for Youth Development, 99*, 9–15. https://doi.org/10.1002/yd.51

Walsh, M. (2018). *Malady mongers: How drug companies sell treatments by inventing diseases. Yahoo News*. https://www.yahoo.com/news/malady-mongers-drug-companies-sell-treatments-inventing-diseases-100040360.html

Waters, R. (2005). Medicating Amanda. *Mother Jones*. https://www.motherjones.com/politics/2005/05/medicating-amanda/

Weiss, R. (2005). Many scientists admit to misconduct. *Washington Post,* p. A03. https://www.washingtonpost.com/archive/politics/2005/06/09/many-scientists-admit-to-misconduct/6baa5d04-d20d-447a-9130–09cd93941c6b/

Willman, D. (2003, December 7). Stealth merger: Drug companies and government medical research. *Los Angeles Times*, p. A1.

Willman, D. (2004, December 22). The National Institutes of Mental Health: Public servant or private marketer? *Los Angeles Times*.

Wilson, M. (1993). *DSM-III* and the transformation of American psychiatry: A history. *American Journal of Psychiatry, 150*(3), 399–410.

World Bank. (2019). *Current Health expenditure (% of GDP)*. https://data.worldbank.org/indicator/SH.XPD.CHEX.GD.ZS

Wortis, J. (1954). *Fragments of an analysys with Freud.* Simon and Schuster.

Zadra, A., & Stickgold, R. (2021). *When brains dream: Exploring the science and mystery of sleep.* W. W. Norton & Company.

Index

About the Authors

Sue Harris obtained her PhD in psychology from Columbia University Teachers College. She has been in private practice in New York City since 1968. She has developed and implemented clinical programs at various institutions, including as ward director at Bronx State Hospital, clinical director of Astor Group Homes, and director of the psychology department at Covenant House. At the Richmond Fellowship in England, she served as consultant and clinical supervisor for a halfway house for long-term chronic patients. There she helped develop the therapeutic use of cooperative group living in building self-confidence through community membership. Harris has published in various journals, including *Psychiatry*, "Schizophrenics' Mutual Glance Patterns: A Study of the Frequency of Mutual Glances Between Schizophrenic Patients, Their Parents, Hospital Attendants and Peers." She also authored "A Theoretical Approach to the Halfway House," a chapter in *The Therapeutic Community Outside the Hospital*, edited by Elly Jansen of the Richmond Fellowship. She presented on the use of group experience in a halfway house at the Midwestern Scholars Conference and lectured on the individual personality and the collective in Kursk and Minsk. Her work on the therapeutic collective experience at the Komsorg Camp was sponsored by the psychology department of the Kursk Pedagogical Institute.

Janet R. Mayes obtained her PhD in psychology from Ferkauf Graduate School of Psychology, Yeshiva University. In addition to her private practice in New York City, Mayes served as director of mental health services for several foster care agencies; as department chairperson and consultant to colleges and universities, focusing on interpersonal approaches to overcoming adult learning obstacles; and as president/director of a nonprofit clinic for children and adults. She was adjunct lecturer of psychology at various colleges and universities, including Montclair State University and Kean University, and was a faculty member of the SEEK (Search for Education, Elevation and Knowledge) department at the City College of New York,

The City University of New York, a summary of which is in the chapter on learning in this volume. She also presented her work on social facilitation of learning, "The Study Group Program: Helping Students Kick the Failure Habit," at, among others, the Pennsylvania Association of Two-Year Colleges Annual Meeting. Mayes's other professional presentations include "Overcoming Resistance to Change: Working with Disturbed Adolescents and Their Parents," "Hope and Despair: Working with the Sense of Self," and a paper on educating emotionally disturbed adolescents at the Association of New York State Educators of the Emotionally Disabled Annual Conference. While a faculty member of the counseling department at York College, The City University of New York, she served on the Editorial Board of *The New York State Personnel and Guidance Journal.*

Marilyn Miller (1939–2020) obtained her MA degree in psychiatric mental health nursing from New York University and was a New York State certified clinical nurse specialist in adult psychiatric and mental health nursing. In addition to her private practice in New York City, she served as clinical instructor in psychiatry at Columbia University's School of Nursing baccalaureate program; assistant professor at the State University of New York and the Health Science Center at Brooklyn College of Nursing; assistant professor at Albert Einstein College of Medicine; and director of psychiatric nursing at Martland Medical Center. Miller's journal articles and conference presentations in the United States and Latin America have focused on the development of the need for tenderness, the therapeutic relationship, and critical thinking across health care disciplines, all from an interpersonal theoretical perspective. She co-authored a chapter, "Development of the Need for Tenderness as a Theoretical Model for Caring: Application to Nursing Education," in *Ethical and Moral Dimensions of Care*, edited by Madeleine M. Leininger.

David Singer obtained his PhD in psychology from New York University and his MA in economics from New School University. In addition to his private practice in New York City, he serves as clinical psychologist at Abbott House and as adjunct assistant professor, Department of Sociology, at John Jay College for Criminal Justice. He was also an instructor at Downstate University of the State University of New York and New York University. He has treated and supervised the treatment of children, adolescents, and adults at various foster care agencies, group homes, and hospitals. He also served as senior psychologist for Family Court for the State of New York. Singer's published articles include *Monthly Review*, "The Health Care Crisis in the United States"; *Journal of Personality and Social Psychology*, "An Experimental Analysis of the Contrast Effect and Its Implications for Intergroup Communication and the Indirect Assessment of Attitude" (co-author); and *New Politics*, "The Political Economy of Psychotherapy," which has been updated and reprinted in this volume. His professional presentations include "Perceived Dissimilarity: An Internal Basis for the Actor Observer Divergence" (co-presenter) at the American Psychological Association Convention.

www.ingramcontent.com/pod-product-compliance
Ingram Content Group UK Ltd.
Pitfield, Milton Keynes, MK11 3LW, UK
UKHW041450071026
15587UKWH00010B/717

9 781666 927504